THE MUSCULOSKELETAL SYSTEM

Basic Processes and Disorders

SECOND EDITION

Edited by

FRANK C. WILSON, M.D.
Professor and Chairman
Division of Orthopaedics
University of North Carolina School of Medicine
Chapel Hill, North Carolina

18 Contributors

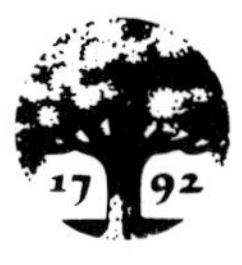

J.B. LIPPINCOTT COMPANY
Philadelphia • Toronto

The authors and publisher have exerted every effort to ensure that drug selection and dosage set forth in this text are in accord with current recommendations and practice at the time of publication. However, in view of ongoing research, changes in government regulations, and the constant flow of information relating to drug therapy and drug reactions, the reader is urged to check the package insert for each drug for any change in indications and dosage and for added warnings and precautions. This is particularly important when the recommended agent is a new or infrequently employed drug.

Sponsoring Editor: Darlene D. Pedersen
Manuscript Editor: Rosanne Hallowell
Designer: Rita Naughton
Production Supervisor: N. Carol Kerr
Production Coordinator: Charles W. Field
Compositor: Waldman Graphics, Inc.
Printer/Binder: Halliday Lithograph

2nd Edition

For information address J. B. Lippincott Company, East Washington Square, Philadelphia, PA 19105

1 3 5 6 4 2

Library of Congress Cataloging in Publication Data
Main entry under title:
The Musculoskeletal system.
Bibliography
Includes index.
1. Musculoskeletal system. 2. Musculoskeletal system—Diseases. I. Wilson, Frank Crane, 1929-
[DNLM: 1. Musculoskeletal system. WE 100 M985]
QP321.M9 1982 612′.7 82-138
ISBN 0-397-52096-4 AACR2

THE MUSCULOSKELETAL SYSTEM

This book is dedicated to students of the musculoskeletal system—past, present, and future—without whose stimulus it would not have been written.

Contributors

William H. Bowers, M.D.
Formerly, Associate Professor of Orthopaedics
University of North Carolina
School of Medicine
Chapel Hill, North Carolina

H. Robert Brashear, M.D.
Professor of Orthopaedics
University of North Carolina
School of Medicine
Chapel Hill, North Carolina

Philip L. Cohen, M.D.
Assistant Professor of Medicine
Division of Rheumatology
University of North Carolina
School of Medicine
Chapel Hill, North Carolina

Robert A. Eisenberg, M.D.
Assistant Professor of Medicine
Division of Rheumatology
University of North Carolina
School of Medicine
Chapel Hill, North Carolina

Michael A. Friedman, M.D.
Formerly, Fellow in Rheumatology
Department of Medicine
University of North Carolina
School of Medicine
Chapel Hill, North Carolina

Walter B. Greene, M.D.
Assistant Professor of Orthopaedics
University of North Carolina
School of Medicine
Chapel Hill, North Carolina

Stephen A. Grubb, M.D.
Assistant Professor of Orthopaedics
University of North Carolina
School of Medicine
Chapel Hill, North Carolina

Colin D. Hall, M.D.
Associate Professor of Neurology
University of North Carolina
School of Medicine
Chapel Hill, North Carolina

Charles W. Hooker, Ph.D.
Professor of Anatomy
University of North Carolina
School of Medicine
Chapel Hill, North Carolina

George Johnson, Jr., M.D.
Professor of Surgery
University of North Carolina
School of Medicine
Chapel Hill, North Carolina

Gary E. Ragan, M.D., Ph.D.
Formerly, Fellow in Rheumatology
Department of Medicine
University of North Carolina
School of Medicine
Chapel Hill, North Carolina

R. Beverly Raney, M.D.
Chairman Emeritus, Division of Orthopaedics
University of North Carolina
School of Medicine
Chapel Hill, North Carolina

Timothy N. Taft, M.D.
Associate Professor of Orthopaedics
University of North Carolina
School of Medicine
Chapel Hill, North Carolina

Roy V. Talmage, Ph.D.
Professor of Orthopaedics
University of North Carolina
School of Medicine
Chapel Hill, North Carolina

Carole J. VanderWiel, Ph.D.
Assistant Professor of Orthopaedics
University of North Carolina
School of Medicine
Chapel Hill, North Carolina

Frank C. Wilson, M.D.
Professor and Chairman
Division of Orthopaedics
University of North Carolina
School of Medicine
Chapel Hill, North Carolina

John B. Winfield, M.D.
Professor of Medicine
Chief, Division of Rheumatology
University of North Carolina
School of Medicine
Chapel Hill, North Carolina

Paul H. Wright, M.D.
Formerly, Assistant Professor of Orthopaedics
University of North Carolina
School of Medicine
Chapel Hill, North Carolina

Preface

The Musculoskeletal System: Basic Processes and Disorders has been written to acquaint the reader with the structure and function—normal and abnormal—of the musculoskeletal system and to relate these basic precepts to the principles of diagnosis and treatment.

The book is divided into nine parts, beginning with a section on the normal development of the musculoskeletal system. After reviewing the gross anatomy of the limbs and back, each of the tissues of the musculoskeletal system—bone, muscle, cartilage, and synovium—is considered individually with respect to microscopic structure, physiology and biochemistry, and pathology. The final section is devoted to trauma, proceeding from the systemic and local response of the organism to injury to a consideration of the principles of diagnosis and treatment.

Each chapter is preceded by two items: the chapter's goals and objectives and an outline. The goals state what we hope to accomplish, and the list of specific educational objectives represents our effort to define exactly what is considered important. Given a well-motivated student and clearly stated educational objectives, the precise methods by which learning takes place are probably unimportant. By serving as a study guide, the objectives can make the learning process more efficient; in addition, they permit the reader to determine his rate of progress through self-testing.

The second edition of this text retains the organizational format of the first edition; however, the section on metabolic bone disease includes many new concepts in mineral metabolism; the chapters on arthritis are more comprehensive, incorporating the immunologic aspects of rheumatoid and infectious arthritis; the clinicopathologic aspects of neuromuscular disorders are considerably expanded; and the biochemistry and physiology of bone and cartilage are presented in greater depth than in the first edition. In addition, the integration of basic and clinical material has been strengthened by having a basic scientist and a clinician coauthor most of the chapters.

I owe much to many, but wish to express particular gratitude to Martha Thomas for her careful and tireless work in the preparation of the manuscript, to Gwynne Moore for having illustrated, in such a clear manner, what we have not been able to put completely into words, and to Felton Parker for his meticulous preparation of the index.

FRANK C. WILSON, M.D.

Contents

THE MUSCULOSKELETAL SYSTEM

Introduction to the Musculoskeletal System

The musculoskeletal system includes the bones, joints, and muscles of the body together with their associated structures such as ligaments, tendons, and bursae. Comprising as it does over 70% of the body, it is subject to a great many disorders. These disorders often result in pain, deformity, or malfunctions of joints, and are more likely to interfere with the quality than the length of life.

Most musculoskeletal pathology can be classified as adults' disorders, children's disorders, or traumatic disorders. Adults' disorders include metabolic diseases of bones and joints, bone tumors, affections of the spine, infections of bones and joints, neuromuscular diseases, foot and hand problems, and attritional disorders. Children's disorders include inborn errors of metabolism and genetic defects, congenital deformities, and prenatal and perinatal disorders such as cerebral palsy. The traumatic disorders include all types of injury to the bones, joints, muscles, tendons, and associated structures.

The importance of the musculoskeletal system as a source of disability (and as an unusual educational opportunity for the learner) is evident from data showing that musculoskeletal conditions rank second in the nation's overall medical expenses, second in frequency of reasons for visiting a physician, and fifth as a cause of hospitalization. Musculoskeletal disabilities cause more limitation of activity than disorders in any other system of the body in all age groups. Impairments of the back alone have been shown to produce a month of activity reduction and 9 days of bed disability per year in every 100 persons between the ages of 25 and 44 years. Arthritis is also a major cause of disability. In 1976, it was estimated that about 13 million persons in the United States had moderate or severe osteoarthritis and 5 million were affected by rheumatoid arthritis, resulting in a total cost for arthritis in the United States of over $13 billion annually. Trauma, another major category of musculoskeletal disorders, requires medical care or activity limitation in about one of every ten Americans each year.

The wide variety of musculoskeletal disorders justifies a comprehensive coverage of basic principles as outlined in the following list of goals and objectives.

GOALS AND OBJECTIVES

Goals:

1. To acquaint the reader with the normal development, structure, and function of the musculoskeletal system

2. To introduce the reader to the normal physiology and biochemistry of bone cartilage, synovium, and muscle

3. To introduce the pathological conditions altering the normal structure, function, biochemistry, and physiology of the musculoskeletal system

4. To help the reader acquire the information and skills necessary to evaluate a patient with injury or disease of the musculoskeletal system

5. To help the reader apply his knowledge to the diagnosis and treatment of patients with musculoskeletal pathology

Objectives: On completion of the course material, and using the text as a standard reference, one should be able to describe, list, and recognize the following:

1. Normal development, structure (gross and microscopic), and function of the musculoskeletal system
2. Normal physiology and biochemistry of bone, cartilage, synovium, and muscle
3. Changes produced in bone, cartilage, synovium, and muscle by injury or disease
4. Essential findings in the evaluation of a patient with a given injury or disease affecting the musculoskeletal system, and how these findings are related to treatment of the condition

Part One

DEVELOPMENT

Chapter 1

Normal Development of the Musculoskeletal System

Charles W. Hooker
and Walter B. Greene

GOALS AND OBJECTIVES

Goals: To introduce the reader to the development of the skeleton and its articulations and the development of the muscles as organs, as a background for both the appreciation of the organization of these systems in the adult and the anticipation of variations and malformations

Objectives: On completion of this unit, and using the text as a standard reference, one should be able to evaluate, describe, list, or recognize the following:

1. The major events in the origin and gross development of the muscular and skeletal systems and their components, and the abnormalities resulting from faulty development
2. The evidence bearing on the site of origin of the categories of skeletal muscles (limb, trunk, and branchiomeric) and bones (membranous and endochondral)
3. The patterns of innervation of groups of muscles as based on developmental events
4. A simple classificaion of joints on the basis of structure and function

OUTLINE

I. The somites
II. Development of the skeleton
   A. Vertebral column, ribs, and sternum
   B. Limbs
   C. Skull

- D. Joints
- E. Sesamoid bones

II. Development of the muscles
- A. Cellular differentiation
- B. Deep muscles of back and neck
- C. Prevertebral muscles
- D. Innervation of somitic muscles
- E. Origin of thoracolumbar fascia
- F. Muscles not clearly somitic in origin
- G. Muscles of the limbs
- H. Arteries of the limbs
- I. Trapezius and sternocleidomastoid muscles
- J. Ventrolateral muscles of neck and trunk
- K. Muscles of the head
- L. Tendons
- M. Fasciae

THE SOMITES

The skeleton and skeletal muscle develop from the mesoderm, a thin layer of cells in the early embryo situated between the ectoderm and the endoderm and interrupted in the midline by the notochord (Fig. 1-1*A*). With the formation of the neural groove, the mesoderm on each side of the notochord thickens to form a longitudinal mass, the paraxial mesoderm. Each paraxial mass thins into lateral plate mesoderm, which is in turn continuous with the extra-embryonic mesoderm (Fig. 1-1*B*).

Beginning around the 21st day of development, the paraxial mesoderm segments into paired, more or less cuboid and later pyramidal masses, the *somites*. The first somites formed are the first occipital somites, situated at the cranial end of the notochord. Subsequent pairs of somites appear caudally next to the previously formed pair. In the human embryo, paraxial mesoderm continues as more or less diffuse mesenchyme as far forward as the rostral end of the future brain plate, but no somites form rostral to the first occipital pair. A total of some 42 to 44 pairs of somites are formed between the 21st and the 30th days of development. The lateral plate mesoderm remains largely unsegmented and is attached to the ventrolateral angle of each somite by a continuous tract, the intermediate mesoderm, which later forms the nephrogenic cord.

In the neck and trunk, each somite develops into three more or less recognizable portions (Fig. 1-1*C*): laterally a *dermatome*, destined to differentiate into dermis; medially and ventrally a *sclerotome*, from which develop the vertebrae, the intervertebral discs, and the ligaments of the vertebral column; and, between the dermatome and sclerotome, a *myotome*, which gives rise to muscles, tendons, and fasciae. In the head and caudal region the somites degenerate, develop atypically, or fail to form.

DEVELOPMENT OF THE SKELETON

Vertebral Column, Ribs, and Sternum

Beginning about the 4th week of development, sclerotome cells from each pair of somites migrate medially, meeting in the midline around the notochord and separating it

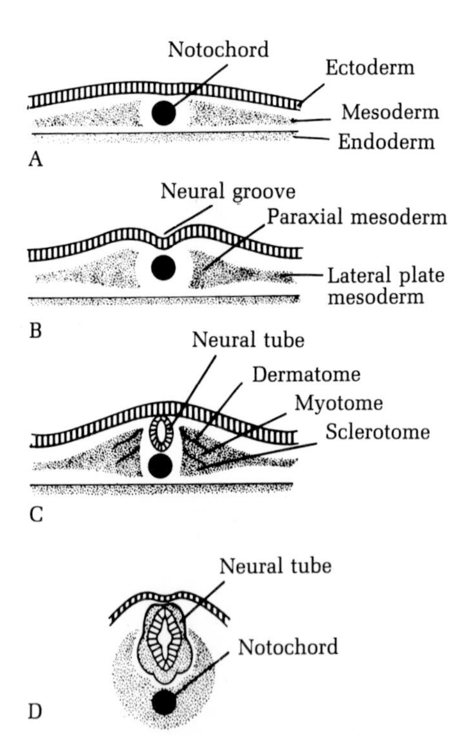

Fig. 1-1. Development of the somite. (*A*) Initially, the mesoderm exists as a sheet of cells between the ectoderm and the endoderm. (*B*) The mesoderm thickens along the notochord to form the paraxial cords of mesenchyme. (*C*) The somite is shown composed of dermatome, myotome, and sclerotome. (*D*) The cells of the sclerotome have migrated around the notochord to form the primordium of a vertebra.

from the neural tube dorsally and from the gut ventrally (Fig. 1-1*D*). The notochord now lies in a segmented, longitudinal condensation of sclerotomal mesenchyme, and segmental artery lies at each intersegmental level (Fig. 1-2*A*). Beginning in cervical sclerotome 3 and continuing caudalward, each of these segmental masses of mesenchyme soon exhibits a condensed layer of cells near its caudal border with distinctly less condensed mesenchyme both cranial and caudal to it (Fig. 1-2*B*). The condensed layer now appears to migrate cranially to the level of the middle of the adjacent myotome (Fig. 1-2*C*) and in time differentiates into the anulus fibrosus of an intervertebral disc. The caudal, less condensed portion of each sclerotome fuses with the rostral, less condensed portion of the succeeding sclerotome to form the primordium of a vertebra. Thus, the skeletal portions of the somites cease to correspond to the original segmentation, which is, however, retained by the myotomes. As a result of the shift in segmentation of the sclerotome, segmental muscles developing from myotomes span intervertebral joints instead of being coextensive with individual vertebrae. As another consequence of the shift, the originally intersegmental arteries come to be related to the midpoints of the verte-

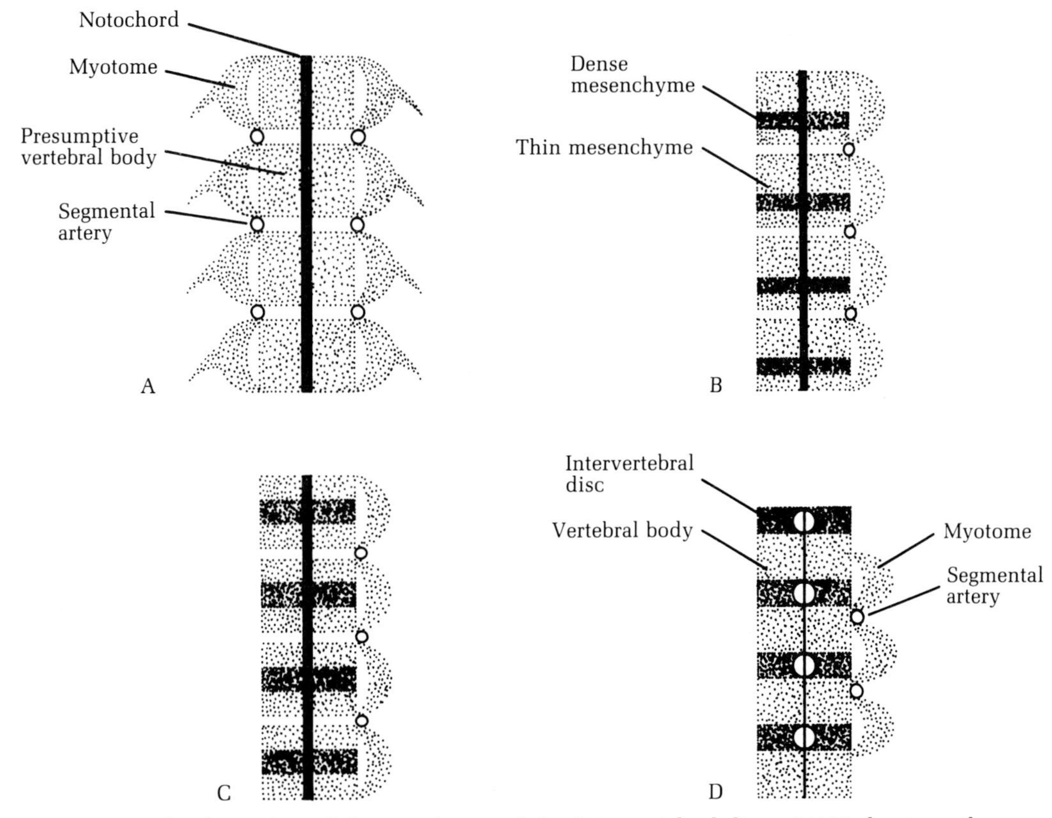

Fig. 1-2. Events in the formation of the vertebrae and the intervertebral discs. (*A*) Early stage: the sclerotome is segmented and each sclerotomal segment is paralleled by a pair of myotomes; the sclerotomal segments surround the notochord, and a segmental artery courses between myotomes. (*B*) Each sclerotomal segment contains condensed mesenchyme in its caudal portion. (*C*) The condensed mesenchyme of the sclerotome has migrated forward and lies midway between the cranial and caudal borders of the myotome. (*D*) The condensed mesenchyme of the sclerotome is becoming an intervertebral disc; the notochord is disappearing in the vertebral body, but has enlarged in the intervertebral disc as the nucleus pulposus; the myotome extends from one vertebral body to the next.

brae instead of being situated between vertebrae.

The portion of the mesenchymal vertebral primordium surrounding the notochord becomes the vertebral body. The more dorsally situated portions of the primordium extend further dorsally to surround the neural tube, becoming the neural arch. The lateral portions of the primordium become the transverse processes and, in the thoracic region, the ribs. As the vertebral body develops, the portion of the notochord within it becomes thinner and ultimately disappears. Between vertebral bodies the notochord persists and enlarges in the developing intervertebral disc, becoming the nucleus pulposus of the adult disc (Fig. 1-2*D*).

Chondrification begins while the mesenchymal vertebral primordia are still growing (Fig. 1-3). Two centers appear in each body and soon fuse across the midline to form a cartilaginous body. A similar center appears in each lateral half of the neural arch; it expands dorsally to fuse, during the third month, with its fellow dorsal to the neural tube. It expands ventrally to unite with the cartilaginous body, and laterally between the dorsal and ventral masses of the myotome (see "Development of the Muscles") to form the transverse processes. In the thoracic region, the lateral projection forms the cartilaginous rib as well as the transverse process. In the cervical region, the lateral projection forms both the dorsal and ventral roots of the transverse process, the latter being a reduced cervical counterpart of a rib.

The cartilaginous model of the vertebra thus formed is a single piece. At about 9 weeks, *ossification* begins, with the appearance of centers in the bodies of the lower thoracic and upper lumbar vertebrae. Such centers successively appear both caudally and cranially. Ossification centers for each arch are paired and usually arise in a craniocaudal sequence; centers for the arches are said to antedate those of the bodies in cervical vertebrae.

At birth, the usual vertebra consists of three bones joined by cartilage, and osseous union is achieved over a period of years. Usually during the 16th year, secondary centers of ossification appear in the cartilage that still exists over the cranial and caudal ends of the vertebral bodies; these centers of ossification form disclike epiphyses that unite with the bony bodies by the 25th year. Other secondary centers appear during adolescence and fuse later.

Variations from this general plan of development occur at the two ends of the vertebral column. At the cranial end, intervertebral discs do not develop between the skull and the atlas or between the atlas and axis. During formation of the atlas, a body appears, but it is soon appropriated by the axis to form the dens. As a consequence, the atlas is essentially a neural arch that is closed ventrally to form a ring. At the caudal end, the sacral and coccygeal vertebrae have reduced arches. Between puberty and approximately the 25th year, the sacral vertebrae unite into a single bony mass; a somewhat similar fusion occurs between coccygeal vertebrae.

When ossification of the thoracic vertebrae begins, the cartilaginous union with costal processes is replaced by a joint in which a depression on the body of the vertebra receives the head of the rib; at much the same

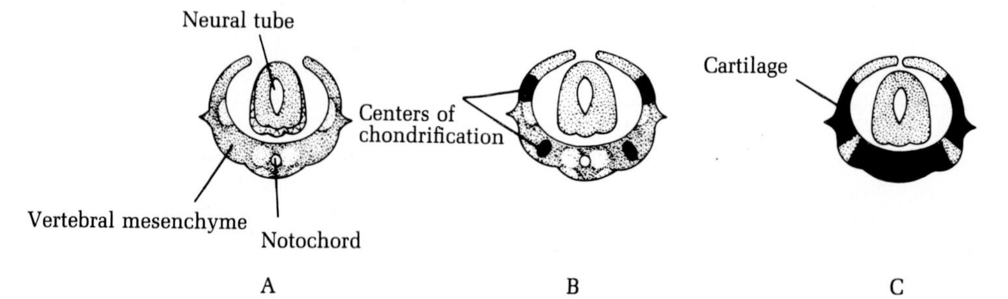

Fig. 1-3. Development of a vertebra. (*A*) The mesenchymal primordium. (*B*) Two centers of chondrification are shown in the body, and a center of chondrification is shown in each lateral half of the future arch. (*C*) Extension of chondrification.

time, the transverse process reaches the rib and forms a joint with the tubercle. In the ninth week, a center of ossification appears near the future angle of the rib, and the cartilaginous rib is converted into bone except for the distal end. At the 15th year, two secondary centers of ossification arise in the tubercle and one in the head.

Ribs manifest the greatest development in the thoracic region; in the cervical region they remain small and unite with the bodies and transverse processes, creating the transverse foramina; in the lumbar region, they are short and are fused to the transverse processes; and in the sacral region, they are represented by large, fused masses forming the pars lateralis of the sacrum. The first coccygeal vertebra retains the only trace of a rib in this region.

Several congenital deformities of the vertebral column appear to be consequences of disturbance of early events in development. Local failure of the paraxial mesoderm to segment could account for fused (blocked) vertebrae. Partial failure of segmentation laterally could result in a unilateral, unsegmented bar of bone; the affected side of the vertebra involved fails to grow, and growth of the vertebrae on the side opposite the bar may produce scoliosis (lateral curvature of the vertebral column). Partial failure of segmentation anteriorly could result in anterior fusion of vertebral bodies; continued growth of the posterior portions of the partially fused vertebrae could result in kyphosis (anterior curvature of the vertebral column).

Unilateral failure of formation of a sclerotome, failure of medial migration of sclerotomal cells, or failure of differentiation of sclerotomal cells could result in a wedge-shaped hemivertebra and scoliosis. Two or more hemivertebrae on the same side are likely to result in scoliosis that progresses as the child grows. On the other hand, when two hemivertebrae exist on opposite sides, scoliosis may be slight. Failure of development of the anterior portion of one or more vertebrae results in kyphosis.

These malformations have no clear-cut genetic basis, and, indeed, the cause of the developmental error is unknown. Inasmuch as the basic error occurs quite early in the development of the embryo, one may expect other anomalies to accompany these malformations. The relatively high incidence of renal anomalies in patients with congenital vertebral deformities is perhaps related to the fact that the kidney develops from mesoderm adjacent to the somites. Abnormal curvatures of the spine may, for mechanical reasons, result in problems that are not themselves malformations: in addition to disfigurement, scoliosis may lead to pulmonary dysfunction, cor pulmonale, and back pain; kyphosis may result in paralysis from the stretch imposed upon the spinal cord.

Failure of the primordia of the two laminae to unite leaves the vertebral canal open dorsally (*spinal rachischisis, or spina bifida*). It has also been suggested that such an opening may be caused by swelling of the spinal cord. In either event, the dorsal body wall may or may not be intact over the open vertebral canal. If the meninges protrude through the opening in the vertebral canal, the condition is termed a *meningocele;* if the spinal cord also protrudes, the condition is called *meningomyelocele.* The latter condition is usually accompanied by damage to the spinal cord and nerve roots, resulting in neurologic deficits that correspond to the level of the lesion. Related to spina bifida is the condition known as *diastematomyelia,* in which the spinal cord is split by a bony spicule or a fibrous band, with each portion surrounded by a dural sac. As the child grows, a long spicule of bone or a fibrous band may tether the spinal cord and produce neurologic deficits.

In the abnormality known as *spondylolysis,* which commonly involves the fifth lumbar vertebra, a defect passes between the superior articular process and the remainder of the lamina. When the condition is bilateral, the superior articular processes are attached to the body by the pedicles, but most of the lamina and the spinous and inferior articular processes are detached. This defect does not appear to be an acute fracture, but compelling evidence of an embryologic origin is lacking. As a consequence of the defect, the body of the involved vertebra may displace anteriorly (*spondylolisthesis*).

The number of the thoracic vertebra may be increased by formation of ribs related to the first lumbar vertebra. Such an event would, of course, reduce the number of lumbar vertebrae, a circumstance that can also be a consequence of fusion of the fifth lumbar vertebra to the sacrum. These anomalous vertebrae are known as *transitional vertebrae*.

The *sternum* is first indicated at about the sixth week of embryonic development by a pair of longitudinal bands of mesenchyme in the ventrolateral body wall. Following attachment of the cartilaginous ribs to these bands, they unite in a craniocaudal direction. At 9 weeks the bands are fused and are cartilaginous. Ossification begins toward the end of the fifth month, but is not complete until late in childhood.

Limbs

The paired limb buds make their appearance late in the fourth embryonic week, the upper limb buds at the level of the pericardial swelling and the lower limb buds just caudal to the level of the umbilical cord. Both the upper and the lower limbs undergo early descent from their largely cervical and lumbar levels. In the condition known as *Sprengel's deformity* (undescended scapula), the scapula is attached to cervical vertebrae by bone, cartilage, or fibrous tissue. This attachment is presumably established early in development and prevents descent of the scapula to its customary thoracic level. The deformity is usually unilateral, although it may be bilateral.

Each limb bud is initially a lateral swelling that consists of mesenchyme covered by ectoderm of the lateral body wall. Some of the mesenchyme of the limb bud is undoubtedly mesenchyme of the lateral body wall, and some of it may have migrated early or later into the limb bud from adjacent somites. Despite much experimental study, there is still uncertainty as to whether and how extensively somitic mesoderm migrates into the limb bud. The distal end of each bud flattens as a beginning stage in the formation of hand or foot, and is marked from the remainder of the bud by a constriction. A later constriction at the location of future elbow or knee distinguishes the forearm or leg from the arm or thigh. The distal, flattened plate develops ridges, separated initially by grooves, that become the digits. The lower limb lags behind the upper limb throughout its development.

The limbs may fail to develop or may be represented by mere stubs, a condition known as *amelia*. The distal portion of a limb may fail to develop and may taper to a stump, while the proximal portion develops normally *(hemimelia)*. On the other hand, the proximal portion of a limb may be deficient, with the hand or foot appearing to project directly from the trunk *(phocomelia)*. The basis of these malformations when they occur spontaneously is unknown. A rare and spectacular anomaly is *sympodia* (the mermaid condition), in which the lower limbs are fused. The condition is apparently a consequence of failure of development of the wedge-shaped mass of mesenchyme of the trunk that serves to press the lower limb buds apart.

Anomalies of numerous types occur in the hand and foot, in keeping with their complexity. One is *syndactyly* (webbing or fusion of two or more digits), a result of failure of early interdigital tissue to degenerate. Another is *polydactyly*, one or more supernumerary digits, most often a postminimus (an extra little finger). Polydactyly is one of the few anomalies of the limbs with a genetic basis, usually involving autosomal dominant transmission. The digits may be abnormally short *(brachydactyly)*, a consequence of short or missing phalanges; in *hyperphalangism*, supernumerary phalanges are present in the digit(s). A rare anomaly is absence of a digit, an extreme form of which is cleft hand *("lobster claw" hand)*. In this deformity, the phalanges of the middle finger, and sometimes the corresponding metacarpal, are absent, and a cleft in the plane of the missing digit and metacarpal separates the hand into medial and lateral portions; the digits on either side of the cleft may exhibit various degrees of fusion.

When they first appear, the limb buds are somewhat conical in shape. They shortly flatten anteroposteriorly and come to resemble flippers that project inferiorly. Perhaps associated with descent toward their definitive locations, they soon project laterally, almost at right angles to the trunk. Having attained this orientation, they then bend ventrally at the sites of the future elbows and knees, leaving these future joints pointing laterally and the palms and soles facing medially. At this stage, the thumbs and the radial sides of the upper limbs, and the great toes and the tibial sides of the lower limbs form the superior borders of the four limbs.

Each limb is commonly thought to undergo a rotation of 90° in its long axis, that of the upper limb being an external, or lateral, rotation, and that of the lower limb being an internal, or medial rotation. In consequence of this rotation, the flexed elbow now points inferiorly and the flexed knee now points superiorly. In the standing anatomical position, then, the elbow projects posteriorly, the palm faces anteriorly, and the radial side of the upper limb is its lateral surface. Similarly, the knee points anteriorly, the sole faces dorsally when plantar flexed, and the great toe, or tibial, side of the lower limb is its medial surface.

These orientations, especially that of the lower limb, are not fully attained until after birth, and in the adult the distribution of nerves, the arrangement of dermatomes, and the configuration of certain ligaments attest to the occurrence of these rotations during development.

Certain bones of the adult limbs exhibit torsion that is readily apparent when dried specimens of these bones lie on a flat surface. In relation to their heads, the torsion of the humerus is external and that of the femur is internal, circumstances consistent with the direction of developmental rotation of the two limbs. The fact that the degree of torsion in both bones is greater in the fetus than in the adult seems inconsistent with the supposition that the torsion is a manifestation of developmental rotation of the limbs. Moreover, the torsion of the adult tibia is external, whereas developmental rotation of the lower limb as a whole is internal. Findings in experimental studies have in the main supported the premise that the torsions are a consequence of the pull of muscles rather than an aspect of developmental rotation of the limbs.

The skeleton of upper and lower limbs, here considered to include the bones of the pectoral and pelvic girdles, appears to arise from unsegmented mesoderm rather than from somites, but there is experimental evidence that mesenchyme from adjacent somites enters the early limb bud and contributes to the development of the cartilages in both substance and pattern. At 5 weeks, mesenchymal condensations are present at the sites of the future pectoral and pelvic bones and within the limb buds themselves. The several primordia are well along in chondrification at 7 weeks; the largest ones begin ossification in the eighth week, with differentiation generally occurring in a proximodistal direction. As an aspect of earlier differentiation in the upper limb as compared with the lower limb, it is not until the second year after birth that the lower limb becomes longer than the upper limb.

The skeleton of the limbs is, of course, incompletely ossified at birth, and portions such as the carpals, the patella, the navicular, the cuneiforms, and often the cuboid bone, are entirely cartilaginous. Secondary ossification centers arise between birth and the 20th year; fusions of these secondary centers with the main bones usually occur in late adolescence.

The presence of a secondary center of ossification in the lower end of the femur and the upper end of the tibia at about the time of birth, and the appearance of primary centers of ossification in the calcaneus and talus in the sixth to the eighth fetal month (or earlier), and in the cuboid at or soon after birth, are data useful in the medicolegal decision as to whether a newborn child is a full-term fetus.

Along the length of the limbs, perhaps the most frequent anomaly is partial or total absence of the fibula (fibular hemimelia), usually accompanied by deficiency in the lateral side of the foot and deficiency in the muscles on the peroneal side of the leg. In consequence of this condition, the involved limb is usually shortened, and the foot is in the equinovalgus position.

Skull

The skull consists of both endochondral and membrane bone. Much of the former constitutes the floor of the cranial cavity and—stated very simply—develops from four cartilaginous masses: (1) a plate that extends from the caudal end of the hind brain, dorsal to the notochord, to the nasal region and gives rise to much of the ethmoid and sphenoid bones; (2) two otic capsules, each surrounding a developing internal and middle ear, that give rise to the petrous portions of the temporal bones; and (3) the fused sclerotomes of occipital somites 2, 3, and 4 that become much of the occipital bone. Except for the foramen magnum, most of the foramina in the base of the skull are situated along the curved line of junction of the otic capsule with the other cartilaginous masses. The bones of the cranial vault (frontal, parietal, and the interparietal portion of the occipital) are membrane bones. Most of the other bones of the skull develop from mesenchyme of the first and second pharyngeal arches, mesenchyme that may be derived from cells of the neural crest. These bones, including the ossicles of the ear, the mandible, the maxilla, and the squamous temporal, appear to be membrane bones.

Ossification of the chondrocranium begins early in the third month, and differentiation of membrane bone to form the frontal and parietal bones may begin even earlier. Union of the parietal bones with adjacent bones is delayed until several months after birth, the membranous gaps being the fontanelles.

Joints

Speaking generally, two varieties of joints may be recognized: *synarthroses,* which permit limited movement or no movement and which lack a joint cavity and a synovial membrane; and *diarthroses,* which are freely movable and have a joint cavity lined by synovial membrane.

In the development of a synarthrosis, the mesenchyme between the prospective bones, and between ossified portions of a single bone, differentiates into a connecting tissue. The connecting material may be (1) fibrous tissue, in which event the joint is a *syndesmosis* (e.g., the cranial sutures and the stylohyoid joint where the stylohyoid ligament is the connecting fibrous tissue); (2) cartilage, in which case the joint is a *synchondrosis* (e.g., an intervertebral disc, the pubic symphysis, a costosternal joint); or (3) bone, in which case the joint is *synostosis,* (e.g., an ossified epiphyseal line).

In the development of a diarthrosis, or synovial joint (Fig. 1-4), the mesenchyme between the prospective bones exhibits peripheral clefts during the third month. The clefts enlarge and meet, creating a joint cavity and often leaving no tissue between the cartilaginous ends of the participating bones. In certain joints, one or more bands of mesenchyme connecting the participating bones persist and differentiate into ligaments, such as the cruciate ligaments of the knee joint and the ligament of the head in the hip joint. The caps of cartilage over the ends of the

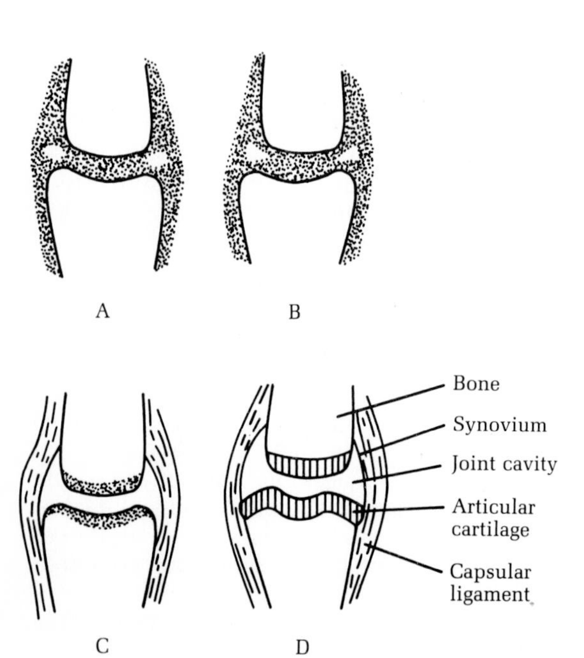

Fig. 1-4. Major events in the development of a synovial joint. (*A*) The cartilaginous models of the two participating bones are surrounded by condensed mesenchyme. Small clefts in the dense mesenchyme between the bones will enlarge to form the joint cavity. (*B*) Progress in the formation of the joint cavity. (*C*) The clefts have coalesced to form the joint cavity; the mesenchyme surrounding the joint has become the joint capsule lined with synovium. Mesenchyme persists over the ends of the two bones. (*D*) The mesenchyme over the ends of the two bones has disappeared, leaving the bones covered with articular cartilage.

participating bones persist as articular cartilage. The sleevelike capsular ligament develops from the mesenchyme external to the synovial cavity and is continuous with the perichondrium (and later the periosteum) of the two bones. The innermost portion of the capsular mesenchyme facing the joint cavity becomes the synovial membrane. The outermost portion of the capsular mesenchyme around many joints thickens to form ligaments such as the tibial and fibular collateral ligaments.

Certain synovial joints have an articular disc between the participating bones. Here two joint cavities arise, and the intervening mesenchyme differentiates into a fibrocartilaginous disc. In the knee joint the menisci are, in effect, incomplete articular discs projecting from the capsular ligament as crescentic discs that incompletely subdivide the joint cavity.

Anomalies of joints that may be attributed to errors in development are uncommon. An interesting one that has been observed in several sites is congenital fusion of bones. Perhaps the most common such anomaly is *congenital radioulnar synostosis* in the proximal third of the forearm. Such a fusion prevents pronation and supination but has little effect upon flexion and extension.

Sesamoid Bones

Sesamoid bones develop in relation to tendons and joints. Most of them arise in the early joint capsules and may pass through a cartilaginous stage.

DEVELOPMENT OF THE MUSCLES

Cellular Differentiation

In the development of skeletal muscle, the progenitor cell is the mesenchymally derived myoblast. Initially cylindrical, myoblasts soon become spindle-shaped and arranged in parallel bundles, meanwhile multiplying rapidly by mitosis. Myofibrils appear first at about 4 weeks in the periphery of the myoblast and increase in number, possibly at least partially by splitting. In the third month, cross-striations of the fibrils become aligned. There seems to be no agreement as to the means or events by which long, multinucleated muscle fibers develop from myoblasts, although study of developing amphibian muscle with the electron microscope has lent support to the theory that the muscle fiber is a syncytium resulting from fusion of many cells.

Deep Muscles of the Back and Neck

The deep muscles of the back and many of the neck muscles are clearly somitic in origin. At 5 weeks the myotomes have begun to fuse superficially and are beginning to be subdivided along the plane of the primitive transverse processes into a dorsal, epaxial portion and a ventral, hypaxial portion (Fig. 1-5). The developing myoblasts are longitudinally oriented. The epaxial column subdivides further into a more superficial, fused portion situated laterally, and a more me-

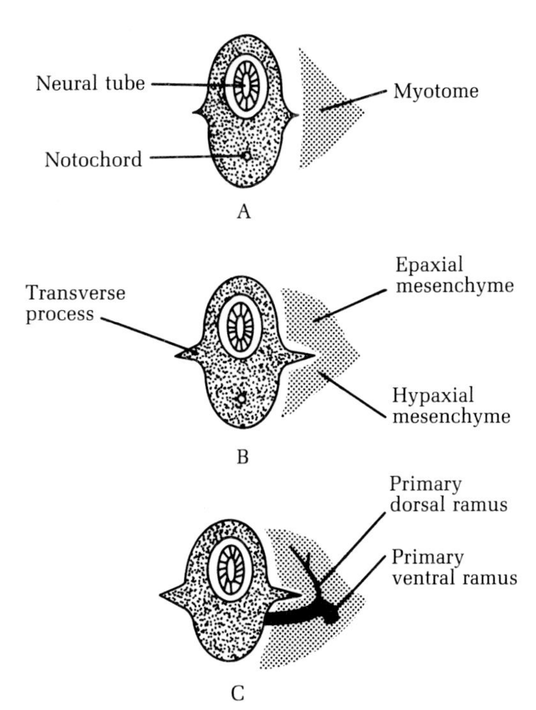

Fig. 1-5. Development of the myotome. (*A*) The myotome in an early stage. (*B*) The transverse process and early fascia have separated the myotome into a dorsal epaxial portion and a ventral hypaxial portion. (*C*) A spinal nerve with its primary dorsal ramus growing into the epaxial portion of the myotome and its primary ventral ramus growing into the hypaxial portion.

dial, discontinuous portion. The superficial portion gives rise to the long muscles of the back and neck: the iliocostalis, longissimus, and splenius muscles. The deeper portion gives rise to the shorter, largely intervertebral muscles: the semispinalis, multifidus, rotator, interspinalis, intertransversarius, obliquus capitis, and rectus capitis muscles. Any muscle derived from epaxial portions of lower sacral and coccygeal myotomes regresses and is represented by dorsal sacral ligaments.

Prevertebral Muscles

The hypaxial column of mesenchyme differentiates into prevertebral muscles: rectus capitis lateralis, rectus capitis anterior, longus capitis, and longus cervicis muscles, the scalene muscles in the neck, and the psoas major and minor and quandratus lumborum muscles in the lumbar region.

Innervation of Somitic Muscles

Certain corollaries of the subdivision of the myotomes into epaxial and hypaxial portions are of more than a little significance. In terms of plan of innervation, a typical spinal nerve early exhibits a primary dorsal ramus and a primary ventral ramus. The primary dorsal rami enter the epaxial portions of myotomes and the primary ventral rami enter the hypaxial mass (Fig. 1-5C). Each primary dorsal ramus typically subdivides further into a lateral and a medial branch. The primary dorsal rami innervate skin and the muscles derived from epaxial portions of the somites, the lateral branches supplying the more lateral muscles and the medial branches supplying the more medial muscles. Each long muscle derived from the superficial epaxial mesenchyme is supplied by several spinal nerves; each of the short muscles is likely to receive a single spinal nerve. The primary ventral rami supply the prevertebral muscles derived from hypaxial mesoderm and the muscles of the body wall. In addition, primary ventral rami form the brachial and lumbosacral plexuses and innervate the limbs.

Origin of Thoracolumbar Fasica

The connective tissue that, along with the transverse processes, separates the epaxial portions of myotomes from the hypaxial portions is a lateral extension of the mesenchyme that differentiates into transverse processes. This connective tissue becomes the middle layer of the thoracolumbar fascia.

Muscles Not Clearly Somitic in Origin

The developmental history of many of the other muscles, especially the superficial muscles of the back and the muscles of the head, anterior neck, trunk, pelvic floor, and limbs, is less certainly known. For many years the prevailing concept has been that all of the muscles except those arising from the pharyngeal arches develop from myotomal mesenchyme. Both the fact that the spinal nerves grow into the myotomes and the dictum that the most reliable clue to the site of origin of a muscle is its innervation support this view. However, the superficial muscles of the back (latissimus dorsi, rhomboid, and serrati posteriores muscles) present a difficulty for this concept inasmuch as these muscles are innervated by primary ventral rami of spinal nerves but are located superficial (dorsal) to the deep muscles that are innervated by primary dorsal rami. This difficulty can be circumvented by supposing that the superficial muscles arise from mesenchyme of hypaxial portions of myotomes that migrate, carrying with them nerves from primary ventral rami. Such migration would have to be extensive for the rhomboid and latissimus dorsi muscles, especially for the latissimus dorsi, whose innervation implies origin from cervical myotomes.

Muscles of the Limbs

Human limb buds arise after most of the somites have appeared. The musculature can be identified early as condensations of mesenchyme, especially near the base of each limb about the terminal ends of nerves growing into the limb. One possibility is that the myogenic mesenchyme in the limb is derived entirely from mesoderm of the lateral body wall with no contribution from adjacent myotomes. Observations made in several experimental studies support this view. Another possibility is that some or all of the myogenic mesenchyme in the limb bud has migrated from adjacent myotomes. Results in other experimental studies support this possibility.

There seems to be less uncertainty concerning the probable myotomal origin of several of the muscles related to the pectoral and pelvic girdles. It has been suggested that the proximal portion of a limb may be a zone of transition from muscle of myotomal origin to muscle that arises *in situ* in the limb. If the suggestion is valid, muscles that span the gap from trunk to limb could have a dual origin.

The upper limb bud lies opposite the lower six cervical and the first two thoracic myotomes, and the lower limb bud is opposite the second to the fifth lumbar myotomes and the upper three sacral myotomes. Branches of nerves supplying these myotomes reach the base of the limb bud and grow into it as it elongates. This growth occurs in such a manner that the muscles of the preaxial border of the upper limb are innervated by the lower five cervical nerves; those of the postaxial border are innervated by the lowest cervical and the first thoracic nerves. Similarly, the preaxial muscles of the lower limb are innervated by the second to fifth lumbar and first sacral nerves; the postaxial muscles receive the first, second, and third sacral nerves. The nerves supplying the limbs divide into the anterior and posterior divisions that supply muscles on the anterior and posterior side, respectively, of the skeleton of the primitive limb. Thus, anterior branches supply primitive flexors and posterior branches supply primitive extensors of the limbs.

Arteries of the Limbs

As is true of blood vessels generally, the blood vessels of the limbs are the surviving components of a network of tentative arteries and veins. The ascending course of the proximal portion of the subclavian artery is a consequence of the descent of the developing heart. This artery projects into the early upper limb bud in an axial position, its proximal portion becoming the subclavian–axillary–brachial trunk, and its distal portion becoming an interosseous artery that intially supplies a plexus of arteries in the primitive hand (Fig. 1-6). A branch of the trunk artery, the median artery, for a time replaces the interosseous artery in supplying the hand. A bit later, the ulnar and then the radial arteries arise as branches of the trunk vessel and assume much of the supply of the forearm and of the superficial and deep palmar arches of the hand that arise from the primitive plexus. The deep branch of the brachial artery and the arteries about the shoulder and elbow arise relatively late as branches of the primary axial vessel.

The placental circulation has been established and the umbilical arteries have attained considerable size when the lower limb bud arises. Where the umbilical artery lies near the root of the limb bud, it gives off a small branch, the ischiadic artery, that serves for a time as the axial artery of the limb (Fig. 1-7). The external iliac artery, arising from the umbilical artery a bit proximal to the ischiadic, soon becomes the chief arterial route of the limb as, successively, the femoral, popliteal, and posterior tibial arteries. An

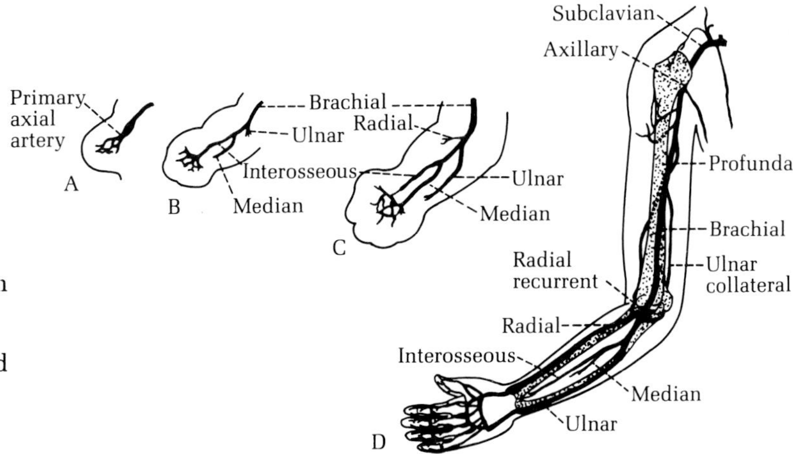

Fig. 1-6. Stages in the development of the arteries of the upper limb. (Redrawn from Patten BM: Human Embryology. New York, P. Blakiston & Son, 1953. Used with permission of the McGraw-Hill Book Company.)

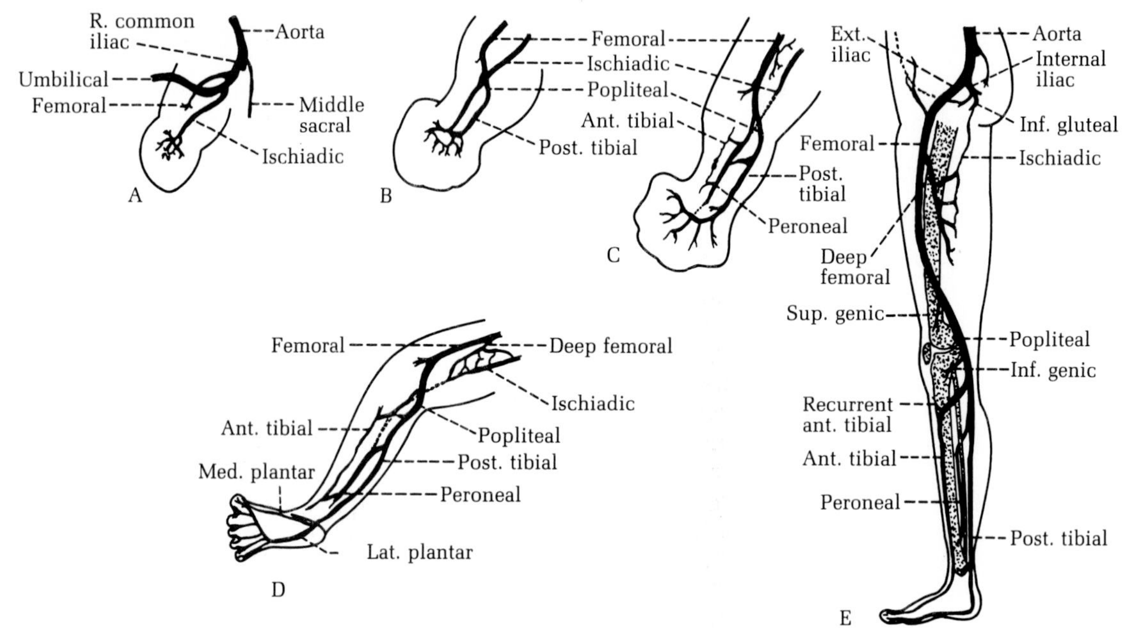

Fig. 1-7. Stages in the development of the arteries of the lower limb. (Redrawn from Patten BM: Human Embryology. New York, P. Blakiston & Son, 1953. Used with permission of McGraw-Hill Book Company.)

anastomosis is formed as the popliteal artery passes near the ischiadic, and the lower part of the ischiadic becomes the peroneal artery. The anterior tibial artery is a new channel paralleling the posterior tibial and peroneal arteries; it is formed by several longitudinal anastomoses that connect small branches extending from the early ischiadic artery toward the anterior surface of the leg. Upon the formation of an anastomosis with the posterior tibial artery, the anterior and posterior tibial arteries become the terminal branches of the popliteal artery. The persisting distal portions of the ischiadic artery become the peroneal and medial inferior genicular arteries. The proximal portion persists as the arteria comitans nervi ischiadici, a branch of the inferior gluteal artery, which lies on the surface of the sciatic nerve and sends branches to anastomose with the lateral and medial femoral circumflex arteries and the first perforating branch of the deep femoral artery—an anastomosis sometimes called the cruciate or crucial anastomosis. The early vascular plexus of the foot is supplied by the ischiadic artery. As this connection regresses, the plexus is supplied by the posterior tibial artery. Later, the new anterior tibial artery reaches the foot and comes to supply the dorsal arcuate artery and its branches, and the posterior tibial artery supplies the plantar arteries.

Trapezius and Sternocleidomastoid Muscles

The developmental history of the trapezius and sternocleidomastoid muscles, innervated by the spinal portion of the accessory nerve, is uncertain. These muscles apparently arise from a common mesenchymal mass that later splits to form the two muscles. Some investigators consider this mass to be of somitic origin; others believe it to be derived from branchial mesenchyme; still others consider it to be of mixed somitic and brachial origin.

Congenital Torticollis (wryneck) is a consequence of unilateral shortening of a sternocleidomastoid muscle, commonly associated with fibrosis of the muscle; it may also involve the platysma and the scalene muscles. Many causes have been suggested for the condition.

Ventrolateral Muscles of Neck and Trunk

The infrahyoid muscles, diaphragm, intercostal muscles, and muscles of the abdominal wall are usually said to develop from ventral extension or migration of hypaxial portions of myotomes. Longitudinal splitting of the mesoderm in frontal and sagittal planes presumably accounts for the geniohyoid and individual infrahyoid muscles. It has also been believed that the muscle of the diaphragm differentiates from ventral extensions of cervical myotomes during or after much caudad migration. The innervation of this muscle by phrenic nerves is consistent with this supposition, but there is no direct evidence supporting such origin. Tangential splitting of hypaxial mesoderm from thoracic myotomes and the first lumbar myotome into three layers is usually said to account for the external, internal, and innermost intercostal muscles, as well as the transversus thoracis of the thoracic wall and for the external oblique, internal oblique, and transversus abdominus muscles of the abdominal wall. The most ventral extension of myotomal tissue is said to give rise to the narrow, longitudinally oriented band that becomes the rectus abdominis. The infrequent sternalis muscle may be a persisting superior portion of this band. Segmental arrangement of muscle is accented in the thoracic wall by the presence of ribs, and the tendinous intersections of the rectus abdominis are a suggestion of segmentation in the abdominal wall.

The pattern of innervation of the muscles of the thoracic and abdominal walls is consistent with myotomal origin of these muscles. Experimental studies in amphibians and mammals seem to support somitic origin of the intercostal muscles. Observations made in experiments employing chick embryos, however, indicate that the ventral portions of the three muscles of the lateral abdominal wall, the entirety of the rectus abdominis muscle, and the ventral portions of the intercostal muscles arise *in situ* from cells of lateral plate mesoderm rather than from somites.

It has been suggested that the levator ani and coccygeus muscles, the voluntary anal sphincters, and skeletal muscle associated with the external genitalia arise from hypaxial portions of the third sacral to first coccygeal myotomes. Innervation and structure in lower mammals seem to support this view.

Muscles of the Head

In respect to their origin, the muscles of the head and the visceral muscles of the neck fall into three categories: branchiomeric muscles, somitic muscles, and muscles arising from general mesoderm of the head.

The muscles of mastication, the mylohyoid muscle, the anterior belly of the digastric muscle, the tensor tympani muscle, and the tensor veli palatini muscle develop, with little migration, from mesenchyme of the first branchial arch. These are innervated by the nerve of that arch, the mandibular division of the trigeminal nerve. The muscles of facial expression (a group that includes the buccinator, occipitofrontalis, auricular, and platysma muscles), as well as the posterior belly of the digastric, the stylohyoid, and the stapedius muscles, develop from mesenchyme of the second arch and are innervated by the facial nerve, the nerve of the second arch. Mesenchyme of the third arch gives rise to only one muscle, the stylopharyngeus, supplied by the nerve of that arch, the glossopharyngeal nerve. The muscles of the pharynx and larynx and most of the muscles of the palate arise from mesenchyme of the fourth, fifth, and sixth arches; these are supplied by the nerves of these arches, the vagus nerve and the cranial portion of the accessory nerve.

The only muscles of the head that may confidently be considered to be somitic in origin are the intrinsic and extrinsic muscles of the tongue. In experimental studies, mesenchyme from occipital somites has been traced into the region of the tongue. Consistent with such origin, these muscles are supplied by the hypoglossal nerve, which appears to follow the migrating mesoderm and to be comparable in its origin and course to motor fibers of spinal nerves.

In respect to their innervation, the ocular muscles are somitic in origin. In man, however, the occipital somites are the most rostral somites, and no evidence is available indicating migration of this mesenchyme into the ocular region. It is possible that paraxial mesoderm in the region of the eye differentiates into the ocular muscles without first segmenting into somites.

Tendons

The tendons also arise from mesenchyme, but they are said to develop independently of the muscle and to be secondarily attached to it and to bone. Aponeuroses, on the other hand, are said to arise through degeneration of muscles or myotomes, or parts of myotomes.

Fasciae

Fasciae arise from mesenchyme between and surrounding the several organ primordia, including muscles; this mesenchyme may be regarded as building material not used in the formation of the organ. For example, the prevertebral fascia of the neck arises from the connective tissue (epimysium) surrounding each of the pervertebral and scalene muscles. The superficial layer of the deep cervical fascia arises from the connective tissue surrounding the mesenchymal sheet that forms sternocleidomastoid and trapezius muscles; the separation of this sheet into the two muscles leaves the superficial layer of fascia covering the posterior triangle of the neck. Anteriorly, this layer of fascia invests the infrahyoid muscles, or, put another way, it fuses with the epimysia of these muscles.

The origin of the thoracolumbar fascia from the connective tissue between epaxial and hypaxial division of the myotomes has already been mentioned. Like other fasciae, this layer comes to provide attachments for muscles. Apparently in response to mechanical stress, the fascia takes on the structural character of an aponeurosis. Fascia about a muscle mass in one region usually becomes continuous with fascia of a homologous muscle in an adjacent region.

SELECTED REFERENCES

Agnish ND, Kochhar DM: The role of somites in the growth and early development of mouse limb buds. Dev Biol 56:174, 1977

Arey LB: Developmental Anatomy, pp. 396–438. Philadelphia, WB Saunders, 1966

Bardeen CR, Lewis WH: Development of the limbs, body-wall and back in man. Am J Anat 1:1, 1901

Coventry MB et al: The intervertebral disc: Its microscopic anatomy and pathology. Part I: Anatomy, development and physiology. J Bone Joint Surg 27:105, 1945

Ehrenhaft JL: Development of the vertebral column as related to certain congenital and pathological changes. Surg Gynecol Obstet 76:282, 1943

Gardner E, Gray DJ: Prenatal development of the human shoulder and acromioclavicular joints. Am J Anat 92:219, 1953

Haines RW: The development of joints. J Anat 81:33, 1947

Hamilton WJ, Boyd JD, Mossman HW: Human Embryology, pp 389–425. Baltimore, Williams & Wilkins, 1962

Lewis WH: The development of the arm in man. Am J Anat 1:145, 1902

Noback CR, Robertson GG: Sequences of appearance of ossification centers in the human skeleton during the first five prenatal months. Am J Anat 89:1, 1951

Sensenig EC: The early development of the human vertebral column. Carnegie Contributions to Embryology 33:21, 1949

Shands AR Jr, Steele MK: Torsion of the femur: A follow-up report on the use of the Dunlap method for its determination. J Bone Joint Surg 40A:803, 1958

Straus WL Jr, Rawles ME: An experimental study of the origin of the trunk musculature and ribs in the chick. Am J Anat 92:471, 1953

Streeter GL: Developmental horizons in human embryos: A review of the histogenesis of cartilage and bone. Carnegie Contributions to Embryology, 33:149, 1949

Winter RB, Moe JH, Eilers VE: Congenital scoliosis: A study of 234 patients treated and untreated. Part I: Natural history. J Bone Joint Surg 50A:1, 1968

Chapter 2

Congenital Malformations

Charles W. Hooker and Walter B. Greene

GOALS AND OBJECTIVES

Goals: To summarize the developmental and genetic basis of malformations; to describe certain congenital malformations of the musculoskeletal system and to review their causation

Objectives: On completion of this unit, and using the text as a standard reference, one should be able to recognize, describe, or explain the following:

1. The hereditary patterns of autosomal dominant, autosomal recessive, and sex-linked traits
2. The pattern of inheritance in a family pedigree
3. Chromosomal abnormalities
4. Autosomal malformations
5. Familial disorders
6. Nongenetic malformations
7. Deficiencies in the limbs

OUTLINE

I. The developmental substrate
II. Basic genetic considerations
III. Chromosomal abnormalities
IV. Autosomal malformations
   A. Achondroplasia
   B. Multiple epiphyseal dysplasia
   C. Multiple cartilaginous exostoses
   D. Osteogenesis imperfecta
   E. Marfan's syndrome
   F. Mucopolysaccharidoses
V. Sex-linked disorders: hypophosphatemic vitamin D-resistant rickets
VI. Multifactorial disorders
   A. Congential dislocation of the hip

- B. Clubfoot
- C. Spina bifida

VII. Nongenetic influences
- A. Radiation
- B. Infection
- C. Chemicals
- D. Maternal trauma

VIII. Deficiencies in the limbs

The term *congenital malformations* is generally understood to denote deformities or abnormalities, usually anatomic in nature, that can be recognized at birth. The magnitude of this problem is suggested by the estimate that one or more malformations are present in 10% of all live births.

A concern with malformations antedates written history. Certain physical abnormalities are depicted in the carvings and rock drawings of primitive peoples. Prophetic significance was attached to them by Chaldean diviners and early Romans, and throughout the Middle Ages; explanations have included the wrath of an offended god, hybridity with another species, and maternal impression. The hybridity hypothesis, widespread in the Dark Ages, persisted with cruel consequences in colonial New England; belief in maternal impression has not yet disappeared.

This chapter, in summary fashion, describes and reviews the genesis of a few of the malformations of the musculoskeletal system that create clinical problems.

THE DEVELOPMENTAL SUBSTRATE

A striking attribute of the development of the embryo is the ostensible simplicity of the highly significant and orderly morphologic events that constitute the early phases of the development of individual organs and organ systems. For example, an apparently simple infolding of the dorsal surface of the very young embryo produces a mid-line, longitudinal tube that, with appropriate proliferation and differentiation of the cells of its wall, becomes both the spinal cord and the brain, into and out of which grow the spinal nerves and most of the cranial nerves. A minute deviation or error in such an early developmental event or a deviation from the exquisitely programmed schedule of events can have consequences that range from the undetectable to the catastrophic. Additionally, the demonstrated influence of one developing tissue or organ upon the differentiation of another* makes it possible for a single small error to result in more than one disturbance in development. Inasmuch as the basic steps in the formation of organs occur early, the errors that result in malformations must in many instances also occur early, and factors that provoke profound errors in development must be operative in the quite young embryo.

Upon completion of the early morphologic events involved in the formation of organ primordia, further development involves, in addition to proliferation of cells, cell differentiation with its morphologic and biochemical components. Thus, differentiation of the primordia of most of the components of the skeleton involves, in ordered sequence, formation of collagenous fibers, formation of the amorphous matrix of cartilage, and ultimately osteogenesis—all directed in such a way as to produce the morphologic attributes and specializations of each individual bone. A significant aberration in any of these events can result in a defective or malformed bone, and the cause could be failure of one specific enzyme or its substrate to appear at the scheduled time. In short, the malformation is morphologic, but its immediate nature may be biochemical.

The numerous small but significant events in development provide opportunities for many errors, a situation that could account for the sporadic and unpredictable occurrence of individualized malformations. Analysis of such errors, irrespective of cause, is at best an uncertain undertaking because of insufficient precise information concerning the identity and *modus operandi* of the influences that govern normal development. If as currently postulated, however, the details of every aspect of development are encoded in the nucleic acids of the chromosomes of the fertilized ovum, it follows that departures from normal development must be manifestations of the original genetic composition of the fertilized ovum, of modification of the genetic composition by spon-

*Examples of such influence are induction by the optic cup of formation of the lens from body wall ectoderm and many instances of the influence of mesenchyme upon the differentiation of overlying epithelium.

taneous mutation or environmental factors, or of interference with expression of that genetic composition by other genetic influences or environmental factors.

In keeping with this postulate, it has been estimated that as many as 90% of all congenital malformations have a genetic background, and enough information concerning several malformations is at hand to permit formulation of pedigrees and predictions of occurrence that warrant genetic counseling. Of this 90%, about 10% are said to reflect visible abnormalities of the chromosomes, about 20% to involve simple mendelian inheritance, and about two-thirds to have a multifactorial basis.

BASIC GENETIC CONSIDERATIONS

All human cells except spermatozoa and ova and their immediate precursors have an allotment of 23 pairs of chromosomes: 22 pairs of autosomes and one pair of sex chromosomes (Fig. 2-1). In the female, the sex chromosomes are alike (XX); in the male they are unlike (XY). The biologic units of heredity, the genes, are located on the chromosomes and, like the chromosomes, are paired, a member of each pair (termed alleles) being on a member of a pair of chromosomes.

The simplest pattern of inheritance involves a trait whose presence or absence is determined by a single pair of genes. When the paired genes are alike, the organism is said to be *homozygous* for the trait; when the paired genes are unlike, the organism is said to be *heterozygous* for the trait. The member of a heterozygous pair of genes that expresses itself in a trait is said to be a *dominant* gene; the member that does not express itself is said to be *recessive*. The traits determined by dominant genes, on either autosomes or sex chromosomes, will be manifested whether the person is homozygous or heterozygous for the condition. Recessive genes on autosomal chromosomes will be manifested only when the person is homozygous for that gene. If a trait is due to a recessive gene on an X chromosome, that trait will be expressed in a female homozygous for that gene but not in a heterozygous female. Inasmuch as the male has one X chromosome and a Y chromosome, one recessive gene on the X chromosome produces the trait; this circumstance accounts for traits that appear in the male and only rarely in the female. It is clear that the heterozygous female transmits the characteristic to *at least* half of her offspring. Traits transmitted by genes carried only on the X chromosomes are termed *sex-linked*.

A malformation whose transmission depends upon a single gene or a pair of genes may be said to involve simple mendelian in-

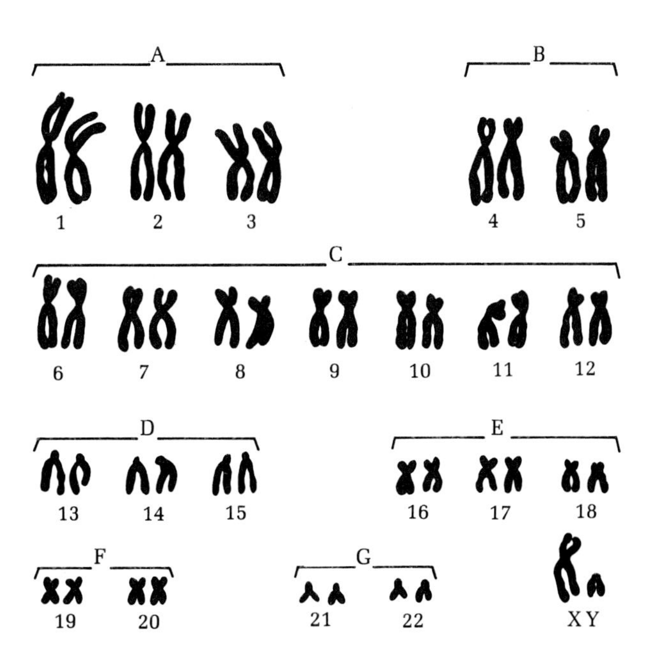

Fig. 2-1. Karyotype of a normal male.

heritance. Depending upon the disorder, the responsible gene may be autosomal dominant (Fig. 2-2), autosomal recessive (Fig. 2-3), sex-linked dominant (Fig. 2-4), or sex-linked recessive (Fig. 2-5). Such inheritance exhibits variable expressivity in the sense that affected members of a family usually manifest different degrees in the severity of the disorder. Generally speaking, dominant disorders have a degree of variability in expression that is greater than that of recessive disorders. The extent of expressivity may be influenced by the responsible gene, by other genes, and by the environment of the embryo.

Many traits in man involve more than one pair of genes, a circumstance that makes genetic analysis more difficult. Complicating the problem are such considerations as the small number of progeny in a crossing, limited information concerning the pedigrees of families, and the high order of genetic heterogeneity of the human being.

CHROMOSOMAL ABNORMALITIES

Chromosomal abnormalities are alterations in the number of chromosomes or visible abnormalities in one or more chromosomes, both of which entail alterations in the genic composition of cells. These abnormalities may be a consequence of mutations, and certain of them are passed on from generation to generation. Although chromosomal abnormalities have been found in roughly 20% of spontaneously aborted fetuses, Carter holds that they account for relatively few of the malformations seen in fetuses examined in the late weeks of gestation.

The most frequently occurring generalized disturbance produced by abnormal chromosomes is Down's syndrome (mongolism, trisomy 21). This disorder is characterized by mental retardation, short stature, eyes with epicanthal folds that confer an oriental appearance, a single flexion crease in the fifth finger, and a simian crease in the distal portion of the palm. Other skeletal abnormalities include small acetabular angles, large ilia, elongated and tapering ischia, and dysplastic middle phalanges of the fifth finger. About 95% of children with Down's syndrome have 47 chromosomes, the extra chromosome being associated with the 21st pair (Fig. 2-6). In others there has been transfer of material from the 21st pair of chromosomes to a chromosomes of the D group (pairs 13 to 15) or to a chromosome of the G group (pairs 21 and 22).

Other recognized abnormalities of autosomal chromosomes are rare and include Trisomy 18 and Trisomy D. Abnormalities that involve the sex chromosomes produce abnormalities in genital development and in other traits associated with genes on the sex chromosomes. One of these is Klinefelter's syndrome, which occurs in one of 800 live births and involves the presence of one or two extra X chromosomes (45/XXY or 45/XXXY). Another is Turner's syndrome, re-

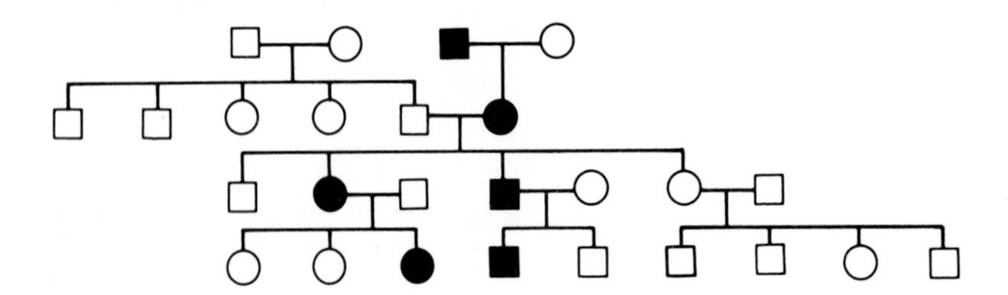

■● Affected male, female
□○ Unaffected male, female

Fig. 2-2. Autosomal dominant pattern of inheritance. The trait is exhibited in each generation; roughly 50% of the offspring of both sexes carry the responsible gene and exhibit the trait. (McKusick VA: Heritable Disorders of Connective Tissue, 3rd ed. St Louis, C. V. Mosby, 1966)

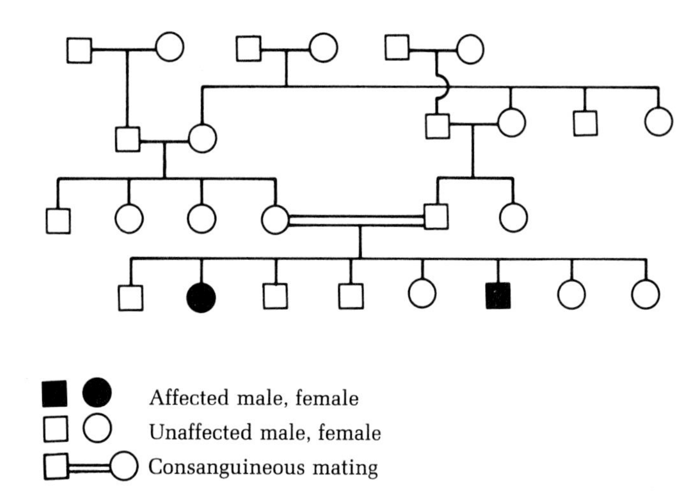

Fig. 2-3. Autosomal recessive inheritance. The trait is absent in one or more generations; occasionally there is a family history of consanguinity. Offspring manifest the trait only when homozygous for the responsible gene; males and females are equally affected. (McKusick VA: Heritable Disorders of Connective Tissue, 3rd ed. St. Louis, C. V. Mosby, 1966)

lated to absence of the second sex chromosome (45/XO), a rare condition in which there may be webbing of the neck and cubitus valgus.

AUTOSOMAL MALFORMATIONS

Achondroplasia is inherited as an autosomal dominant trait, the child of an achondroplastic parent having a 50% chance of inheriting the disorder. Eighty to ninety percent of all persons with this disorder, however, are born to parents who are not achondroplastic, and such parents rarely have a second achondroplastic child. It is presumed in these instances that the disorder is the consequence of a mutation.

Achondroplasia (Fig. 2-7) is a generalized disorder that is a consequence of disturbance of growth of the epiphyseal cartilages of endochondral bones. The limbs are disproportionately short; the head is large, both relatively and absolutely; the forehead is prominent; and the nasal bridge is depressed. In addition to their shortness, the limbs typically exhibit limitation of extension of the elbow, trident hands (increased space between the third and fourth fingers), contractures of flexion of the hip, and genu varum (bowlegs); the long bones are wide, with flaring of the metaphyses. The pelvis is broad and short, with relatively wide iliac wings and horizontal acetabular margins. There is a progressive decrease in the distance between the pedicles of the lumbar vertebrae, with diminution in size of the vertebral canal. Other problems include dental malocclusion, communicating hydrocephalus, arthritis, compression of the lower spinal

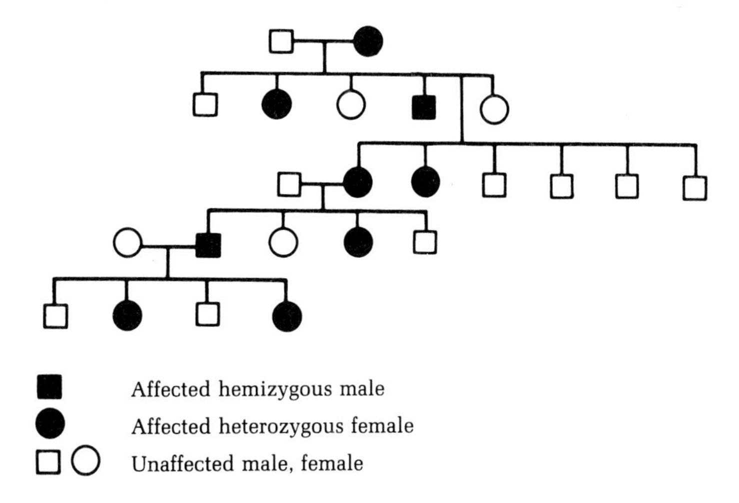

Fig. 2-4. Sex-linked dominant inheritance. Each generation usually exhibits the trait. When the female is the carrier, 50% of the offspring exhibit the trait. When the male is the carrier, all daughters but no sons exhibit the trait, that is, there is no transmission male-to-male. (McKusick, VA: Heritable Disorders of Connective Tissue, 3rd ed. St. Louis, C. V. Mosby, 1966)

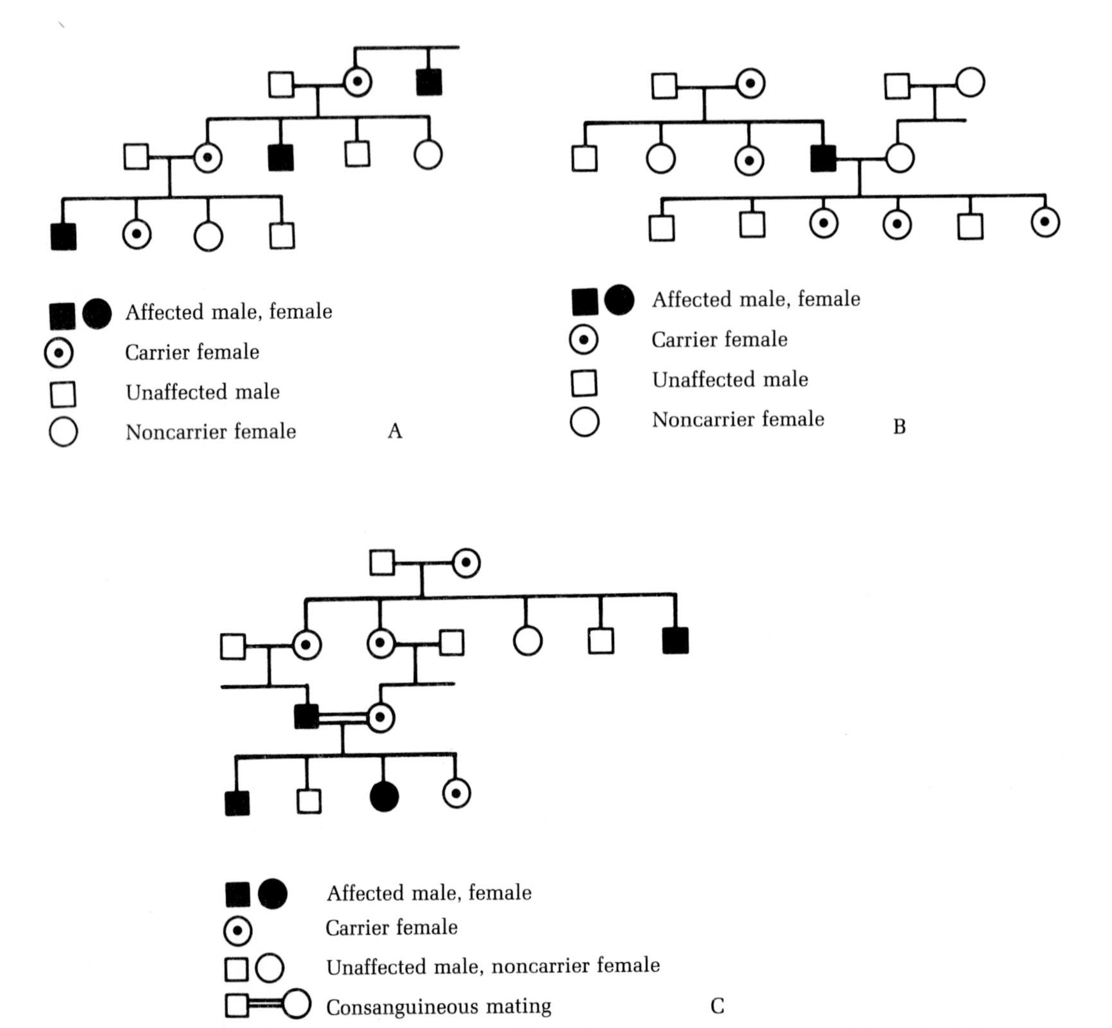

Fig. 2-5. Sex-linked recessive inheritance. When the female is the carrier (A), 50% of the sons exhibit the trait and 50% of the daughters are carriers. When the male exhibits the trait (B), all of the daughters are carriers and the sons are free of the trait. A cross between a male exhibiting the trait and a female carrier (C) results in the trait's being exhibited by 50% of the sons; half of the daughters exhibit the trait and the other half are carriers. (McKusick VA: Heritable Disorders of Connective Tissue, 3rd ed. St. Louis, C. V. Mosby, 1966)

cord by the narrowing of the vertebral canal, and the psychologic problems of short stature.

Achondroplasia is but one of the more than 600 types of skeletal dysplasia, most of which are characterized by short stature and many of which are caused by inherited abnormalities. Short stature is considered to be abnormal when height is less than that of the third percentile for persons of the same age and sex. The term *midget* denotes a person with abnormally short stature and a limb-to-trunk ratio that is normal. *Dwarfs*, on the other hand, have a deformity of the trunk or limbs or both and, in addition, limb-to-trunk ratios that are abnormal.

Skeletal dysplasia may be manifested as arms or thighs that are short relative to the entire limb (rhizomelic dwarfism), disproportionately short forearms or legs (mesomelic dwarfism), or disproportionately short hands or feet (acromelic dwarfism).

Multiple epiphyseal dysplasia is inherited as an autosomal dominant trait with variable expressivity. The disorder is manifested as multiple areas of abnormal

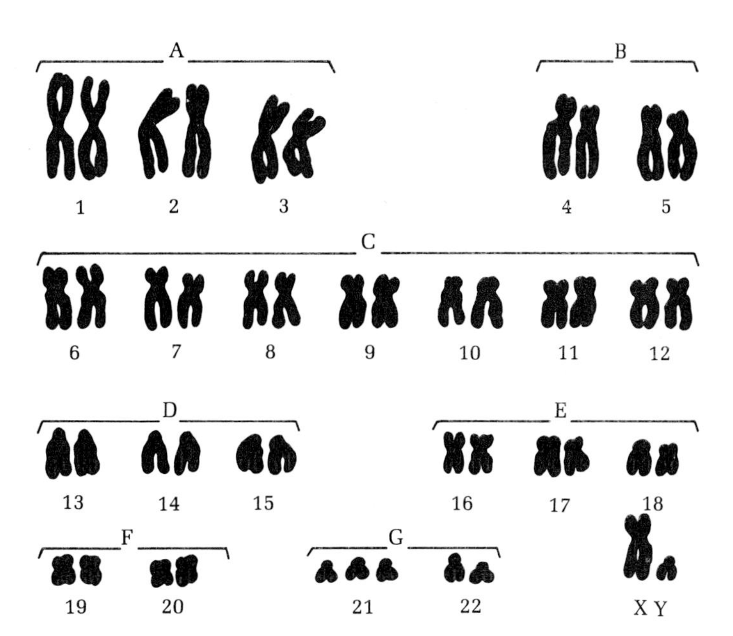

Fig. 2-6. The chromosomes in Trisomy 21 (Down's syndrome). Compare with Fig. 2-1.

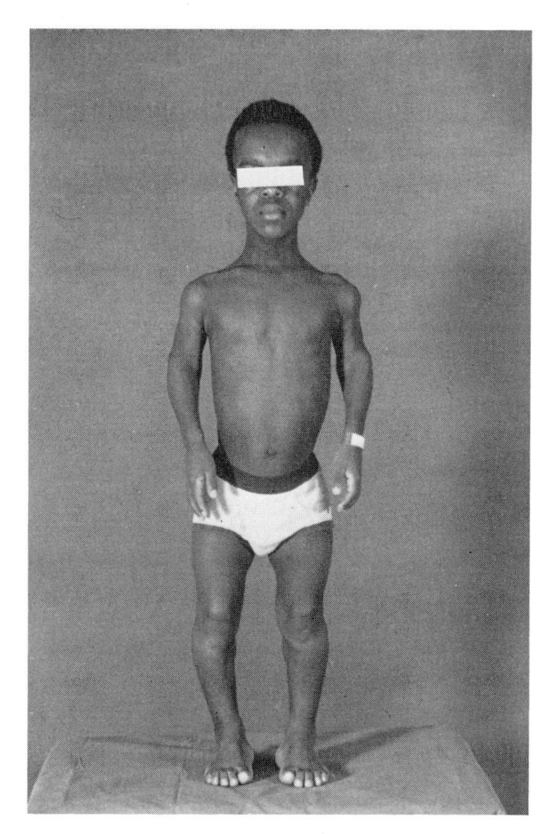

Fig. 2-7. Achondroplasia in a male 14 years of age. Height, 118 cm (47 inches). Note rhizomelic shortening, mild genu varum, and relatively large head.

epiphyseal ossification. The epiphysis involved varies from person to person, but the disorder tends to be bilaterally symmetrical and to affect predominantly the hips, knees, ankles, and wrists. In the severe type of this disorder, the epiphyseal ossification centers are small and frequently fragmented. The irregularities of the joint surfaces often lead to degenerative arthritis, with significant disability by the third or fourth decade.

The condition of *multiple cartilaginous exostoses* is typically inherited as an autosomal dominant trait. The lesions are osteochondromas (projections of bone with cartilaginous caps) that occur in several sites. In over 90% of cases the distal femur, proximal tibia, proximal femur, and proximal humerus are the areas of involvement. The problems include pain owing to fracture or pressure of the exostosis on surrounding soft tissues, neurovascular compromise, interference with the configuration of a joint, and possible sarcomatous degeneration of the osteochondroma.

Osteogenesis imperfecta is usually inherited as an autosomal dominant trait, but there is evidence that it may also be an autosomal recessive trait; the latter usually leads to early death. The outstanding attribute of this disorder is diminished density and increased fragility of bones, leading to multiple fractures and secondary deformities (Fig.

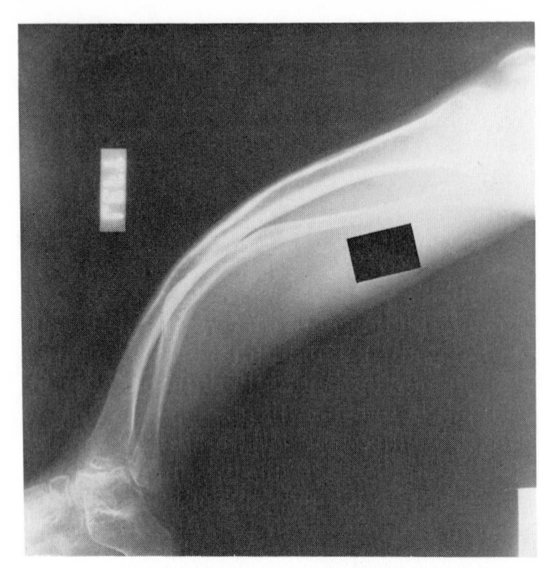

Fig. 2-8. Osteogenesis imperfecta as it appears on a lateral roentgenogram of the tibia. Note the osteopenia and thin cortices. Multiple fractures have resulted in anterior angulation of the tibia, placing the foot in equinus and making walking quite difficult.

2-8). Other problems may include short stature, blue sclerae, middle-ear deafness, laxity of ligaments, and scoliosis. Two forms of the disorder are recognized: osteogenesis imperfecta congenita, characterized by intrauterine fractures, and osteogenesis imperfecta tarda, in which fractures appear when the child begins to walk. The fundamental defect appears to be a disorder of collagen that interferes with calcification.

Marfan's syndrome is inherited as an autosomal dominant trait with variable expressivity. It is characterized by long, thin limbs and by laxity of ligaments. Related problems may include scoliosis, recurrent dislocation of the patella, flat feet, flexion deformities of the fingers and toes, and hypotonia of muscle. Associated abnormalities include dislocation of the lens, retinal detachment, aortic regurgitation, and abdominal aortic aneurysm. There is evidence that this is a disorder of collagen.

Mucopolysaccharidoses are characterized by a defect in the metabolism of one or more mucopolysaccharides, with resulting excessive accumulation of these substances in the extracellular spaces of the connective tissues. One such disorder is *Morquio's syndrome* (Fig. 2-9), inherited as an autosomal recessive trait. In addition to short stature, skeletal problems associated with this disorder include instability of the cervical portion of the vertebral column due to hypoplasia of the dens, either scoliosis or kyphosis or both, a keel-like sternum (pectus carinatum), laxity of the joints, knock-knees, and dysplastic hips. Other problems include corneal opacity and abnormal dentition. Keratan sulfate accumulates in the tissues.

Another member of this group of disorders is *Hurler's syndrome* (Fig. 2-10), also inherited as an autosomal recessive trait. This rare disorder is characterized by a facial structure described as gargoylism, which includes a low forehead, widely separated eyes, a saddle nose, and a large tongue. There may also be a shoe-shaped sella turcica and a lower thoracic or upper lumbar hump (gibbus) produced by hypoplasia of the anterior portions of vertebral bodies and spatulate ribs. The faulty metabolism of mucopolysaccharides results in accumulation of dermatan sulfate and heparin sulfate in tissues and high levels of these substances in the urine.

SEX-LINKED DISORDERS

Hypophosphatemic vitamin D-resistant rickets is one of the few disorders inherited as a sex-linked dominant trait. As in other sex-linked dominant diseases, the degree of expressivity varies, and there may be incomplete penetrance. In some affected patients, the disorder is manifested only by a low serum phosphorus; in others there is also widening of epiphyseal plates and bowing of the legs. The classic picture is short stature, bowing of the lower limbs (especially at the knees), and typical rachitic changes in the long bones. Recent studies suggest that the basic defect is faulty renal reabsorption of phosphate. Serum phosphorus is low, serum calcium is usually normal, and serum alkaline phosphatase is elevated when turnover of bone is increased.

MULTIFACTORIAL DISORDERS

Several disorders have a familial incidence significantly higher than that dictated by chance and a genetic basis that is multifac-

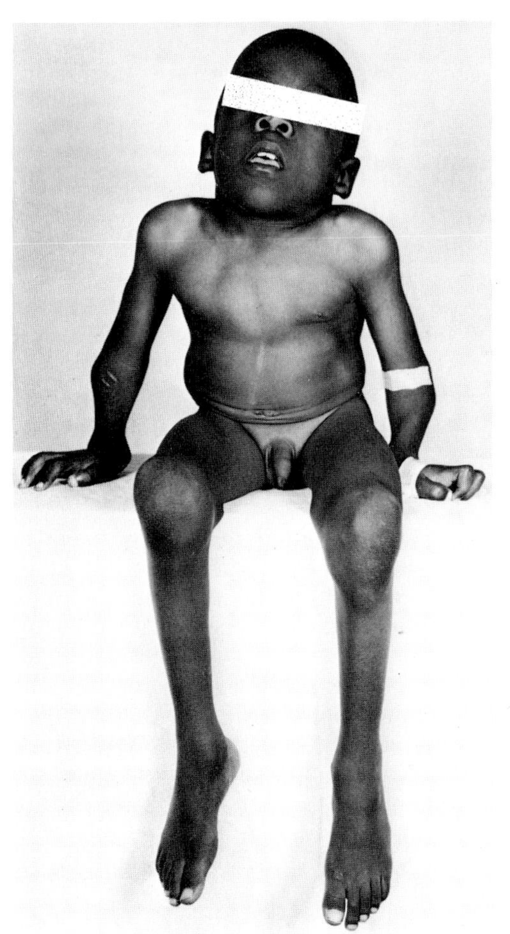

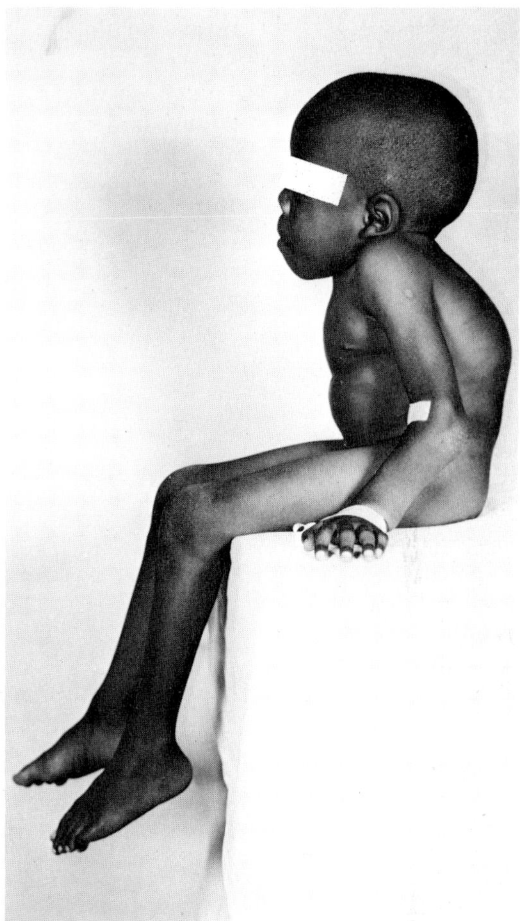

Fig. 2-9. Morquio's syndrome.

torial (polygenic). In some, a genetic predisposition is influenced by factors in the environment.

In *congenital displacement of the hip*, there is subluxation or dislocation of the head of the femur from the acetabulum. In one study, the incidence was 1.6 per 1000 live births, and it occurred six times as often in females as in males. There is reported concordance in 40% of monozygotic twins but in only 5% of dizygotic twins; it occurs 10 to 50 times more often in siblings of affected children than in the general population. It is generally supposed that instability of the hip joint is a consequence of laxity of the ligaments, perhaps genetically determined, and that displacement of the femoral head results from such environmental influences as breech delivery or restraint of the hips in a position of extension and adduction.

In patients with *congenital talipes equinovarus* (clubfoot), the foot is plantar-flexed and inverted. The condition has an incidence of one per 1000 live births. It occurs twice as often in males as in females, and in half of affected persons the condition is bilateral. The chance that siblings of an affected child will have the disorder is 3%; the chance that offspring of an affected parent will have the deformity is 8% to 11%. Both members of a pair of monozygotic twins have the deformity more often than both members of a pair of dizygotic twins. The nature of the genetic basis for the disorder has not been established, but it has been suggested that the usual hereditary pattern is recessive, although in some families it appears to be dominant with reduced penetrance.

Spina bifida reflects local failure of the vertebral arch to enclose the vertebral canal.

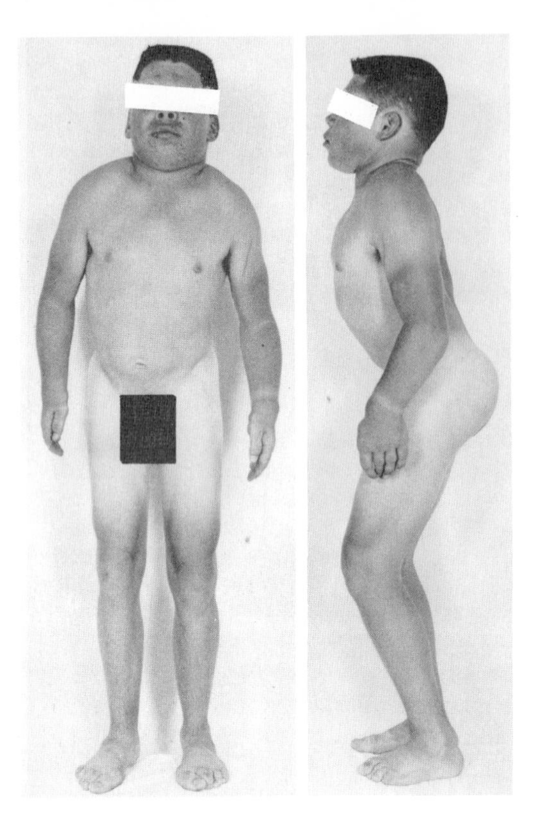

Fig. 2-10. Hurler's syndrome.

In spina bifida occulta, the defect involves primarily bone, but the skin may be attached to the dura, the spinal cord, or nerve roots by fibrous bands. In spina bifida cystica, neural tissue may be exposed (myeloschisis), the meninges may protrude (meningocele), or nerve roots or spinal cord may protrude with the meninges (meningomyelocele). There is a 6% probability of occurrence in siblings of children with spina bifida cystica, and there is some concordance in monozygotic twins. The condition may be due to an autosomal recessive gene with low penetrance. It has also been suggested that this condition results from a polygenic inheritance that interacts with intrauterine environmental factors.

The data at hand show that the foregoing and certain other congenital malformations of the musculoskeletal system have a genetic basis that has been analyzed to some extent. It is apparent, however, that in most instances the specific developmental error or errors have not been identified in more than a general way—if, indeed, specific errors are operating.

Although not categorized as congenital because they are not recognized at birth, several other disorders have a demonstrated genetic basis. An example is Duchenne's muscular dystrophy, usually diagnosed at age 4 or 5 when muscular weakness begins to create problems in running and walking.

Inherited disorders of other organ systems may create problems in the musculoskeletal system. An example is the arthropathy that results from hemophilia.

NONGENETIC INFLUENCES

Many agents, called teratogens, have been shown to provoke a wide variety of congenital malformations in experimental animals. In producing their effects, teratogens appear to act as mutagens, as environmental factors affecting the expression of genic determination, as promoters of abnormal growth or differentiation, or as lethal agents preventing survival of specific embryonic tissues or organ primordia. Agents that have produced malformations in man include radiation, extraneous chemicals, infections, and maternal trauma.

Radiation as a possible cause of malformations must be considered in terms of the dose and duration of radiation and the time of its delivery to the germ cells or conceptus. High levels of radiation may kill or damage the germ cells, often resulting in sterility or alterations in the chromosomes.

Irradiation of the conceptus may cause multiple anomalies; the effects appear to be related to the amount and duration of exposure and to the stage of development. It is reported that irradiation of experimental animals after conception and prior to implantation does not provoke abnormalities; the conceptuses survive intact or are stillborn, as in nonirradiated animals. On the other hand, irradiation late in gestation, unlike most other teratogens, has produced malformations in animals, most often involving the central nervous system. There is no evidence that exposure to background or diagnostic radiation during pregnancy results in increased incidence of malformations in man.

Therapeutic radiation during pregnancy, however, constitutes a serious hazard: in one study, as many as one-third of such infants were born with abnormalities, most frequently microcephaly. The classic exposure to massive radiation during pregnancy occurred with the use of atomic bombs in Japan. The most frequent malformation in children born subsequent to the explosions was microcephaly, its frequency being related to the proximity of the mothers to the explosion. Many other anomalies occurred in these children, but none in higher incidence than that expected in an unexposed population.

The nature and magnitude of the hazards of irradiation to future generations are unknown, but they have been the subject of much concern and discussion.

The most familiar example of *infection* as a cause of malformations is *rubella*. When the disease occurs in the first trimester of pregnancy, the defects that may occur in the infant include deafness, cataracts, microcephaly, mental retardation, cardiac anomalies, thrombocytopenia, retarded growth, and metaphyseal abnormalities. The infant with *congenital syphilis* may have pseudoparalysis of a limb as a consequence of separation of an epiphysis; the long bones show irregular, sclerotic epiphyseal lines.

The most thoroughly documented production of malformations by a *chemical compound* taken by the mother is that by the drug *thalidomide*. When this drug is taken during the first trimester, there is an especially high incidence of malformations, particularly of the limbs, ranging from partial to complete amputation (Fig. 2-11). Administration of the folic acid antagonist *aminopterin* during the first trimester may result in a baby with anomalies of the skeletal system that include small size, a small skull, and clubfeet.

Maternal trauma early in pregnancy may rupture the amnion, leaving the chorion intact. When this rupture occurs, bands of amnion may encircle a developing limb or digit.

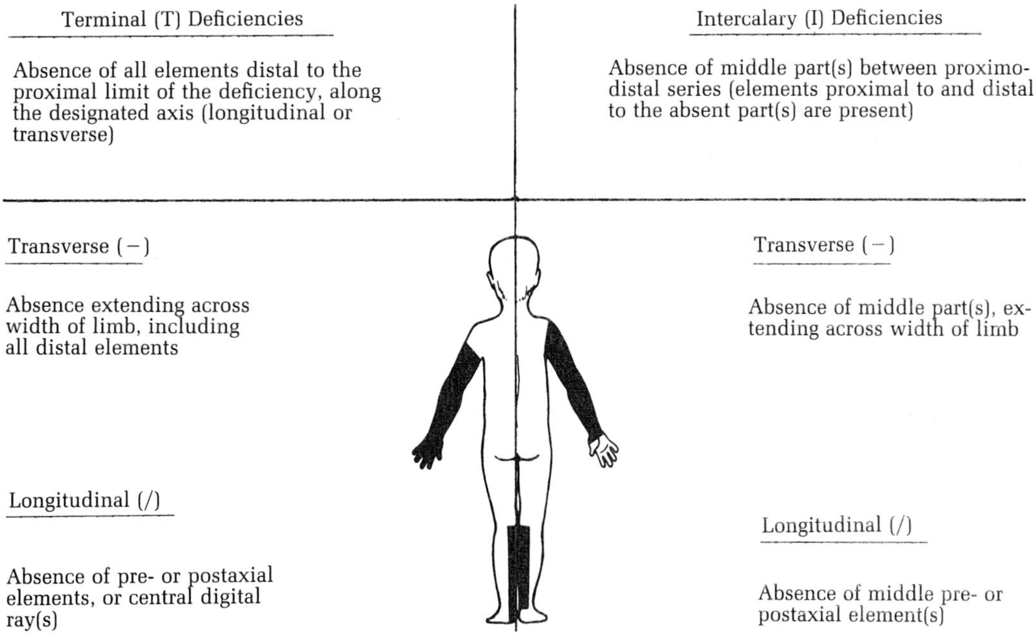

Terminal (T) Deficiencies

Absence of all elements distal to the proximal limit of the deficiency, along the designated axis (longitudinal or transverse)

Intercalary (I) Deficiencies

Absence of middle part(s) between proximo-distal series (elements proximal to and distal to the absent part(s) are present)

Transverse (−)

Absence extending across width of limb, including all distal elements

Transverse (−)

Absence of middle part(s), extending across width of limb

Longitudinal (/)

Absence of pre- or postaxial elements, or central digital ray(s)

Longitudinal (/)

Absence of middle pre- or postaxial element(s)

Fig. 2-11. A system of classification for congenital skeletal limb deficiencies. Complete absence of a free limb is referred to as amelia; partial absence as meromelia. (Modified from Burtch RL, Hall CB, Lambert CN, O'Rahilly R, Swinyard CA: Nomenclature for congenital skeletal limb deficiencies, a revision of the Frantz and O'Rahilly classification. Artificial Limbs 10:24, 1966)

If the resulting constriction is tight, the limb or digit may be amputated. If the encirclement is not initially constrictive, the limb or digit may exhibit congenital banding (Streeter's dysplasia), and postnatal growth may lead to constriction that limits circulation distal to the band. Surgical release of the tight band permits normal growth and blood flow. It has also been reported that constriction may occur in the absence of amniotic bands. Indeed, dermatoglyphic evidence suggests that many persons with apparently normal hands had a prenatal postminimus (supernumerary little finger) that was lost before birth by amputation, apparently without intervention of amniotic bands. Consistent with this possibility is the view that the pisiform bone is a vestige of an ancestral postminimus.

DEFICIENCES IN THE LIMBS

The limbs exhibit a variety of congenital deficiences that are usually sporadic, with no genetic or other documentable cause. They can be conveniently classified as primarily transverse or longitudinal deficiences. The former involve absence of a complete transverse segment of the limb; the latter refer to absence of preaxial or postaxial portions of the limb. In both, the deficiency may be the absence of the distal portion of the limb (terminal deficiency), or it may consist of absence of an intermediate portion of the limb (intercalary deficiency) with preservation of the portions of the limb proximal and distal to the deficiency (Fig. 2-11).

Examples of transverse deficiency are *amelia* (total absence of the limb) and *hemimelia* (absence of the distal portion of the limb), both of which are terminal transverse deficiences. *Phocomelia,* in which the proximal portion of the limb is absent and the hand or foot projects directly from the trunk, is an intercalary type of transverse deficiency. The production of these malformations by thalidomide was mentioned earlier.

Longitudinal deficiencies include fibular hemimelia, tibial hemimelia, radial hemimelia, and ulnar hemimelia (Fig. 2-12). The most common of these deficiencies is fibular hemimelia, in which the fibula is partially or completely absent. When this defect is intercalary, the foot is normal. More often, fibular hemimelia includes deficiency in the postaxial muscles of the leg and in the lateral rays of the foot; the limb involved is short, and the foot is plantar-flexed and everted (equinovalgus).

SELECTED REFERENCES

Carter CO: Congenital defects. Proceedings of the Royal Society of Medicine 61:991, 1968

Cowen D, Geller LM: Long-term pathological effects of prenatal X-irradiation on the central nervous system of the rat. J Neuropathol Exp Neurol 19:488, 1960

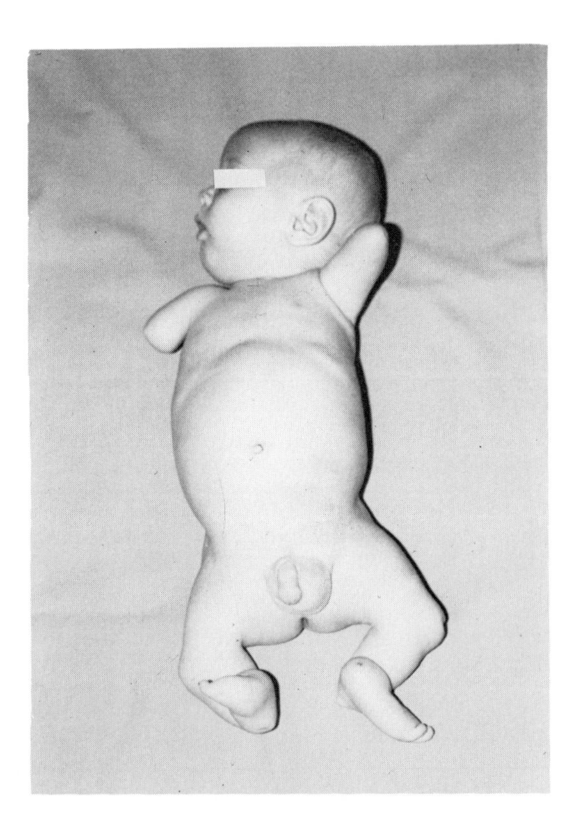

Fig. 2-12. Multiple congenital limb deficiency. The right upper limb demonstrates terminal transverse deficiency, mid-humerus. The left upper limb shows terminal longitudinal deficiency with absence of radius and preservation of ulna (not seen in photograph). Bilateral tibial hemimelia is evident in the lower limbs, with equinovarus position of the feet and absence of medial rays.

Frantz CH, O'Rahilly R: Congenital skeletal limb deficiences. J Bone Joint Surg 43A:1202, 1961
Grüneberg H: The Pathology of Development. New York, John Wiley & Sons, 1963
McKusick VA: Heritable Disorders of Connective Tissue, 3rd ed. St Louis, CV Mosby, 1966
Muller HJ: Radiation damage to the genetic material. In Baitsell GA Science in Progress, 7th series, Chap 4. New Haven, Yale University Press, 1951
Murphy DP: The outcome of 625 pregnancies in women subjected to pelvic radium or the roentgen irradiation. Am J Obstet Gynecol 18:179, 1929
Torpin R: Fetal Malformations Caused by Amnion Rupture During Gestation. Springfield, Charles C Thomas, 1968
Warkany J: Congenital malformation in the past. J Chronic Dis 10:84, 1959
Wilson JG: Experimental studies on congenital malformations. J Chronic Dis 10:111, 1959

Part Two

ANATOMY

Chapter 3

The Upper Limb

Frank C. Wilson
and Charles W. Hooker

GOALS AND OBJECTIVES

Goals: To review the gross anatomy of the upper limb, including the anatomical relationships and function of muscle groups, bones, joints, vessels, brachial plexus, and nerves; to indicate how the knowledge of anatomy may be applied to an understanding of the biomechanics, kinesiology, and function of the upper limb, especially the hand; and to correlate the gross and roentgenographic anatomy of the upper limb in health and disease

Objectives: On completion of this unit, and using the text as a standard reference, one should be able to evaluate, describe, list, or recognize the following:

1. Formation and divisions of the brachial plexus
2. Functional deficits and deformities produced by interruption of the major nerves or muscles of the upper limb
3. Pathways of collateral circulation about the shoulder, elbow, and wrist following interruption of the axillary, brachial, or radial and ulnar arteries
4. Probable deformities following fracture of the tubular bones of the upper limb as determined by the muscular forces acting on the fracture fragments
5. Components of scapulohumeral rhythm
6. Lesions and anatomical changes associated with swan-neck deformity, boutonnière deformity, clawhand, the hand of benediction, carpel tunnel syndrome, Volkmann's ischemic contracture, and Colles' fracture
7. Normal surface and roentgenographic anatomy of the upper limb

OUTLINE

I. The axilla and shoulder
   A. Bones: clavicle, scapula, proximal humerus
   B. Joints: glenohumeral, scapulothoracic, acromioclavicular, sternoclavicular
   C. Muscles: rotator cuff, internal rotators, scapular stabilizers, deltoid
   D. Surface and roentgenographic anatomy

E. Pathological conditions: fracture of the clavicle, glenohumeral dislocation, acromioclavicular injury, "bursitis"

II. The arm
  A. Humeral shaft
  B. Muscles: biceps, brachialis, triceps
  C. Relationships of muscles, brachial vessels, and major nerves
  D. Surface and roentgenographic anatomy
  E. Pathological conditions: fracture of the humeral shaft

III. The elbow
  A. Bones: humerus, radius, ulna
  B. Joints: humeroulnar, humeroradial
  C. Surface and roentgenographic anatomy
  D. Pathological conditions: supracondylar fracture, dislocation of the elbow

IV. The forearm
  A. Bones: radius and ulna
  B. Joints: proximal radioulnar, interosseous, distal radioulnar
  C. Muscles: flexors, pronators, extensors, supinators
  D. Surface and roentgenographic anatomy
  E. Pathological conditions: expected displacement with fractures of the radius and ulna

V. The wrist
  A. Bones: radius, ulna, carpals
  B. Joints: radiocarpal, intercarpal
  C. Surface and roentgenographic anatomy
  D. Pathological conditions: Colles' fracture, scaphoid fracture, dislocation of the lunate, carpal tunnel syndrome

VI. The hand
  A. Bones: metacarpals and phalanges
  B. Joints: carpometacarpal, metacarpophalangeal, interphalangeal
  C. Muscles: intrinsics and extrinsics
  D. Surface and roentgenographic anatomy
  E. Pathological conditions: fracture of the metacarpals and phalanges, swan-neck and boutonnière deformities

VII. The brachial plexus and nerves of the upper limb
  A. Axillary, radial, median, ulnar, musculocutaneous
  B. Pathological conditions: deformity and sensory deficit produced by division of major nerves (clawhand, hand of benediction)

VIII. The arteries of the upper limb
  A. Axillary, brachial, radial, ulnar
  B. Pathological conditions: Volkmann's contracture

This presentation of the anatomy of the upper limb is necessarily incomplete. Emphasis is placed on anatomic considerations of major functional and clinical importance. More detailed descriptions of the anatomy of the upper limb are available in the references cited at the end of this chapter.

Man is a biped mammal whose upper limbs differ from his lower limbs in that they are adapted to mobility and prehension rather than stability and locomotion. The upper limbs articulate with the trunk at the sternoclavicular joints; the lower limbs are more firmly united to the axial skeleton at the sacroiliac joints.

THE AXILLA AND THE SHOULDER

The *axilla* is the pyramidal space above the armpit. It has four muscular walls, a skeletal apex, and a base of skin and fascia. Its major contents are the vessels and nerves of the upper limb.

The *shoulder*, or shoulder girdle, is composed of three bones, four joints, and the muscles and ligaments that bind them together into a functional unit (Fig. 3-1).

Bones

The bones of the shoulder are the clavicle, scapula, and proximal humerus.

The *clavicle* is an S-shaped bone that serves as a protector of the brachial plexus and acts as the strut that provides, at the sternoclavicular joint, the only bony connection between the upper limb and the thorax. It is the "boom" from which the upper extremity is suspended. Because of its subcutaneous location, the clavicle is frequently injured. Fractures usually occur in the middle third with characteristic upward displacement of the medial fragment produced by the sternocleidomastoid muscle. The lateral fragment is pulled downward by the weight of the limb acting through the coracoclavicular ligaments.

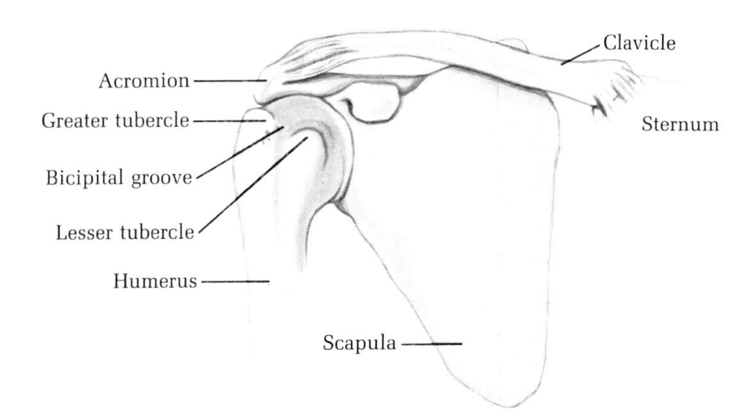

Fig. 3-1. Shoulder girdle.

The *scapula* serves primarily for muscle attachment and is without any bony connection to the thorax. It provides two palpable bony landmarks: the acromion and the coracoid process.

The *proximal humerus* ossifies from four centers: head, shaft, and both tubercles, which unite at age 19 to 20. Fractures in adult life tend to occur along old epiphyseal lines. A depression between the tubercles, the bicipital groove, contains the long head of the biceps. The tubercles also serve as points of insertion for the rotator cuff, with the subscapularis inserting on the lesser tubercle and the supraspinatus, infraspinatus, and teres minor inserting from anterior to posterior on the three facets of the greater tubercle.

Joints

The joints of the shoulder are the glenohumeral, acromioclavicular, sternoclavicular, and scapulothoracic.

The *glenohumeral joint* is a universal joint permitting a greater range of motion than any other joint in the body. It is shallow, resembling more a grapefruit in a saucer than a ball in a socket. The lack of bony stability and the wide range of motion permitted by loose ligamentous and capsular reinforcement account for the fact that the glenohumeral is the most frequently dislocated joint in the body.

The *acromioclavicular joint* is situated between the clavicle and the acromion. It permits motion in three planes: anteroposterior gliding of the acromion during protraction and retraction of the scapula; tilting of the acromion during abduction and adduction of the arm; and rotation of the clavicle. Rotation also occurs during abduction and adduction of the shoulder. The joint is reinforced by two sets of ligaments: the horizontally directed *acromioclavicular ligaments* and the stronger, vertically directed *coracoclavicular ligaments*. The coracoclavicular ligaments are the suspensory ligaments of the upper limb. Tears of the acromioclavicular and coracoclavicular ligaments (as might be produced by a fall on the point of the shoulder) allow the upper limb to drop away from the clavicle, producing separation of the acromioclavicular joint.

The *sternoclavicular joint* is inherently more stable than the acromioclavicular joint. Because of this stability and its more protected medial location, it is injured less frequently than the acromioclavicular joint.

Shoulder girdle motion also occurs between the scapula and posterior thoracic wall. When the arm is abducted to 180°, there is approximately 1° of *scapulothoracic motion* for every 2° of glenohumeral motion.

Each of the bones and joints is definable topographically. The clavicle is subcutaneous throughout its course. The acromion is the most superior bony prominence of the shoulder; just beneath it is the greater tubercle of the humerus, which provides the normal rounded contour of the shoulder. The coracoid process can be palpated through the anterior deltoid muscle one to two finger breadths below the outer portion of the clavicle. One finger breadth lateral to the coracoid is the glenohumeral joint, so the coracoid process is an important bone landmark in locating the glenohumeral joint for aspiration or injection. The acromioclavicular joint may be felt as a shallow depression between the outer end of the clavicle and the

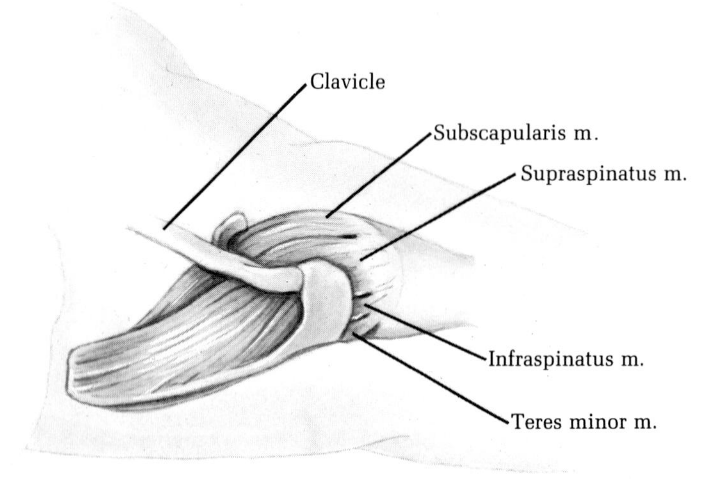

Fig. 3-2. Rotator cuff as seen from above. (Adapted from an original painting by Frank H. Netter, M.D., from Moseley HF: Disorders of the shoulder. Clin Symp 11(3):76, 1959. Copyright by CIBA Pharmaceutical Company, Division of CIBA-GEIGY Corporation. All rights reserved.)

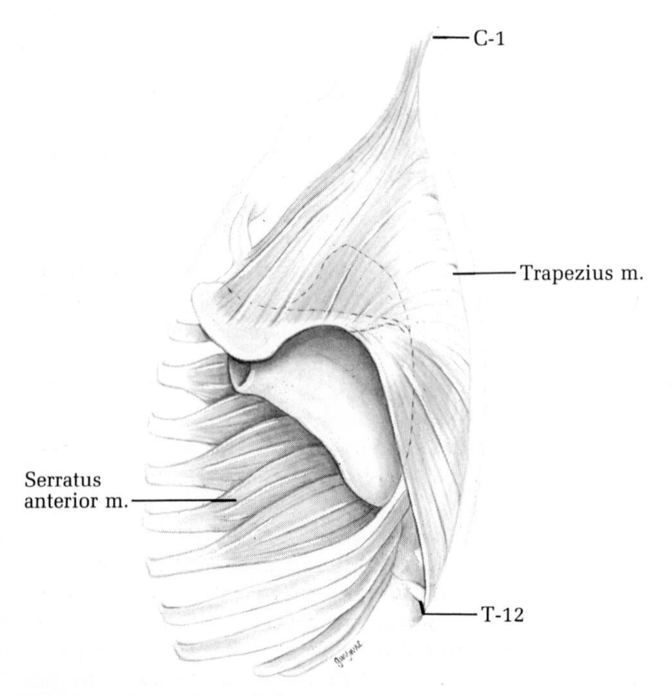

Fig. 3-3. Scapular stabilizers.

acromion. The anteriorly directed bicipital groove is also palpable, and the tendon of the long head of the biceps can be rolled beneath the palpating finger as it passes through this channel between the tubercles.

Muscles

There are four major muscle groups about the shoulder.

The *rotator cuff* or *musculotendinous cuff* (Fig. 3-2) is the name given to the common tendon covering the top, front, and back of the humeral head. Four muscles fuse to form this tendon: the *subscapularis, supraspinatus, infraspinatus,* and *teres minor.* The supraspinatus lies directly over the top of the humeral head and is primarily an abductor. The infraspinatus and teres minor cover the back of the humeral head and are external rotators; the subscapularis, which crosses the front of the joint, is an internal rotator and reinforces the anterior aspect of the joint. The supraspinatus and infraspinatus are supplied by the suprascapular nerve, the teres minor by the axillary nerve, and the subscapularis by the subscapular nerve, all from the brachial plexus. The supraspinatus tendon is predisposed to wear-and-tear changes because of its location between the humeral head and the acromion, which compress the tendon during shoulder movement. These attritional changes are manifested as calcific tendinitis ("bursitis") or tears of the rotator cuff.

The *trapezius* and *serratus anterior* (Fig. 3-3) stabilize the scapular base from which the arm operates. The trapezius, which arises from the spinous processes of the cervical and thoracic vertebrae and inserts on the spine of the scapula and acromion, is innervated by the spinal accessory nerve and branches from the third and fourth cervical roots. Its upper fibers shrug the shoulder and aid in suspension of the shoulder girdle; the middle portion aids in adduction and rotation of the inferior angle of the scapula; the lower segments, together with the serratus anterior, clamp the scapula to the chest wall so that it cannot rotate or slip sideways. The serratus anterior arises from the upper eight ribs, inserts on the vertebral border of the scapula, is innervated by the long thoracic nerve, and functions to draw the scapula forward in activities such as fencing or boxing. Paralysis produces a characteristic prominence ("winging") of the vertebral border of the scapula.

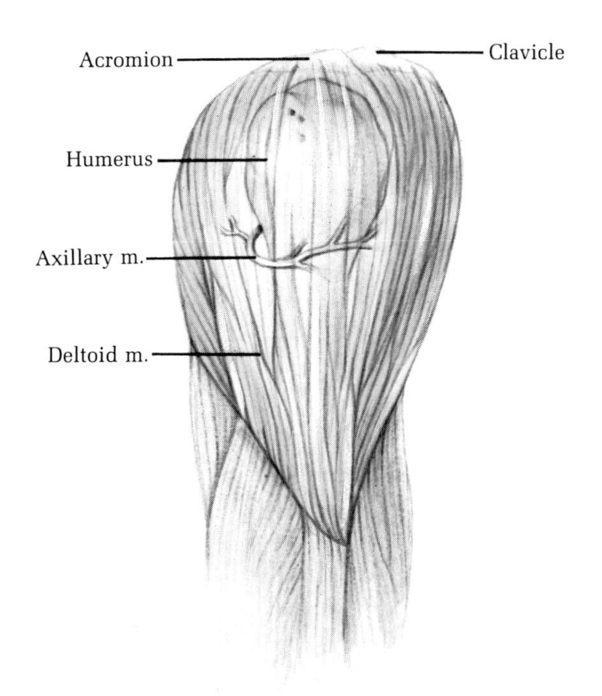

Fig. 3-4. Deltoid muscle

The major function of the *deltoid muscle* (Fig. 3-4) is to abduct the arm. It performs this action after the scapula has been fixed by its stabilizing muscles and the humeral head has been snubbed to the glenoid by the rotator cuff. It is innervated by the axillary nerve.

The major internal rotators (Fig. 3-5) are the *subscapularis, teres major, latissimus dorsi,* and *pectoralis major* muscles. The latissimus dorsi and teres major insert along the medial lip of the bicipital groove and the pectoralis major along the lateral lip. These muscles comprise a larger mass than those that externally rotate the humerus (the posterior deltoid, infraspinatus, and teres minor), which explains the greater power of internal rotation. The internal rotators are suppled by nerves that spring directly from the brachial plexus.

Abduction of the shoulder is a smooth, rhythmic, integrated motion in which all the shoulder joints participate. This motion has

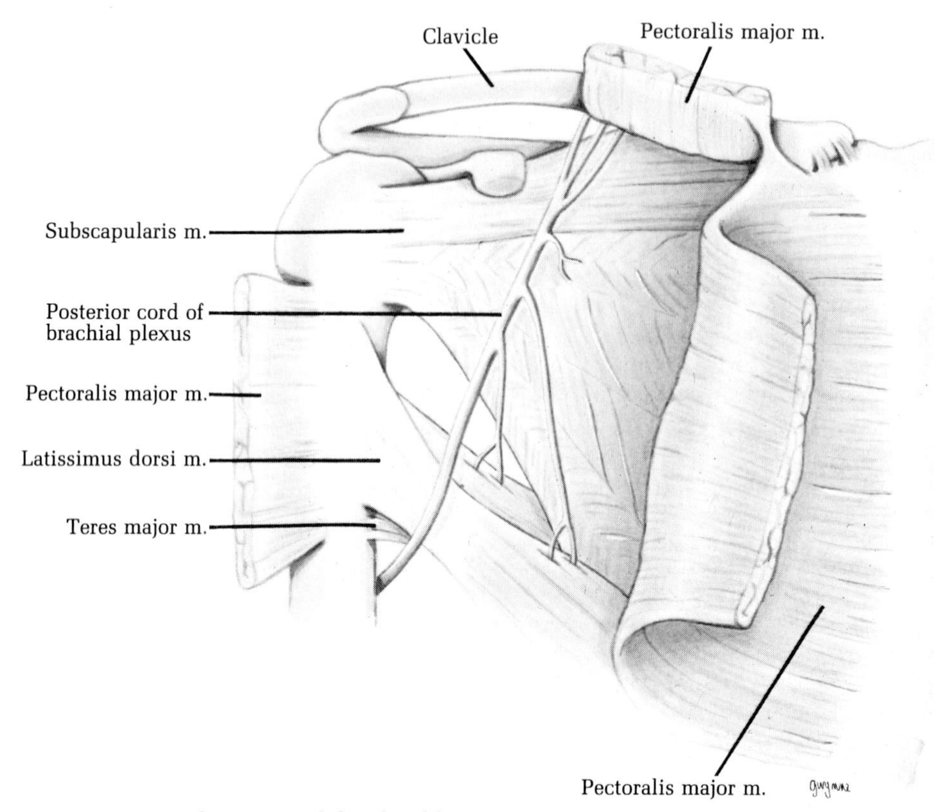

Fig. 3-5. Internal rotators of the shoulder.

been called *scapulohumeral rhythm* by Codman and is significant in that asymmetrical movement usually indicates a pathological disorder of the shoulder. In addition to the two-to-one ratio of movement in the glenohumeral and scapulothoracic joints, the clavicle also plays a part in elevation of the arm, with about 40° of motion occurring at the sternoclavicular joint and 20° in the acromioclavicular joint during full abduction of the shoulder (Fig. 3-6).

THE ARM

The bone that extends from the shoulder to the elbow is called the *humerus*. The region of the humerus just below the tubercles is the narrowest part of the shaft; it is called the *surgical neck* because of the relative frequency of fractures there. The lower half of the humeral shaft is divided into anterior and posterior aspects by the medial and lateral supracondylar ridges, which extend upward from their respective epicondyles and afford attachments for the medial and lateral intermuscular septa. The midlateral aspect of the humerus contains the *deltoid tubercle*. The posterior aspect of the humerus between the deltoid tubercle and the lateral epicondylar ridge is marked by a broad, shallow channel, the *spiral groove*, through which the radial nerve is transmitted to the elbow.

The posterior humeral shaft gives origin to the medial and lateral heads of the triceps muscle, which passes downward to insert on the olecranon, acts to extend the elbow, and is innervated by the radial nerve (Fig. 3-7). The anterior aspect of the humerus is covered, in its lower half, by the origin of the brachialis muscle, which inserts on the tuberosity and coronoid process of the ulna and is the prime flexor of the extended elbow. Superficial to the brachialis muscle is the biceps, which functions more efficiently as a flexor when the elbow is partially flexed. The short and long heads of the biceps arise from the coracoid process and supraglenoid tubercle of the scapula respectively, and insert

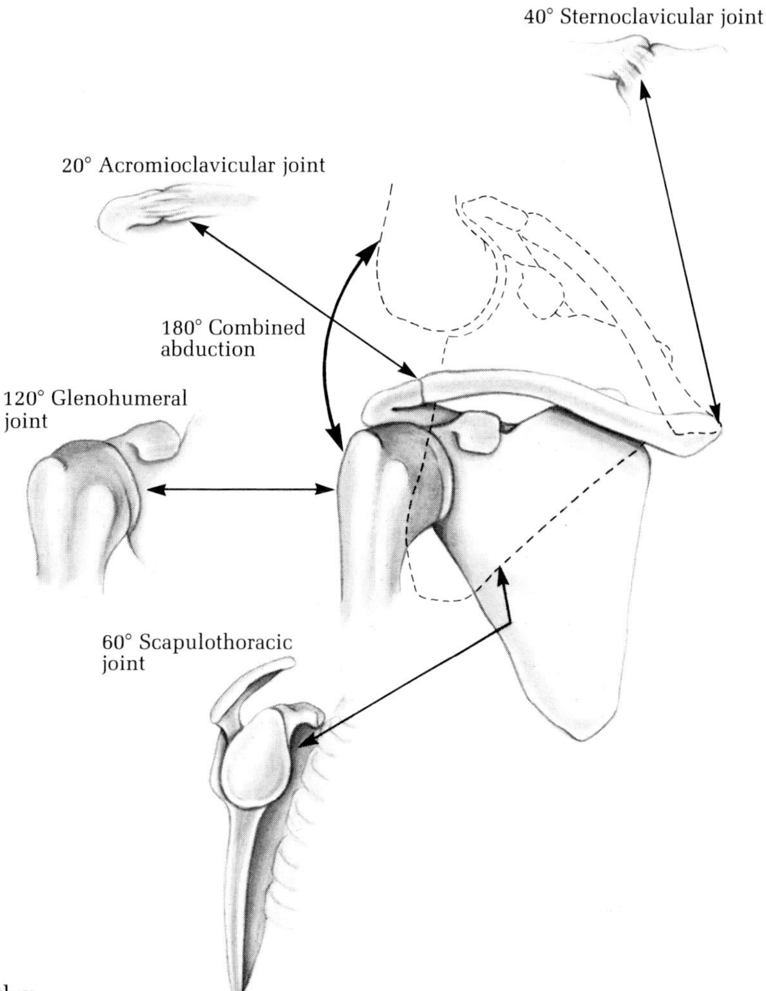

Fig. 3-6. Scapulohumeral rhythm.

on the radial tuberosity. The coracobrachialis also arises from the coracoid process. Its insertion on the medial aspect of the humerus in its midportion enables it to adduct and flex the humerus. Its innervation is from the musculocutaneous nerve just before it pierces the muscle to supply the brachialis and biceps.

Following *fracture of the humerus*, the fracture fragments may be displaced as a result of the pull of the muscles inserting into the two parts. With a fracture of the surgical neck, the upper fragment is usually abducted and externally rotated by the muscles inserting onto the greater tubercle, while the lower fragment is adducted and internally rotated by the internal rotator muscles. In fractures of the shaft, angulation and overriding may result from muscular pull. Fractures of the middle and lower thirds of the humeral shaft are frequently associated with injuries of the encircling radial nerve.

THE ELBOW

The *elbow joint* (Fig. 3-8) is formed by the articulations between the distal end of the humerus and the radius and ulna (flexion and extension) and by the articulation between the proximal radius and the ulna (pronation and supination). A common joint capsule encloses both joints. The lower end of the humerus consists of a spool-shaped pully called the trochlea that articulates in the trochlear (semilunar) notch of the proximal ulna. The lateral portion of the distal humerus, or

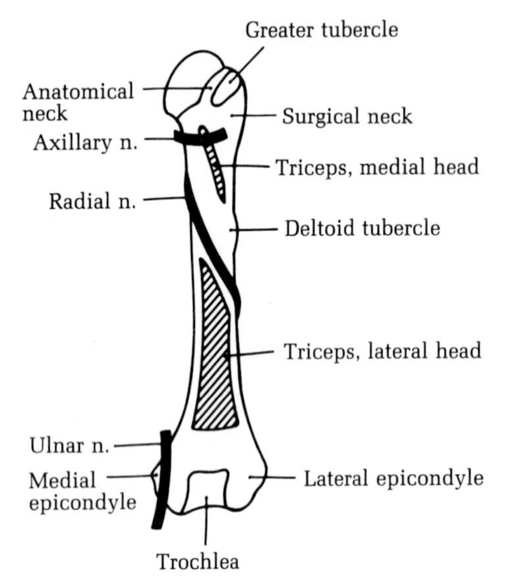

Fig. 3-7. Posterior aspect of right humerus.

capitulum, is convex and articulates with the concave surface of the radial head.

Contact between the radial head and the radial notch of the ulna is maintained by the *annular ligament,* which encircles the head and neck of the radius from the ulna. The median and lateral epicondyles flare proximally from the trochlea and capitulum and serve as sites of origin for the flexor-pronator (median epicondyle) and extensor-supinator (lateral epicondyle) muscles of the forearm and hand. The range of flexion and extension in the elbow is approximately 0° to 140°, with the most useful part of the range between 60° and 120°.

Many important structures cross the elbow (Fig. 3-9). Most of them can be palpated in the antecubital fossa, including the biceps tendon, the brachial artery adjacent to the medial edge of the biceps tendon, the median nerve medial to the artery, and the ulnar nerve behind the medial epicondyle.

Fracture through the region of the humerus just above the condyles is known as a *supracondylar fracture.* It is a potentially dangerous injury because of the possibility of compression or laceration of the antecubital vessels by forward displacement of the proximal fragment. The circulatory deficiency that may result is known as *Volkmann's ischemia* and is recognizable early by pain, pallor, pulselessness, and paresthesias distal to the fracture.

Viewed from behind, the olecranon and the two epicondyles form a straight line in the extended position. When the elbow is flexed to 90°, they form the corners of an isosceles triangle. The shape of this triangle is unaltered in supracondylar fractures of the humerus but is distorted by posterolateral dislocation of the elbow (Fig. 3-10).

THE FOREARM

The bones of the forearm are the *radius* and *ulna;* they lie parallel to each other in supination. During pronation the radius crosses

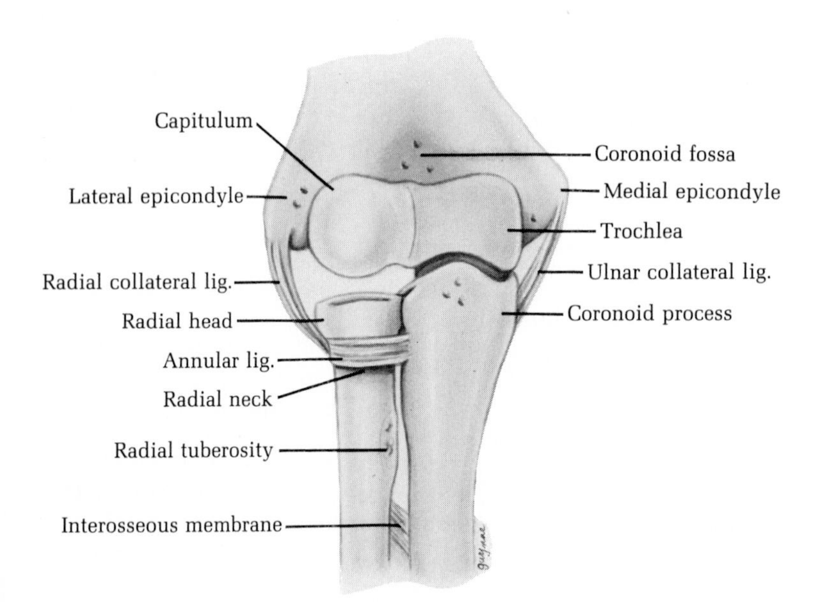

Fig. 3-8. Anterior aspect of the elbow joint.

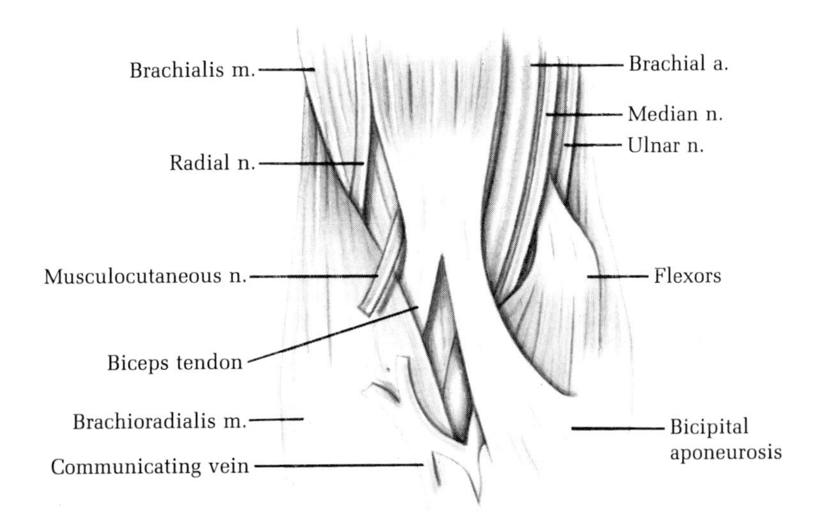

Fig. 3-9. The right antecubital fossa.

the ulna, rotating on an axis that passes from the capitulum through the distal end of the ulna. These bones are joined by the *proximal and distal radioulnar joints* and by the *interosseous membrane,* which is directed obliquely downward from the radius to the ulna (Fig. 3-11). Since the ulna does not articulate with the carpus, the direction of this membrane is important in the transmission of the longitudinal forces from the radius to the ulna.

Both the proximal and the distal radioulnar joints are synovial joints. The proximal joint lies between the head of the radius and the radial notch of the ulna. The distal radioulnar joint is separated from the wrist joint by an articular disc that extends from the base of the ulnar styloid process to the radius. The arc of pronation and supination averages 150° to 160°, with the most useful portion between 80° pronation and 45° supination (0° is the thumb-up position). As a result of proximal displacement of the distal radius, derangement of the distal radioulnar joint occurs frequently following Colles' fractures. Displacement of this joint may produce a wrist with limited and painful rotation.

There are two *muscular compartments* in the forearm: flexor and extensor. The *flexor muscles* are arranged in three layers. The deep muscles that cover the flexor aspect of the bones are the pronator quadratus, the flexor digitorum profundus, and the supinator. The flexor digitorum superficialis comprises the middle layer; the superficial layer is composed of the pronator teres, the flexor carpi radialis, the palmaris longus, and the flexor carpi ulnaris.

Certain differences between the flexor digitorum profundus and the superficialis should be noted. The tendons of the profundus lie side by side at the wrist, whereas the tendons of the superficialis are arranged so

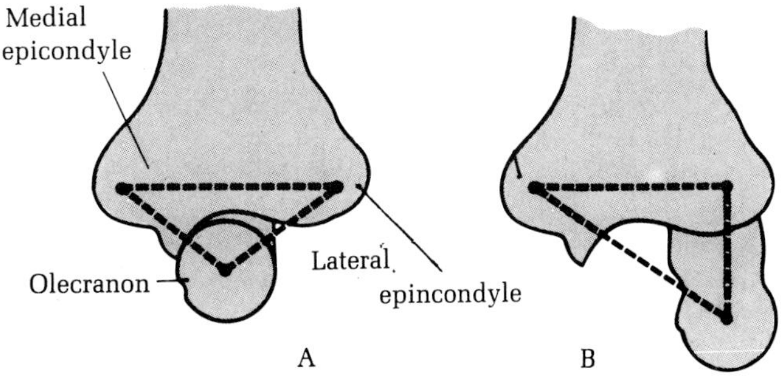

Fig. 3-10. (*A*) Normal relationship of olecranon and epicondyles. (*B*) Relationship of olecranon and epicondyles in posterolateral dislocation of the elbow.

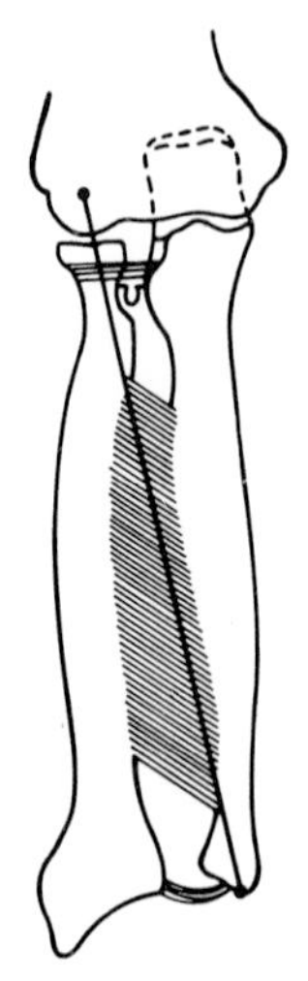

Fig. 3-11. Forearm joints and axis of rotation.

that those for the third and fourth digits are anterior to those of the second and fifth digits. All four of the superficialis tendons are free in the forearm; however, the tendons of the profundus do not divide until they reach the wrist. This arrangement enables the superficialis tendons to act more independently but lends greater power to the profundus tendons. The palmaris longus is continued in the palm as the palmar fascia, a well-defined structure that anchors the palmar skin to the metacarpals. Thickening and contracture of the palmar fascia and skin produces flexion deformities of the fingers, known as *Dupuytren's contracture.*

The muscles of the *extensor region* of the forearm are arranged in two layers, superficial and deep. The superficial muscles arise from a common tendon attached to the lateral epicondyle of the humerus, and divide into lateral and medial groups. The lateral three of these muscles are the brachioradialis and the extensors carpi radialis longus and brevis. The medial group is comprised of the extensor digitorum, the extensor digiti minimi, the extensor carpi ulnaris, and the anconeus. The deep muscles on the back of the forearm are the supinator, abductor policis longus, and extensors pollicis brevis and longus. The latter three muscles to the thumb surface in the furrow between the two groups of superficial muscles. They insert on the thumb at the base of the metacarpal, proximal phalanx, and distal phalanx respectively.

The forearm muscles serve to pronate and supinate the forearm and to move the wrist and fingers. *Pronation* is carried out by the pronator teres and pronator quadratus, whereas *supination* is accomplished by the biceps and supinator muscles. Wrist flexion is provided by the flexors carpi radialis and ulnaris and by the flexors digitorum superficialis and profundus after they have accomplished their primary functions of flexing the proximal and distal interphalangeal joints. All flexor muscles except the flexor carpi ulnaris and flexor digitorum profundus to the ring and little fingers, which are supplied by the ulnar nerve, are innervated by the median nerve. The extensor muscles, which extend the wrist, all metacarpophalangeal joints, and the interphalangeal joint of the thumb, are supplied by the radial nerve.

Fractures of the radius that fall between the insertion of the supinator and pronator teres are difficult to control, since the proximal fragment is strongly supinated by the supinator and biceps, and the distal fragment is pronated by the pronator teres and quadratus (Fig. 3-12). Fractures occurring distal to the insertion of the pronator teres show less rotational displacement (Fig. 3-12). When both bones are fractured, in addition to the rotary forces already mentioned, shortening or telescoping of the fragments is produced by muscles that span the fracture sites.

THE WRIST

The *proximal row of carpal bones* (scaphoid, lunate, triquetral) articulates proximally with the radius and distally with the *distal row of carpals* (trapezium, trapezoid, capitate, and hamate). The eighth carpal bone, the pisiform, is also a member of the proximal row but articulates only with the anterior surface of the triquetral bone (Fig. 3-13).

The *movements at the wrist* are flexion, extension, and radial and ulnar deviation. These movements involve motion at the radiocarpal, midcarpal, and carpometacarpal joints.

The *flexor retinaculum,* or transverse carpal ligament, is a heavy band of fibers that stretches from the hamate and pisiform medially to the scaphoid and trapezium laterally. It converts the volar aspect of the carpal bones into a rigid fibro-osseous tunnel

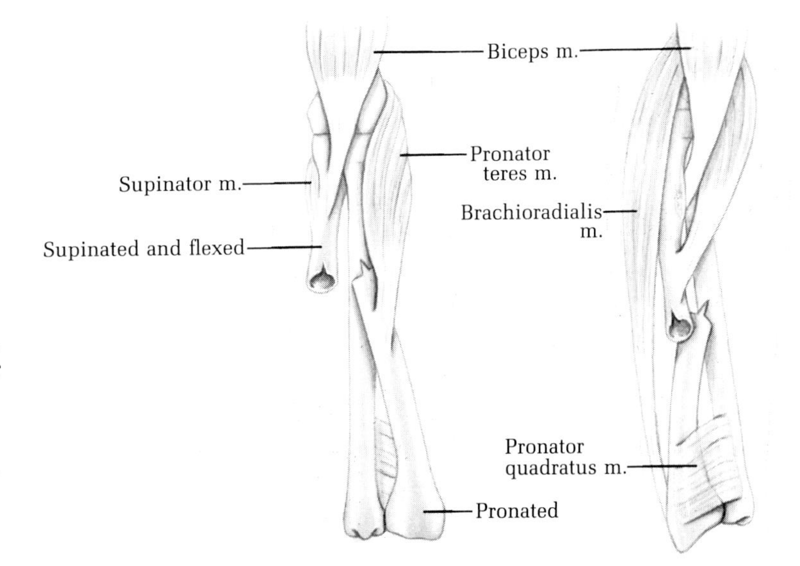

Fig. 3-12. (*A*) Deformity with fracture of the radius proximal to the insertion of the pronator teres. (*B*) Deformity with fracture of the radius between the pronators. (Modified from Hollinshead WH: Anatomy for Surgeons, Vol 3. New York, Hoeber Medical Division, Harper & Row, 1969)

through which pass flexor tendons and the median nerve (Fig. 3-14). A decrease in the size of this canal, or an increase in the volume of its contents, may cause compression of the median nerve, producing pain, sensory disturbance, and weakness in the distribution of the median nerve in the hand. This picture is known as the *carpal tunnel syndrome*.

At the wrist, *Lister's tubercle* is palpable on the dorsum of the radius; it serves as a pulley for the extensor pollicis longus. The *radial* and *ulnar styloid processes* are also palpable, with the tip of the radial styloid process projecting about 1 cm distal to that of the ulna. The distal volar flexion crease crosses the proximal end of the scaphoid and the pisiform and marks the proximal edge of the transverse carpal ligament. The pisiform is palpable and serves to mark the entry, on its lateral aspect, of the ulnar nerve and artery into the hand.

Most *injuries to the wrist* are sustained by a fall on the outstretched hand. Depending upon the age of the patient, the position of the wrist at the time of impact, and the force of the impact, injuries may range from fracture or epiphyseal injury of the distal radius and ulna to fracture or dislocation of the carpus. The carpal bone most frequently fractured is the *scaphoid*, which spans both carpal rows and therefore has less mobility than the other carpals. The most frequently dislocated carpal bone is the *lunate*, which

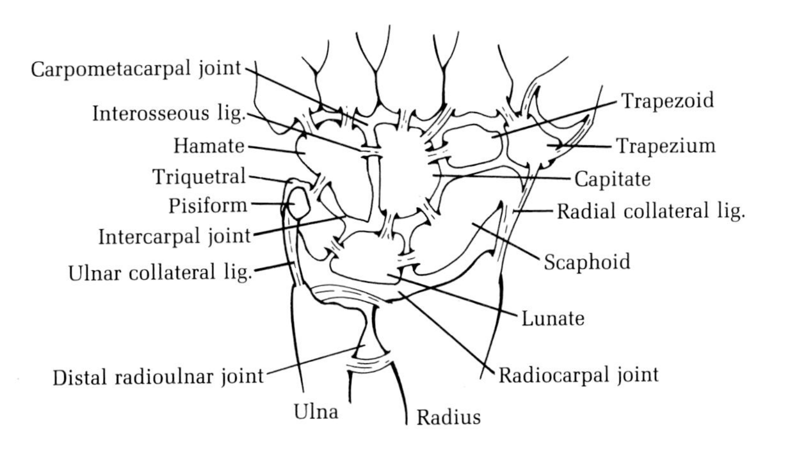

Fig. 3-13. Articulations of the wrist.

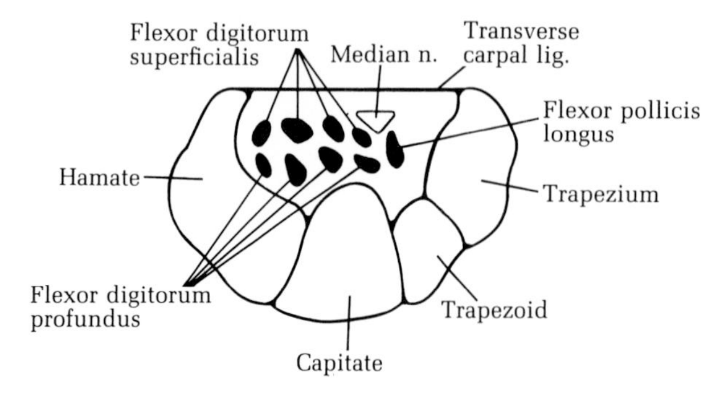

Fig. 3-14. Carpal canal.

displaces volarward with forced dorsiflexion of the wrist. Compression of the median nerve in the carpal canal may be caused by the displaced lunate, producing a carpal tunnel syndrome.

When associated with dorsal tilt and shortening, a fracture in the lower inch of the radius is known as a *Colles' fracture*. This fracture is also caused by forced dorsiflexion of the wrist, producing the characteristic "silver fork" deformity shown in Figure 3-15.

THE HAND

The bones of the hand are the *metacarpals and phalanges*. Each finger has three phalanges; the thumb has only two. Hence, the fingers have distal and proximal interphalangeal joints whereas the thumb has one interphalangeal joint. Both the metacarpophalangeal and interphalangeal joints are primarily hinge joints with a range of motion from 0° to slightly over 90°. The most important joint of the hand is the saddle-shaped carpometacarpal joint of the thumb. The configuration of this joint permits the circumduction movements of the thumb necessary for its opposition to the fingers.

The ability to oppose the thumb is one of the traits that distinguishes humans from the lower primates. Opposition refers to the ability to oppose the pulp of the thumb to the pulp of the fingers. It is actually a composite motion made up of abduction, flexion, and adduction.

There are two groups of muscles in the hand, extrinsic and intrinsic. The *extrinsic muscles* have their origins proximal to the hand and their insertions and actions on the hand. These muscles flex and extend the fingers and thumb and abduct the thumb. Specifically, the radially innervated extensor digitorum, along with the extensor digiti quinti and the extensor indicis proprius, extend the metacarpophalangeal joints. With the metacarpophalangeal joints held in flexion, these muscles are also able to extend the interphalangeal joints of the fingers. The long and short thumb extensors extend the interphalangeal and metacarpophalangeal joints of the thumb respectively. The short exten-

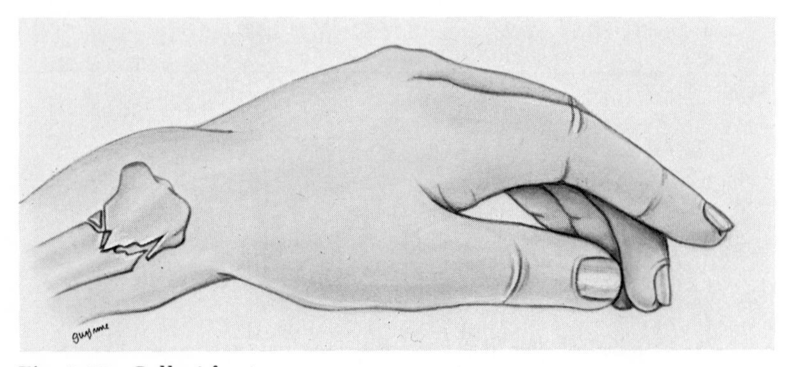

Fig. 3-15. Colles' fracture.

sor lies with the abductor pollicis longus in a common sheath covered by ligaments that hold them against the styloid process of the radius. Occasionally, the friction produced by movement between the sheath and the styloid process leads to a stenosing tenosynovitis known as *de Quervain's disease*. The interphalangeal joint of the thumb is flexed by the flexor pollicis longus, the proximal interphalangeal joints of the fingers by the flexor digitorum superficialis, and the distal interphalangeal joints by the flexor digitorum profundus. Trauma or inflammation of the flexor tendon sheaths may produce a tenosynovitis that leads to cicatricial stenosis of the sheath. Associated proximal swelling and thickening of the tendons interferes with their movement in the sheath, producing a sudden snapping or popping during flexion and extension and occasionally locking the digit in a flexed or extended position. This picture is known as a *trigger finger* (or *trigger thumb*).

The *intrinsic muscles* of the hand are those that both arise and insert within the confines of the hand. They are located in the *thenar* and *hypothenar eminences* and in the space between these eminences. The muscles of the hypothenar eminence are the abductor, flexor, and opponens digiti minimi, and the palmaris brevis. The muscles of the thenar eminence are the abductor pollicis brevis, the flexor pollicis brevis, and the opponens pollicis muscles. The muscles of the hypothenar eminence are innervated by the ulnar nerve. The muscles of the thenar eminence, with the exception of the deep head of the flexor pollicis brevis, which is innervated by the ulnar nerve, are supplied by the median nerve. All thenar and hypothenar muscles, except the abductor minimi, originate partly from the transverse carpal ligament. Their insertions are primarily on the base of the proximal phalanx of the thumb and little finger, except for both opponens muscles, which insert on their respective metacarpals.

The muscles between the hypothenar and thenar eminences are the *interosseous muscles*. They are seven in number: four dorsal and three volar. Their origin is from the metacarpal shafts. The first and fourth dorsal interossei insert on the radial aspect of the index and the ulnar side of the ring fingers; the second and third insert on the radial and ulnar sides of the long finger respectively. By their actions, they abduct the index and ring fingers and adduct the long finger to either side of a line drawn through its longitudinal axis. The first volar interosseous muscle inserts on the ulnar side of the index digit; the second and third insert on the radial aspect of the ring and little fingers. The volar interossei are thus positioned to adduct these digits toward the long finger.

The interossei, along with the four *lumbrical muscles*, also flex the metacarpophalangeal and extend the interphalangeal joints of the fingers. The lumbricales arise from the tendons of the flexor digitorum profundus in the midpalmar area and insert into the radial aspect of the dorsal hood. All interossei and the third and fourth lumbricales are innervated by the ulnar nerve; the first and second lumbricales are supplied by the median nerve.

The arrangement of the tendons on the dorsal surface of the fingers is complex. It consists of a central slip of the extensor digitorum that fuses with the tendons of the interossei and lumbricales to form a *dorsal hood* (Fig. 3-16).

On the volar aspect of the finger, the flexor digitorum superficialis is pierced, just prior to its insertion into the base of the middle phalanx, by the flexor digitorum profundus, which passes through to insert on the distal phalanx (Fig. 3-17). Both long flexor tendons are tightly enclosed in a common tendon sheath; this proximity favors the development of adhesions between the tendons following injury. Meticulous care is therefore necessary in dealing with lacerations of the flexor tendons in the fingers to prevent the loss of independent tendon function that follows the formation of adhesions. The lumbrical muscles prevent proximal retraction of lacerated profundus tendons past the midpalmar area.

The normal balance between the flexor and extensor muscles of the finger permits the synchronous joint motion so necessary for the functional mobility of the hand. Interference with this delicately balanced mechanism may seriously impair hand function. For example, laceration of the flexor superficialis tendon destroys the balance at the proximal interphalangeal joint, producing a hyperextension deformity. Hyperextension

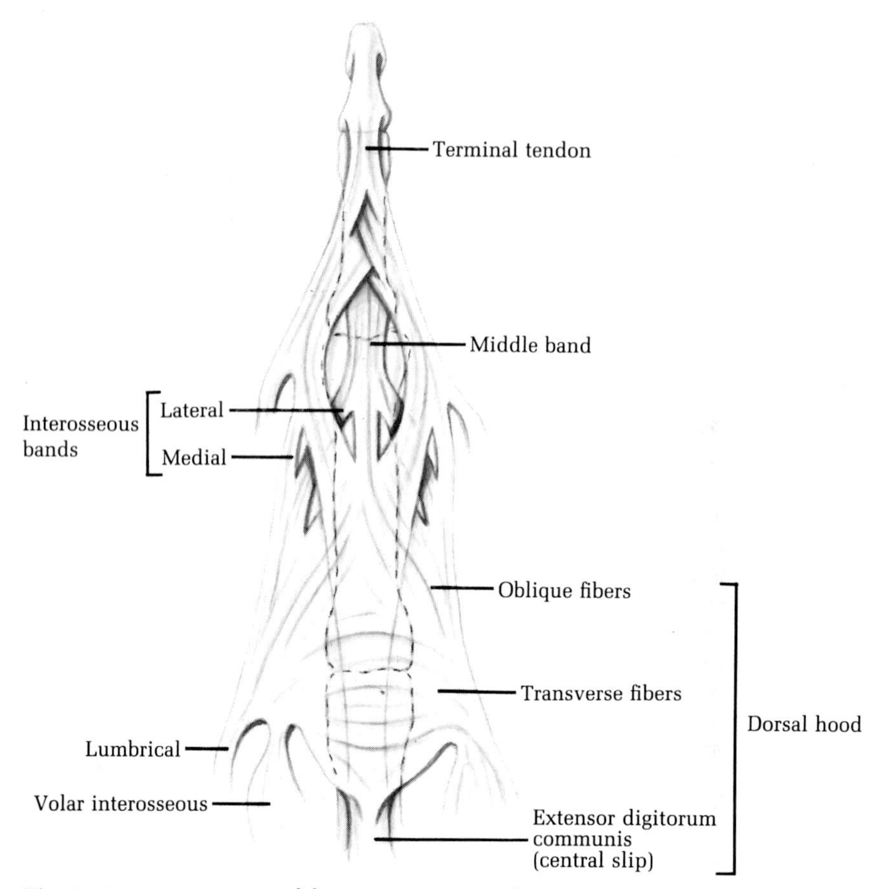

Fig. 3-16. Arrangement of finger extensor tendons.

of this joint may also result from contracture or spasm of the intrinsic muscles, resulting in increased pull on the dorsal hood and production of the so-called *swan-neck deformity,* with proximal interphalangeal joint hyperextension and metacarpophalangeal and distal interphalangeal joint flexion (Fig. 3-18). The opposite picture may be produced by division of the central tendon of the extensor mechanism prior to its insertion into the base of the middle phalanx. This lesion allows the lateral portions of the hood to displace ventrally, producing a *flexion,* or *boutonnière, deformity* of the proximal interphalangeal joint (Fig. 3-19).

THE BRACHIAL PLEXUS AND NERVES OF THE UPPER LIMB

The *brachial plexus* (Fig. 3-20) arises from the anterior primary rami of the fifth, sixth, seventh, and eighth cervical and first thoracic nerves. The upper two and lower two rami unite to form the upper and lower trunks; the seventh nerve remains single as the middle trunk. Each of the three trunks divides into an anterior and a posterior division. The three posterior divisions unite to form a single posterior cord. Of the three anterior divisions, those from the upper and middle trunks unite to form the lateral cord, and the one from the lower trunk continues as the medial cord. Each of the three cords gives off one or more branches and ends by dividing into two major branches. The posterior cord branches into the radial and axillary nerves, the medial cord branches into the ulnar nerve and the medial root of the median nerve, and the lateral cord branches into the musculocutaneous and lateral roots of the median nerve.

Injury to the brachial plexus above the clavicle usually involves the roots and trunks. Lesions of the fifth and sixth roots are usu-

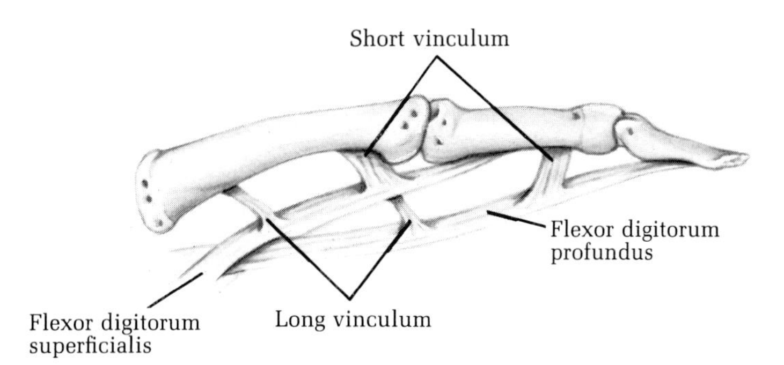

Fig. 3-17. Arrangement of the long flexor tendons of a finger.

ally produced by a widening of the head–shoulder interval. When this injury occurs during delivery, it produces what is essentially a lesion of the axillary, musculocutaneous, and suprascapular nerves known as *Erb's palsy*. The arm cannot be raised, since the deltoid muscles (axillary nerve) and spinati muscles (suprascapular nerve) are paralyzed. Elbow flexion is weakened because of weakness in the biceps and brachialis muscles. If the roots are damaged above their junction, paralysis of the rhomboids and serratus anterior is added, producing weakness in retraction and protraction of the scapula.

Injury to the lower roots (C8 and T1) or lower trunk, which may follow forceful abduction of the shoulder, produces weakness in the intrinsic muscles of the hand as well as the long flexors and extensors of the fingers.

Injury to the brachial plexus below the clavicle usually involves the cords or peripheral nerves. Damage to the posterior cord produces weakness in elbow, wrist, and metacarpophlalangeal joint extension (radial nerve), and in shoulder abduction (axillary nerve). Injury to the lateral cord produces weakness of elbow flexion (musculocutaneous nerve) and wrist flexion (lateral root of median nerve). Division of the medial cord produces a combined median and ulnar nerve deficit.

The *musculocutaneous nerve* (C5, C6) passes through the coracobrachialis, between the biceps and the brachialis, and becomes the lateral antebrachial cutaneous nerve at the elbow. It has only muscular branches above the elbow and only sensory branches below it. A lesion of this nerve produces weakness of elbow flexion and supination, and loss of sensation on the lateral aspect of the forearm.

The *axillary nerve* (C5, C6) passes backward from the posterior cord of the brachial plexus through the quadrilateral space and gives off an anterior branch to the deltoid and a posterior branch to the teres minor. It also has a sensory branch that supplies the skin overlying the deltoid muscle. Injury produces weakness in shoulder abduction and external rotation.

The *radial nerve* (C5, 6, 7, 8, and T1) is the largest and most frequently injured branch of the brachial plexus. In the axilla, it gives off the posterior cutaneous nerve of the arm and supplies the long and medial heads of the triceps. Between the axilla and the spiral groove of the humerus, it distributes a branch

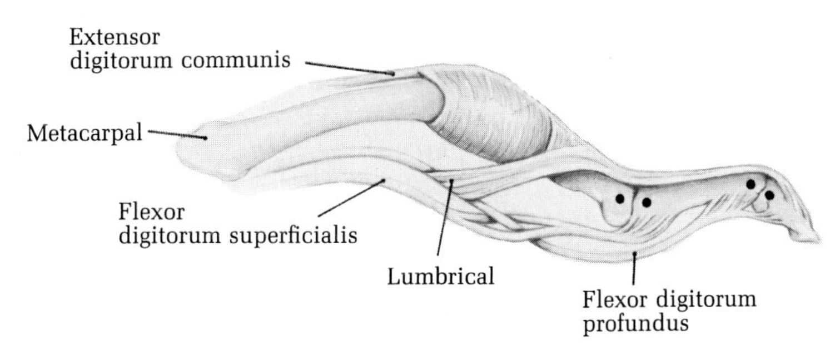

Fig. 3-18. Swan-neck deformity.

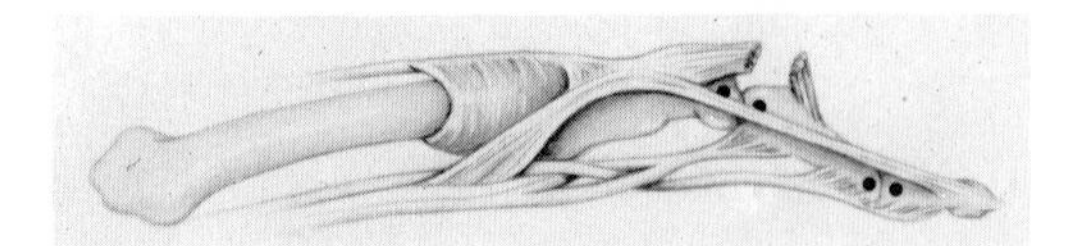

Fig. 3-19. Boutonnière deformity.

to the lateral head of the triceps. After piercing the lateral intermuscular septum and passing to the front of the elbow joint, it gives off a branch to the brachioradialis and the extensor carpi radialis longus. After its division in front of the radial head, the deep or muscular branch passes backward through the supinator to supply the nine muscles on the extensor aspect of the forearm. The superficial or sensory branch passes downward to innervate the dorsal aspect of the first web space and the hand as far ulnarward as the middle of the ring finger and as far distally as the proximal interphalangeal joint. Signs of a radial nerve lesion include the inability to extend or abduct the thumb, proximal phalanges, wrist, or elbow. The hand is pronated and the thumb adducted.

The *median nerve* (C5, 6, 7, 8, and T1) crosses the brachial artery from lateral to medial in the arm, then passes downward on the brachialis, supplying no branches in the arm. It enters the forearm between the two heads of the pronator teres and gives off an anterior interosseous branch, which supplies the flexor pollicis longus, lateral half of the flexor digitorum profundus, and pronator quadratus. It then passes beneath the flexor digitorum superficialis to supply all the muscles on the front of the forearm except the flexor carpi ulnaris and the ulnar half of the flexor digitorum profundus. Signs of a median nerve lesion include weak pronation of the forearm, weak flexion and radial deviation of the wrist, and an "ape hand" with thenar atrophy and the inability to oppose or flex the thumb. The sensory distribution of the median nerve is critical; it supplies the thumb, radial $2\frac{1}{2}$ fingers, and corresponding portion of the palm.

The *ulnar nerve* (C8, T1) passes distally medial to the axillary artery, pierces the medial intermuscular septum halfway down the arm, passes back over the medial head of the triceps, through the groove on the posterior aspect of the medial epicondyle, and enters the forearm between the two heads of the flexor carpi ulnaris. Just below the elbow, it sends branches to the flexor carpi ulnaris and ulnar half of the flexor digitorum profundus.

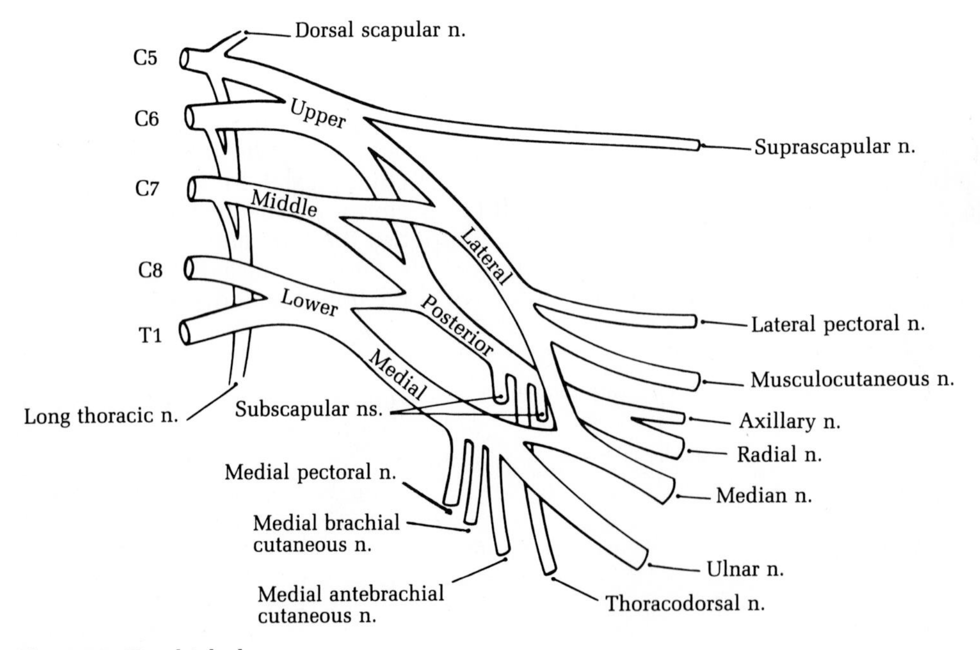

Fig. 3-20. Brachial plexus.

It passes down the forearm under the flexor carpi ulnaris, and gives off a dorsal sensory branch 2 inches above the wrist that supplies the dorsoulnar aspect of the hand and the ulnar $1\frac{1}{2}$ fingers. It has two terminal branches in the palm: a superficial cutaneous branch to the ulnar portion of the palm and the volar surfaces of the ulnar $1\frac{1}{2}$ fingers, and a deep branch, which innervates the hypothenar muscles and follows the deep arterial arch to supply the third and fourth lumbricales, the adductor pollicis, all the interossei, and the deep head of the flexor pollicis brevis. Division of the ulnar nerve at the wrist thus produces paralysis of all the small muscles of the hand except the first and second lumbricales and most of the thenar muscles. Thumb adduction is weakened, and, in attempting to grasp a piece of paper between the thumb and index finger, the thumb is acutely flexed at the interphalangeal joint *(Froment's sign).* If the ulnar nerve is divided below the mid-forearm, an *ulnar clawhand* is produced. With this lesion, the fourth and fifth fingers are hyperextended at the metacarpophalangeal joints by the long extensors but flexed at the interphalangeal joints. This posture is sometimes called the *hand of benediction* (Fig. 3-21). If the ulnar nerve lesion is above the midforearm, clawing of the ulnar two fingers does not occur, because the extrinsic muscles producing interphalangeal joint flexion are also denervated. In a *complete clawhand,* produced by a low lesion of the median and ulnar nerves, the metacarpophalangeal joints are extended and the interphalangeal joints flexed by the still-functional extrinsics (Fig. 3-22).

The sensory distribution of nerves in the right upper limb is shown in Figure 3-23.

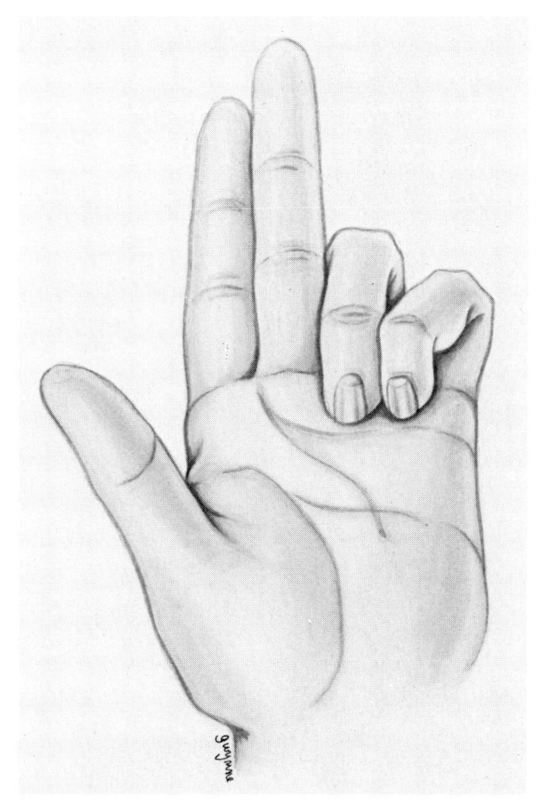

Fig. 3-21. Deformity produced by division of the ulnar nerve at the wrist (hand of benediction).

THE ARTERIES OF THE UPPER LIMB

The stem artery of the upper limb is the *subclavian artery.* It leaves the root of the neck at the first rib to enter the axilla as the *axillary artery.* It leaves the axilla at the lower border of the teres major to enter the arm as the *brachial artery.* The brachial artery bifurcates about 1 inch below the antecubital crease into the *radial and ulnar arteries,* which travel down the forearm to enter the palm and terminate in arterial arches. The ulnar artery is the main contributor to the *superficial palmar arch,* which is completed by the superficial palmar branch of the radial artery. The radial artery, after crossing the floor of the "snuffbox," passes through the first intermetacarpal space to enter the palm as the *deep palmar arch.* This arch is completed by the deep palmar branch of the ulnar artery (Fig. 3-24).

Collateral Circulation. It is safe to ligate either the subclavian or axillary arteries between the thyrocervical trunk and the subscapular artery because of the anastomoses about the scapula. It is usually also safe to ligate the brachial artery distal to the inferior ulnar collateral artery because of the anastomotic pathways around the elbow. Either the radial or the ulnar artery in the forearm may also be sacrificed because these arteries

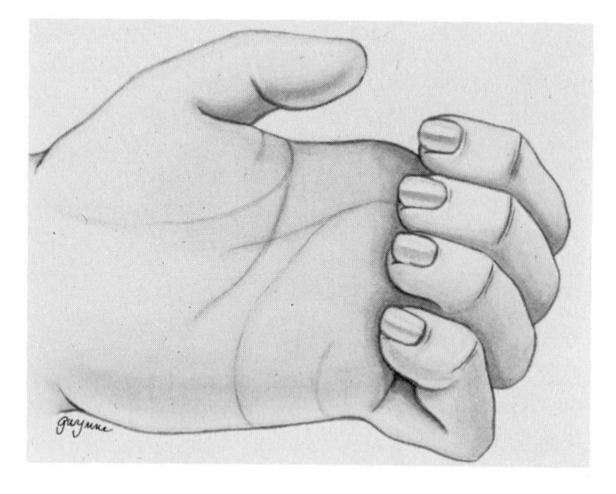

Fig. 3-22. Deformity produced by division of the median and ulnar nerve at the wrist (clawhand).

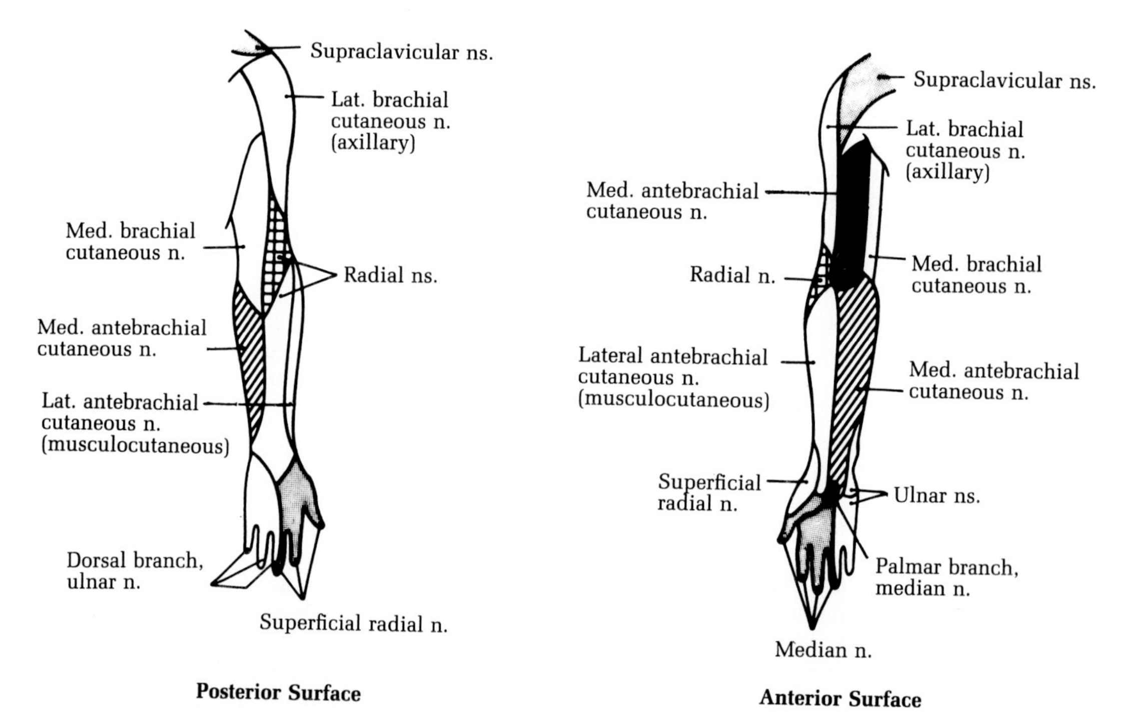

Fig. 3-23. Sensory distribution in the right upper limb. (Flatau E: Neurologische Schemata fur die Artzliche Praxis. Berlin, Springer-Verlag, 1915)

are united by palmar and carpal arches; indeed, the numerous anastomoses about the wrist may preserve the viability of the hand even after ligation of both the radial and ulnar arteries at that level.

SELECTED REFERENCES

Grant JCB, Basmajian JV: Grant's Method of Anatomy, 7th ed. Baltimore, Williams & Wilkins, 1965

Hollinshead WH: Anatomy for Surgeons, Vol 3, pp 207–580. New York, Harper & Row, 1969

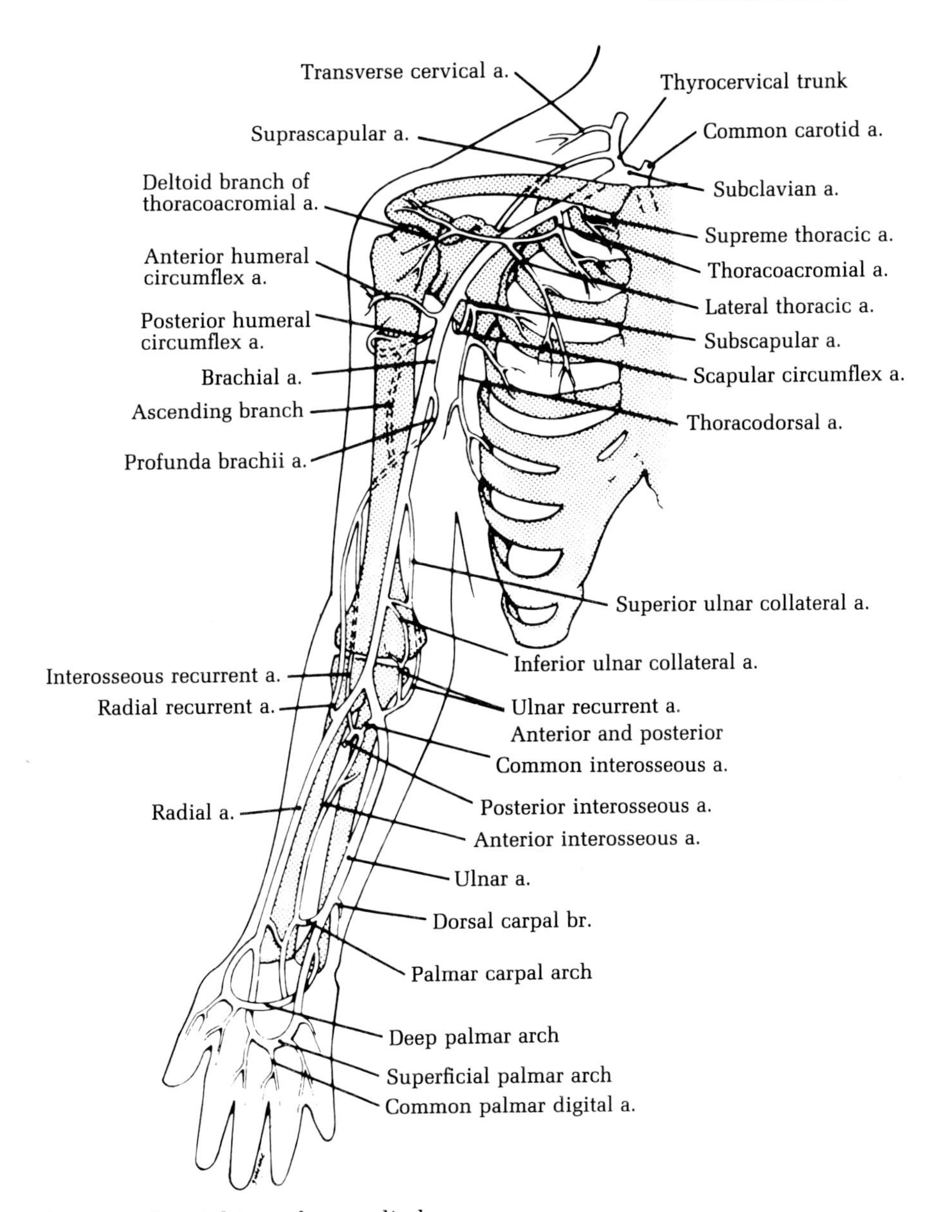

Fig. 3-24. Arterial tree of upper limb.

Chapter 4

The Lower Limb

Timothy N. Taft
and Charles W. Hooker

GOALS AND OBJECTIVES

Goals: To review the anatomy of the lower limb; to relate the structural attributes of the limb to its function; and to introduce the kinesiology of gait

Objectives: Upon completion of this unit, and using the text as a standard reference, one should be able to list, describe, recognize, or evaluate the following:

1. The bones of the lower limb
2. The groups of muscles of the lower limb, their actions, and their innervations
3. The major joints of the lower limb and their movements
4. The biomechanics of the hip and knee joints
5. The composition and divisions of the lumbar and lumbosacral plexuses
6. The plan of vascular supply and the pathways of collateral circulation in the lower limb
7. The components of gait and certain abnormalities of gait
8. Functional deficits and deformities produced by interruption of the major nerves of the lower limb
9. The normal surface and roentgenographic anatomy of the lower limb

OUTLINE

I. The hip and thigh
   A. Hip bone
   B. Upper femur
   C. Hip joint
   D. Forces acting upon the hip joint
   E. Muscles related to the hip joint
   F. Lower femur
   G. Muscles of the thigh
II. The knee
   A. Bones
   B. Capsule and ligaments
   C. Menisci
   D. Synovial membrane and synovial cavity
   E. Movements
   F. Significance of the patella in extension of the knee

III. The leg
  A. Bones and joints
  B. Muscles
  C. Compartments
IV. The ankle
  A. Bones and joint
  B. Ligaments
V. The foot
  A. Bones and arches
  B. Joints
  C. Ligaments
  D. Muscles
VI. The nerves
  A. Lumbar and lumbosacral plexuses
  B. Motor innervation
  C. Cutaneous innervation
VII. The blood vessels
  A. Arteries of gluteal region
  B. Femoral artery and its derivatives
  C. Collateral circulation
  D. Veins
VIII. Gait
  A. Components
  B. Abnormal patterns

In contrast to the upper limb, the lower limb is adapted for stability and locomotion rather than mobility and prehension. The anatomic and biomechanical attributes most essential to these considerations, and hence of the greatest clinical significance, are the concerns of this summary.

THE HIP AND THIGH

Unlike the upper limb, the lower limb has a strong osseous connection with the trunk. The bones of this region are the *os coxae*, or hip bone, and the *femur*, the bone of the thigh. In the adult, the former is a single bone formed by firm fusion of three previously separate bones, the ilium, ischium, and pubis. The *ilium* forms a joint with the sacrum that provides the attachment of the limb to the vertebral column; the *ischium* presents a tuberosity for weight bearing in the seated position; the *pubis* unites at the pubic symphysis with its counterpart of the other hip bone to close the bony pelvis anteriorly. The three bones are fused in the *acetabulum*, the depression in the hip bone that receives the head of the femur to form the hip joint. Prior to skeletal maturity, the area of union of the three separate bones is identifiable in roentgenograms as the *triradiate cartilage*.

The curved and triangular sacrum is wedged between the two ilia, an arrangement that transmits weight from the vertebral column to the hip bone and limb. Although the two *sacroiliac joints* are synovial joints, movement is greatly restricted by the interlocking irregularities of the articular surfaces of the participating bones and by the thickness and strength of complex *sacroiliac ligaments*, especially those over the posterior surface of each joint. The bodies of the two pubic bones are connected to each other by the *pubic symphysis*, a synchondrosis, that virtually prohibits movement at the joint. (In the latter weeks of pregnancy, however, both the sacroiliac joints and the pubic symphysis often become distinctly looser. Such change in the interpubic joint is striking in the burrowing mammals; without it, delivery of the young in these animals would be impossible.)

Several bony prominences in the area are readily palpable and serve as guides to underlying structures. They are the iliac crest, the arched upper border of the ilium; the anterior superior and posterior superior iliac spines at the anterior and posterior ends, respectively, of the iliac crest; and the pubic tubercle, an elevation on the anterior surface of the body of the pubis (in the adult about 3 cm from the midline of the body). The *inguinal ligament*, the inferior border of the aponeurosis of the external abdominal oblique muscle, is attached to the anterior superior iliac spine and to the pubic tubercle and lies in the gutter between the anterolateral abdominal wall and the thigh.

The *femur* extends to the knee joint from a rounded head that fits into the acetabulum to form the hip joint. The upper end consists of the head, a neck, and greater and lesser trochanters at the junction of the neck with the body. The four portions develop from separate ossification centers, with union at skeletal maturity. The head forms roughly two-thirds of a sphere whose surface is articular except for a posteromedial pit (fovea capitis femoris) where the ligament of the head is attached. The neck extends inferolaterally from the head to meet the shaft of the femur at an angle of about 125°. The angle varies somewhat with age, stature, and width of the pelvis, being less in the adult, in persons with short limbs, and in women. When this angle is greater than 135°, the condition is known as coxa valga; when less than 120°, coxa vara (Fig. 4-1). The femoral neck is parallel to neither the frontal plane of the body nor the plane of the femur. Instead, the head is located anterior to the midline of the shaft of the femur and is thus said to be anteverted. In the adult, this angle of the neck with the shaft is usually between 5° and 15°. When it is greater than 15°, increased *femoral anteversion* is present; when less than 5°, the condition is termed *femoral retroversion* (Fig. 4-2). The greater trochanter is a large prominence projecting upward from the shaft on the lateral aspect of the junction of the neck and the body of the femur. The lesser trochanter is a smaller protuberance on the posteromedial side of the junction of the neck and the body. Posteriorly an elevation, the intertrochanteric crest, extends between the two trochanters. A wide, rough intertrochanteric line stretches from the greater to the lesser trochanter on the anterior side of the femur.

Fractures of the proximal femur are quite common, especially in elderly women. These fractures are usually a result of a fall, and most often involve either the intracapsular neck of the femur or the extracapsular intertrochanteric region. With either of these fractures, the limb appears shortened and is externally rotated in consequence of gravity and the force of muscles acting upon the fragments.

At the hip joint, the globular head of the femur fits into the cuplike acetabulum to form a classical ball-and-socket joint that permits a wide range of motion, including circumduction. The mechanical demands upon this joint are great; it must be capable of bearing the weight of the body, as in standing on one foot, and of transferring the weight to the femur with rapid alternation of the hip joints during walking and running. To this end, the socket holding the head of the femur is deep, the fibrous capsule is strong and tense, and the controlling muscles insert at some distance from the axis of movement—all in contrast to circumstances at the shoulder joint. The articular surface of the acetabulum faces downward and forward as well as laterally and is shaped somewhat like a horseshoe, with a deep notch below, as though designed for standing. The acetabulum is made deeper by a fibrocartilaginous lip firmly attached to its bony rim and to the transverse ligament that bridges the acetabular notch.

A strong fibrous capsule encloses the joint and the greater part of the neck of the femur. Reinforcing the *capsular ligament* are three additional ligaments: (1) the triangular *iliofemoral ligament*, attached above to the anterior inferior iliac spine and the adjacent acetabular rim, and below to the intertrochanteric line; (2) the *pubofemoral ligament*, attached to the pubic portion of the acetabular rim and the superior ramus of the pubis, and to the inferior surface of the neck of the femur; and (3) the *ischiofemoral ligament*, attached to the ischial wall of the acetabulum and to the neck of the femur medial to the base of the greater trochanter. The first two of these ligaments lie in the front of the hip joint; the last is largely above and behind the joint. The orientation of the fibers of the capsule and of the three ligaments is such that they "wind up tightly" when the femur is fully extended. An additional ligament, of uncertain significance, is the intraarticular ligament of the head of the femur. This liga-

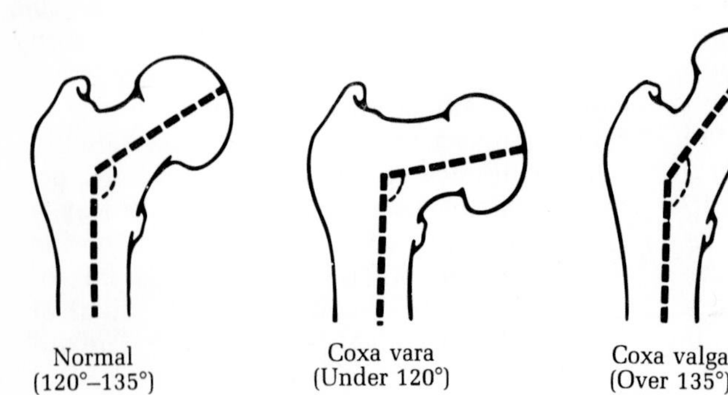

Fig. 4-1. The angle between the neck and the shaft of the femur.

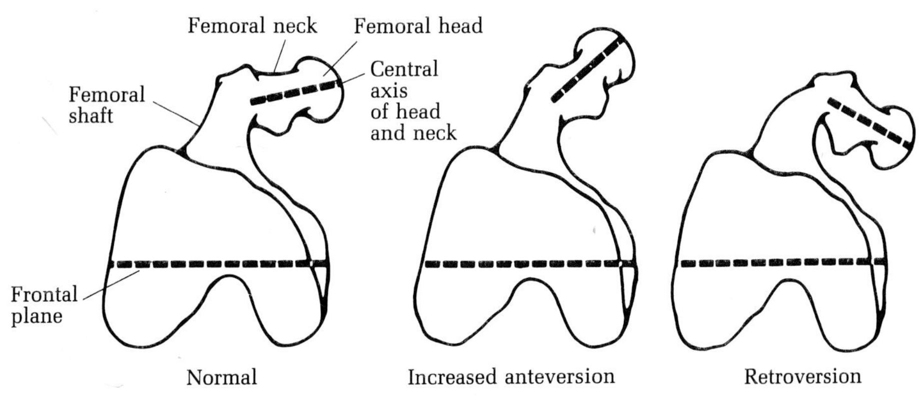

Fig. 4-2. Torsion of the femur as seen from its distal end.

ment is triangular in shape, with its base attached to the transverse ligament and the ischial margin of the acetabular notch, and its apex attached in the pit on the head of the femur. The arrangement of the bones and ligaments confers such stability that dislocation of hip joint requires application of great force.

The muscles of the region may be considered in functional groups. The chief flexor of the hip joint is the *iliopsoas* (Fig. 4-3), which inserts on and at the lesser trochanter. This is, in reality, two muscles, the *psoas major,* arising chiefly from lumbar vertebrae and intervertebral discs, and the *iliacus,* arising mainly from the floor of the iliac fossa. Other significant flexors are the *tensor fasciae latae,* arising from the anterior part of the iliac crest and inserting into the iliotibial band; the *pectineus,* arising from the superior ramus of the pubis and inserting on the femur just below the lesser trochanter; and the *adductor brevis,* arising from the body and inferior ramus of the pubis and inserting on the upper posterior femur.

The chief extensor is the *gluteus maximus* (Fig. 4-4), with an extensive origin from the posterior portion of the ilium, the thoracolumbar fascia, the dorsal surface of the sacrum and coccyx, and the surface of the sacrotuberous ligament. It inserts into the posterolateral surface of the upper one-third of the femur and into the iliotibial tract. Assisting as extensors of the hip joint are the

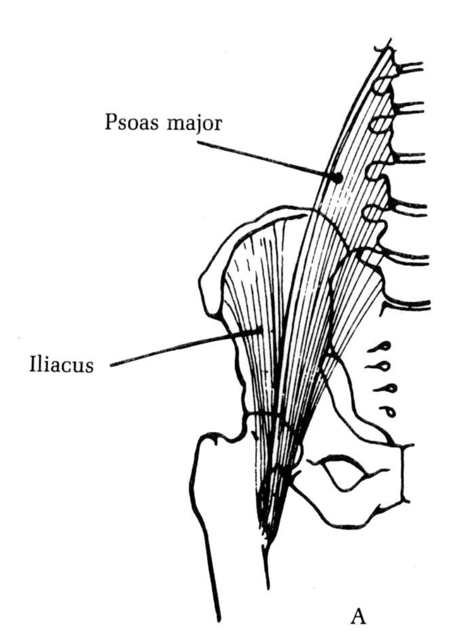

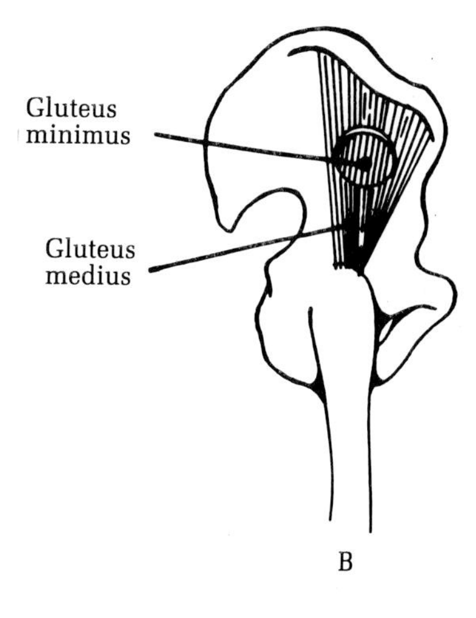

Fig. 4-3. (*A*) Iliopsoas muscle. (*B*) Gluteus medius and gluteus minimus muscles.

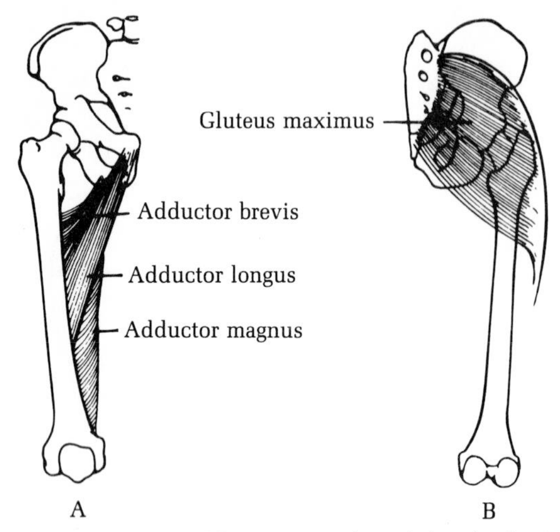

Fig. 4-4. (*A*) Adductor muscles of the thigh. (*B*) Gluteus maximus muscle.

hamstring muscles in the posterior compartment of the thigh that take origin from the ischial tuberosity.

The abductors of the thigh are the *gluteus medius* and *gluteus minimus* (Fig. 4-3). Both muscles arise from the outer surface of the wing of the ilium and insert on the greater trochanter, the gluteus medius lying superficial to the gluteus minimus. Weakness of these muscles manifests itself by a sagging of the contralateral side of the pelvis when standing on the affected limb (positive Trendelenburg sign).

The adductors of the thigh (Fig. 4-4) take origin from the body and inferior ramus of the pubis and from the ramus of the ischium, and insert on the medial side of the femur. They are the *adductors longus, brevis, and magnus* and the *gracilis*.

Serving as lateral, or external, rotators of the thigh are the gluteus maximus (Fig. 4-4) and several small muscles (the *internal and external obturators*, the *gemelli*, the *piriformis*, and the *quadratus femoris*) that arise from the pelvic surface of the sacrum and from the hip bone and insert on or about the greater trochanter. The chief medial or internal rotators are the gluteus minimus and the *tensor fasciae latae*.

Many of the muscles about the hip have more than one action. As examples, the gluteus maximus is both an extensor and a lateral rotator; the glutei medius and minimus are abductors (the former is a medial rotator and the latter is a lateral rotator); the adductor magnus is both an adductor and an extensor; the adductors longus and brevis are adductors and flexors; the tensor fasciae latae is a flexor and an abductor. Moreover, several of the muscles of the thigh produce movement at the hip joint in addition to movement at the knee joint. In addition to the hamstring muscles already mentioned, such muscles are the gracilis, an adductor of the thigh, and the sartorius, a lateral rotator of the thigh.

A broad range of forces acts upon the hip joint. In standing with the weight of the body equally distributed to the lower limbs, the weight on each femoral head is half of the body weight above the hips. In one-legged stance, as in walking, the head of the femur serves as a fulcrum. Body weight presses the pelvis downward medial to this fulcrum, and, in maintaining a level pelvis, the glutei medius and minimus pull the pelvis downward lateral to the fulcrum. The upward opposing force is that of the fulcrum, the head of the femur, a force that is the sum of the two downward forces. These considerations are shown in Figure 4-5.

Contractures about the hip joint produce an apparent but not real difference in length of the two limbs. An abduction contracture causes the affected limb to appear to be longer than the opposite limb, and an adduction contracture causes the affected limb to appear shorter (Fig. 4-6). In both circumstances, the apparent difference in length is a consequence of pelvic tilt.

The shaft of the femur is slightly twisted and curved with the convexity forward, partially accounting for the fullness of the anterior thigh. It is most nearly cylindrical in its middle third; above and below it is somewhat flattened anteroposteriorly and widened, especially toward the lower end. A rough ridge, the linea aspera, on the back of the middle third has two lips that diverge above and below as the bone widens. At or near the upper end of the linea aspera is a nutrient foramen directed upward; a second nutrient foramen may occur lower.

The muscles of the thigh are arrayed in three functional groups. On the anterior side, four muscles comprising the *quadriceps femoris*, with a common tendon of insertion, serve as extensors of the knee joint (Fig. 4-

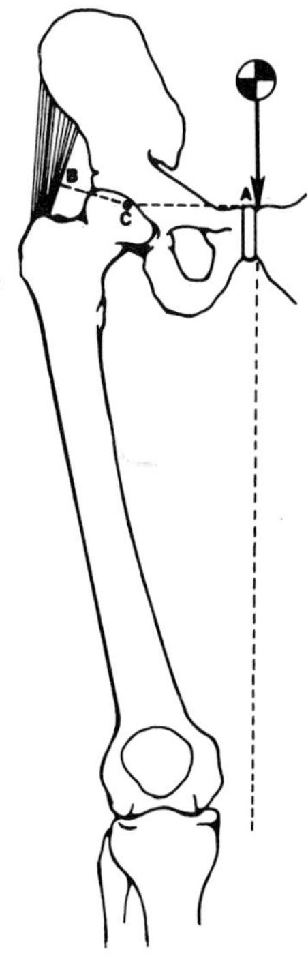

Fig. 4-5. Biomechanics of the hip joint during stance on that limb. The length of lever arm AC is $2\frac{1}{2}$ times that of lever arm BC. If the weight of the body minus that of the weight-bearing limb is 100 lbs, the downward force medial to the joint is $100 \times 2\frac{1}{2}$, or 250 lbs, which must be opposed by the abductors to keep the pelvis level. The *total* force on the hip joint is this abductor force plus the superimposed body weight of 100 lbs, or 350 lbs.

7*A*). Three of the four muscles arise from the femur; the fourth, the rectus femoris, arises from the anterior inferior iliac spine and serves as a flexor of the hip as well as an extensor of the knee. On the posterior side are three muscles, the so-called *hamstrings*, which arise primarily from the ischial tuberosity and serve as flexors of the knee and extensors of the hip (Fig. 4-7*B*). The muscles on the medial side are primarily adductors of the thigh, arising from the anterior portion of the bony pelvis and inserting on the medial side of the femur.

The muscles of the thigh are encased by a heavy layer of fascia, the *fascia lata*. This fascia is thickened on the lateral side as the iliotibial band and serves as a tendon for the tensor fasciae latae and the gluteus maximus.

The relationship of the nerves and vessels to the muscles of the thigh is shown in Figure 4-8.

THE KNEE

The *knee joint*, the largest and probably most complex joint in the body, is primarily a hinge joint, but it also permits rotation when the knee is partially flexed. It must possess stability, especially in extension, that does not interfere with freedom of movement, a requirement met not by the structural attributes of the bones but by a combination of ligaments and muscles, with the muscles serving also as ligaments.

The bones forming the joint are the femur, the tibia, and the patella. Inasmuch as

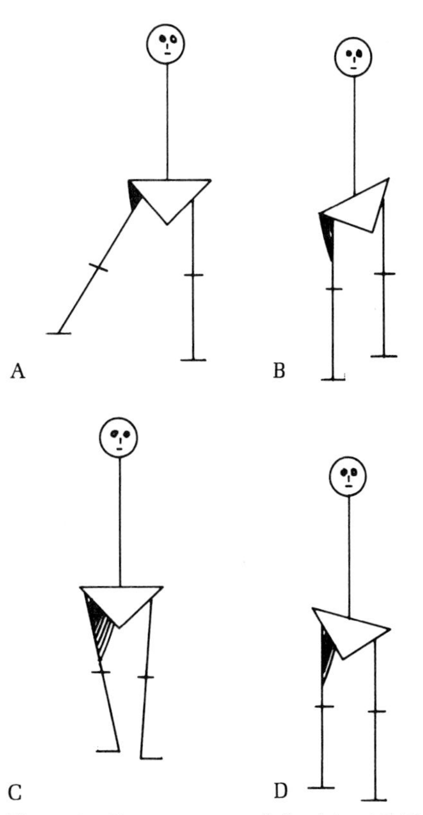

Fig. 4-6. Contractures of the hip. (*A,B*) abduction contracture; when the limbs are parallel (*B*), the affected one appears to be longer than the other. (*C,D*) adduction contracture; with the limbs parallel (*D*), the affected one appears to be shorter than the other.

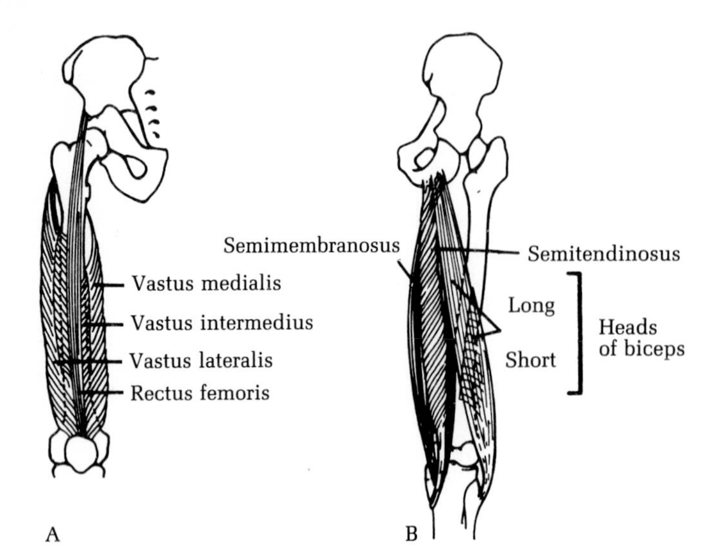

Fig. 4-7. Muscles on the anterior (*A*) and posterior (*B*) sides of the thigh.

the two femurs converge toward the knee and each tibia is nearly vertical, the femur and tibia meet at an angle of some 5° to 12°. A greater angle results in genu valgum (knock-knee); a lesser angle results in genu varum (bowleg).

The *femur* ends in two rounded condyles joined anteriorly to form the patellar articular surface and separated posteriorly by a deep intercondylar fossa. The condyles are almost in line with the front of the shaft, but they project backward well beyond the shaft, as in the letter J, a circumstance of significance in movement of the joint. The medial condyle is larger, more curved, and projects further than the lateral condyle, accounting for the angle between femur and tibia. The sides of the condyles are roughened and

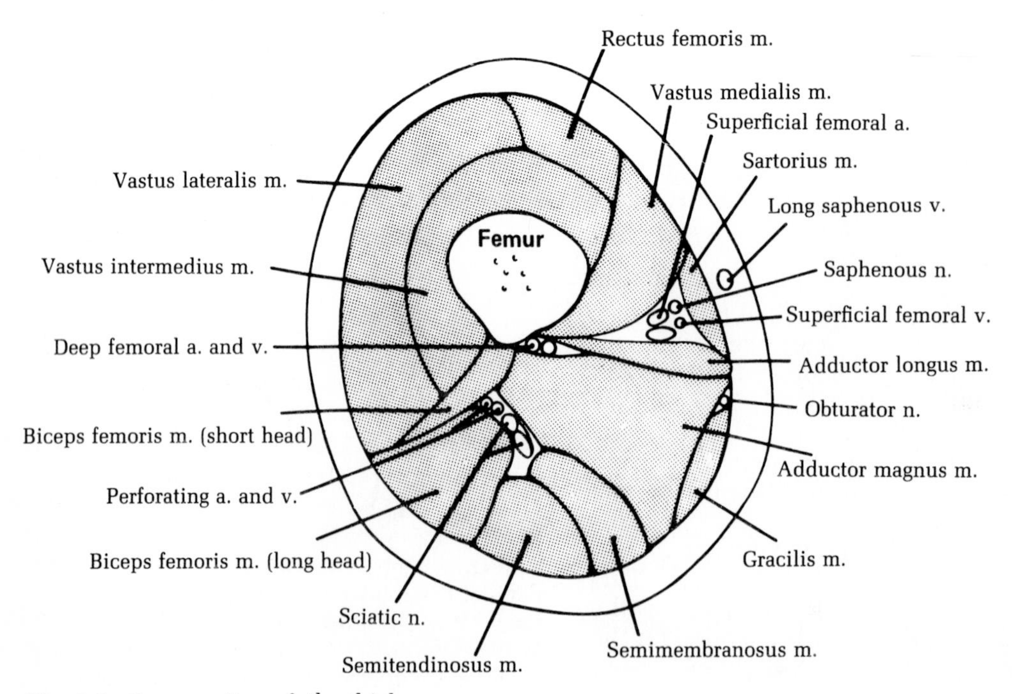

Fig. 4-8. Cross section of the thigh.

project somewhat as the medial and lateral epicondyles.

On its expanded upper end, the *tibia* has two slightly concave condyles separated by an intercondylar eminence and the sloping areas in front and behind it. A low elevation, the tibial tuberosity, for insertion of the quadriceps muscle, is situated at the junction of the anterior border of the shaft with the expanded upper end of the tibia.

The *patella*, a sesamoid bone in the tendon of the quadriceps muscle, has a smooth posterior surface divided by a rounded, vertical ridge into a larger, lateral portion for articulation with the lateral condyle and a smaller medial portion for articulation with the medial condyle of the femur.

Instead of being a thick and continuous ligamentous sheath joining the femur and tibia, much of the capsule is formed by tendons and their expansions. Anteriorly, the tendon of the quadriceps muscle, the patella and the *ligamentum patellae*, supplemented by an expansion of the iliotibial band, serve as the capsular ligament. Many of the bundles of tendon fibers course vertically; others course obliquely. On the posterior side of the joint, a fairly thin capsule extends from the level immediately above the femoral condyles to the posterior border of the upper end of the tibia. Its central region is supplemented by an expansion of the tendon of the semimembranosus that projects upward and laterally as the *oblique popliteal ligament*. The lower portion is supplemented by the *arcuate popliteal ligament*, extending from the posterior portion of the head of the fibula over the tendon of the popliteus muscle to spread over the back of the capsule. Laterally and medially, true capsular fibers extend from the sides of the femoral condyles to the sides of the tibial condyles, blending posteriorly with the ligaments and anteriorly with the tendinous expansion. The *tibial (medial) collateral ligament* is a broad, flat band in the capsular plane, attached above chiefly to the medial epicondyle of the femur and below to the medial surface of the tibia. A *fibular (lateral) collateral ligament* is cordlike and stands free of the thin, lateral part of the capsule. It is attached to the lateral epicondyle of the femur and the head of the fibula, and in its course splits the tendon of the biceps femoris. The medial and lateral collateral ligaments are stretched most tightly in extension of the joint and provide, as their primary function, resistance to valgus and varus stress respectively. Because of the direction of these ligaments—the tibial downward and forward, the fibular downward and backward—they also oppose lateral rotation of the tibia and medial rotation of the femur.

Two intraarticular ligaments, the *cruciate ligaments*, extend from the femur to the tibia. The anterior cruciate ligament extends from the anterior intercondylar area of the tibia upward and backward to the medial side of the lateral condyle of the femur and prevents posterior displacement of the femur on the tibia (or anterior displacement of the tibia on the femur). The posterior cruciate ligament passes upward and forward from the posterior intercondylar area of the tibia to the lateral side of the medial condyle of the femur and prevents anterior displacement of the femur on the tibia (or posterior displacement of the tibia). These ligaments are taut in full extension of the knee joint, and they tend to rotate the tibia laterally.

Projecting into the joint cavity between each of the two articular interfaces is an incomplete articular disc called a *meniscus*, for reason of its crescentic form. Each is attached at its periphery to the capsular ligament on the medial or lateral side of the joint and at its "horns" to the interarticular area of the tibia. Connecting the menisci anteriorly is the transverse ligament. In shape, the medial meniscus resembles a C, whereas the lateral meniscus is more sharply curved and resembles an O that is unclosed medially. The menisci help compensate for the incongruence of the bones, and they appear to be involved in rotation by moving on the tibia. As a result of sufficient stress (usually rotatory in the weight-bearing, flexed knee), either meniscus may be torn within itself or from its peripheral attachment. Inasmuch as the blood supply of the meniscus enters at the periphery, tears in the body of the meniscus do not heal. The detached portion of the meniscus may interfere with movement of the joint and cause recurring pain, locking, or "giving way."

Although the *synovial membrane* is attached all around, above to the articular margins of the femur and below to the articular margins of the tibia, it is not everywhere coextensive with the capsule of ligament and tendons. On the lateral and medial sides of the joint, it lies on the inner surface of the capsular ligament except where it is interrupted by the attachments of the menisci and separated from the capsule on the lateral side by the tendon of the popliteus muscle. It swings anteriorly, covering the deep surface of the tendons lateral to and above the patella, and attaches to the articular margins of the patella. Below the patella it swings over the deep surface of the infrapatellar pad of fat that lies on the deep surface of the ligamentum patellae. From here, a vertical, crescentic fold, the infrapatellar synovial fold, extends downward and backward to attach to the anterior border of the intercondylar notch of the femur, with its edges continuing backward along the lateral and medial borders of the intercondylar fossa. On each side of the infrapatellar fat, a horizontal alar fold may usually be identified. The synovium on the lateral and medial sides of the joint also swings posteriorly and then turns forward as a wide septum that contains the cruciate ligaments. The posteromedial portion of the joint cavity, containing the cruciate ligaments, thus lacks synovial membrane, but these ligaments have synovium on their sides and in front.

Because of the folds of synovial membrane, the synovial cavity is not a simple, short, cylindrical cavity. Behind and above the patella, it is a single cavity that is usually continuous above with the suprapatellar bursa between the tendon of the quadriceps muscle and the femur. Between the femur and the posterior wall of the bursa is a bit of fat and the articularis genu muscle, which arises on the femur and inserts into the posterior wall of the bursa. Below the patella, the synovial cavity is divided into lateral and medial compartments by the infrapatellar synovial fold. Posteriorly, the synovial cavity is divided into two compartments by the fold that contains the cruciate ligaments. The cruciate ligaments, the menisci, and the infrapatellar fat pad are outside the synovial cavity.

For reason of the contour of the femoral and tibial condyles, flexion and extension of the knee joint are not the simple hinge movements that occur at the elbow joint, for example. In full flexion, the posterior portions of the femoral condyles are in contact with the posterior portions of the tibial condyles. As the knee is extended, the femoral condyles roll on the tibial condyles and menisci, the movement resembling that of a rocking chair. There is also some sliding of the femur backward. As extension progresses, the shorter, more highly curved lateral condyle exhausts its articular surface and is checked by the anterior cruciate ligament, whereas the larger and less curved medial condyle continues its forward roll and skids backward, assisted by tightening of the posterior cruciate ligament. The result is a medial rotation of the femur that tightens the collateral ligaments, and the joint is "screwed home", to use mechanical phraseology. Flexion of the extended knee is preceded by lateral rotation of the femur (or medial rotation of the tibia), usually produced by the popliteus muscle, which arises from the lateral surface of the lateral femoral condyle and inserts on the base of the upper portion of the tibia. This rotation relaxes the tension of the collateral ligaments sufficiently to permit flexion.

Inasmuch as the line of gravity passes in front of the knee joints when the body is erect, gravity tends to produce a locking of the knee joint. In ordinary standing, however, the knee joint is not usually locked, but is maintained a bit short of full extension. The quadriceps muscle is relaxed, and the patella can be passively moved from side to side; the hamstring muscles and the gastrocnemius act to maintain the joint in the nearly extended position. In reaching forward, the knee joint usually becomes locked and the quadriceps relaxed.

With extension of the knee joint, the force exerted by the quadriceps muscles is influenced by the patella, which increases the length of the moment arm through which these muscles act. The *moment arm* is the perpendicular distance from the center of rotation to the line of force applied (Fig. 4-9). When the patella is removed, the moment arm is shortened and the force required for extension is increased by 15% to 20%. When the muscles cannot provide the additional force needed, full, active extension of the knee may be impossible.

Readily palpable about the knee are the patella, the tibial and femoral condyles, the

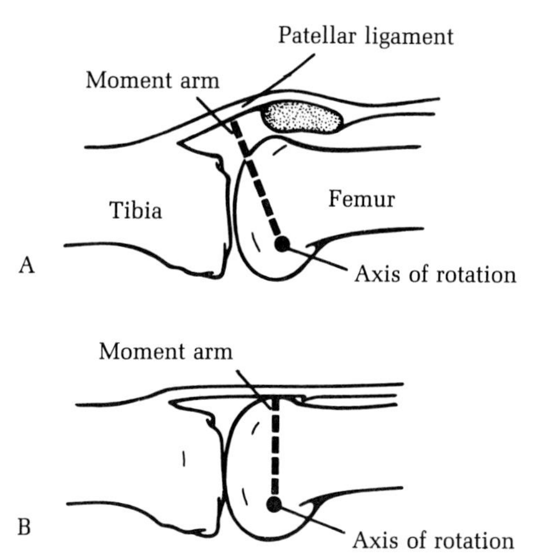

Fig. 4-9. Moment arms of the knee. (*A*) With patella. (*B*) Without patella. (Kaufer H: Mechanical Function of the Patella. J Bone Joint Surg 53A: 1552, 1971)

medial and lateral joint lines, the tibial tubercle, the head of the fibula, the patellar ligament, and the tendons of the semitendinosus and biceps femoris.

THE LEG

The leg is the segment of the lower limb between the knee and the ankle. Its skeleton is formed by two bones: the heavy, weight-bearing tibia, whose upper end has already been described, and the slender, largely non-weight-bearing fibula that parallels the tibia on its lateral side. The extended upper end of the fibula forms a synovial joint with the tibia just below its overhanging lateral condyle, and the expanded lower end of the fibula is joined to the lateral side of the lower end of the tibia by a fibrous joint. The two bones are also connected between the two joints by the interosseous membrane whose fibers extend downward and laterally from tibia to fibula. The lower end of each bone is prolonged downward as the medial (tibial) and lateral (fibular) malleoli of the ankle joint.

The muscles of the leg are sequestered into spatial and functional groups by sturdy membranes (Fig. 4-10). Anterior to the interosseous membrane and lateral to the tibia are the muscles that dorsiflex the ankle and extend the toes (*tibialis anterior, extensor hallucis, extensor digitorum longus, peroneus tertius*). They arise from the lateral side of the tibia, the interosseous membrane, and the fibula.

Behind the interosseous membrane are muscles that plantar flex the ankle, invert the foot, and flex the toes. These muscles are subdivided into superficial and deep groups by a transverse intermuscular septum that

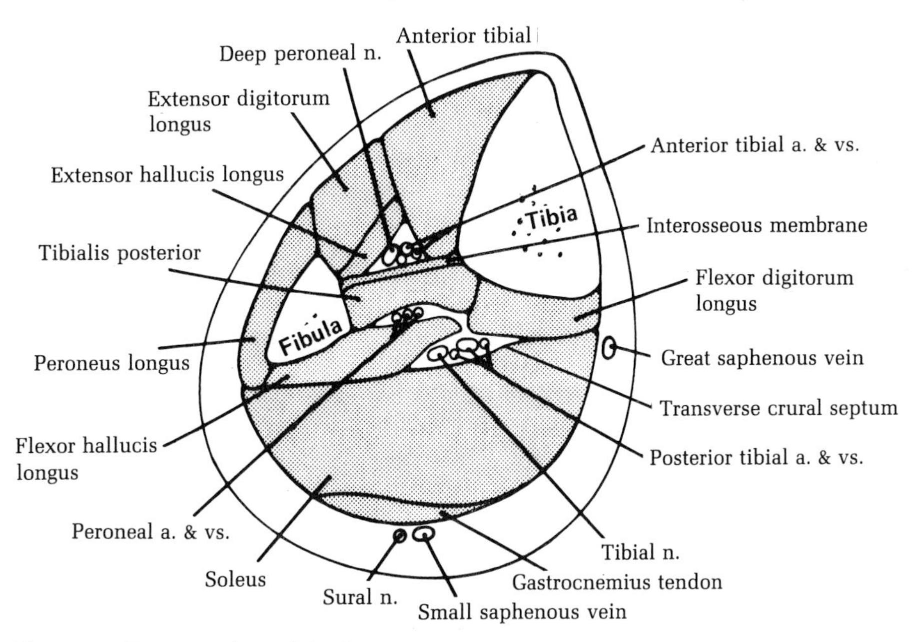

Fig. 4-10. Cross section of the leg.

represents an infolding of the deep (crural) fascia of the leg. The superficial group consists of three muscles that insert on the calcaneus and plantar flex the ankle. The most superficial is the *gastrocnemius*, which arises by two heads from the lateral and medial epicondyles of the femur, forms the muscular mass of the upper part of the leg, and inserts by means of the heavy tendo calcaneus on the posterior end of the calcaneus. The deep muscle is the *soleus*, which arises from the upper part of the fibula and tibia, is prolonged below the inferior margin of the gastrocnemius and inserts into the tendo calcaneus. Between the two muscles is the vestigal *plantaris longus*, which arises immediately above the lateral head of the gastrocnemius and whose long, slender tendon inserts on the calcaneus, occasionally by blending with the tendo calcaneus.

Of the deep group, the *flexor digitorum longus*, the *tibialis posterior*, and the *flexor hallucis longus* arise from the fibula and tibia. Their tendons pass behind the medial malleolus to the plantar surface of the foot. Here, the flexor hallucis longus inserts on the distal phalanx of the great toe and is a flexor of that digit; the flexor digitorum longus divides into four tendons, one to each of the other four toes; the tibialis posterior is primarily an inverter and adductor of the foot. A fourth muscle of this group, the *popliteus*, arises primarily from the lateral surface of the lateral condyle of the femur, within the fibrous capsule of the knee joint and external to the synovial membrane; it inserts on the posterior surface of the upper part of the tibia. Its action in laterally rotating the femur preliminary to flexion of the knee joint has already been mentioned.

Lateral to the fibula and separated from the other muscles by anterior and posterior intermuscular septa that project from the crural fascia to the fibula are the two muscles of the lateral group, the *peroneus longus* and, deep to it, the *peroneus brevis*, both arising chiefly from the fibula. The tendons of both muscles pass behind the lateral malleolus; that of the brevis inserts on the base of the fifth metatarsal, and that of the longus crosses the plantar surface of the foot to insert on the medial cuneiform and the base of the first metatarsal on the medial side of the foot. The chief action of both muscles is eversion of the foot.

Except where the anterior and lateral surfaces of the tibia are subcutaneous, the leg is surrounded by a tough, fibrous layer, the crural fascia, that projects deeply as the several intermuscular septa separating the groups of muscles. Each of the compartments so formed is a closed fascial space in which hemorrhage or edema can compress the blood vessels. The consequence is ischemia and necrosis of muscle that may result in deformity and loss of function, sometimes necessitating amputation.

THE ANKLE

At the ankle the weight-bearing tibia articulates with the spool-like upper surface of the *talus* that, in turn, articulates below with the calcaneus. The joint is a hinge joint of the mortise and tenon variety, with the talus as the tenon and the malleoli projecting downward from the tibia and fibula forming the medial and lateral walls of the mortise. In addition, the malleoli serve as pulleys for tendons reaching the plantar surface of the foot from the posterior and lateral compartments of the leg.

As is usual in hinge joints, the capsular ligament is weak in front of and behind the joint and is reinforced by collateral ligaments at the sides (Fig. 4-11). On the medial side, the heavy *deltoid ligament* is attached above to the medial malleolus and fans out to attach below chiefly to the talus, but also to the navicular bone and the calcaneus. On the lateral side there are three smaller ligaments: the *anterior and posterior talofibular ligaments* and the *calcaneofibular ligament*, which lies between the talofibular ligaments.

The fibrous distal tibiofibular joint, abetted by the interosseous membrane, stabilizes the mortise of the ankle joint to the extent that the malleoli and the collateral ligaments largely limit movement to plantar flexion and extension. The deltoid ligament resists eversion and lateral rotation, and the lateral ligaments resist inversion and internal rotation of the foot. Sudden and forceful eversion, inversion, or rotation of the foot may tear the ligament stressed. Associated talar compression of the opposite malleolus may fracture that malleolus.

As they pass the ankle on the way to the foot the tendons of muscles in the leg have tendon sheaths and are held in place by

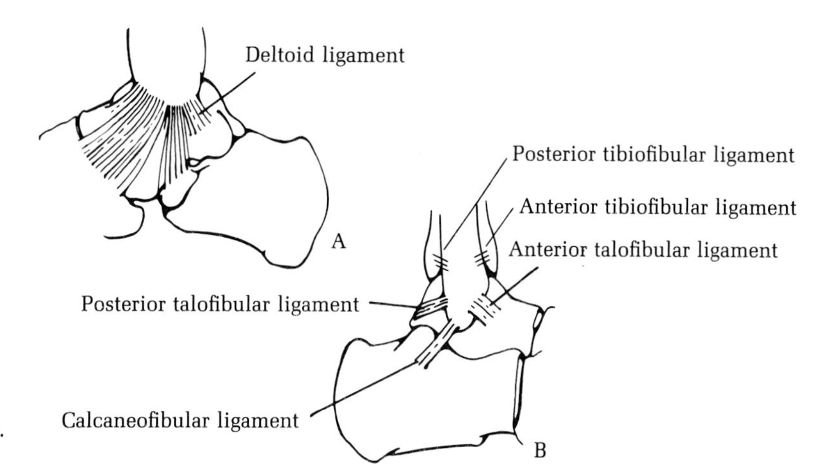

Fig. 4-11. Ligaments of the ankle joint. (*A*) Medial side. (*B*) Lateral side.

thickenings of the crural fascia. On the anterior side, the thin *superior extensor retinaculum* stretches from tibia to fibula a bit above the ankle; at the ankle the heavier *inferior extensor retinaculum* resembles a Y on its side and extends from the lateral side of the calcaneus, one arm attaching to the medial malleolus and the other to the fascia on the medial side of the plantar surface of the foot. On the medial side of the ankle, the *flexor retinaculum* attaches to the medial malleolus and the calcaneus; it gives off three septa that divide the subretinacular space into four compartments, one for each of the three tendons from the posterior leg to the plantar portion of the foot and one for the tibial nerve and posterior tibial vessels. On the lateral side, the *superior peroneal retinaculum* stretches between two areas on the calcaneus; under these pass the tendons of the peroneus longus and brevis.

THE FOOT

In addition to being a weight-bearing entity, the foot serves as a lever to raise the body and to convey thrust in walking and running. Its arched structure provides strength and resilience for the large forces involved, as well as protection of structures in the sole from compression. The bones are so arranged that each foot is half of a dome with its inferior edge extending from the heel along the lateral border of the foot and then medially across the ball of the foot to the ball of the great toe, an arrangement that increases stability in standing.

The skeleton of the foot (Fig. 4-12) is composed of seven tarsal bones comparable to the carpals of the wrist and hand, five metatarsals comparable to the metacarpals of the hand, and the phalanges comparable to those of the hand.

The *talus* is the highest portion of the dome, forms the joint with the tibia and fibula, is supported by the other tarsal bones, and articulates with the calcaneus below and the navicular in front. The *calcaneus*, largest of the tarsal bones, projects backward to form the prominence of the heel, and articulates in front with three wedge-shaped bones, the medial, intermediate, and lateral *cuneiform bones*, which articulate anteriorly with, respectively, the first, second, and third *metatarsals*. The *cuboid* articulates behind with the calcaneus and in front with the fourth and fifth *metatarsals*.

When the bones of the foot are held snugly together, the articular surfaces are so arranged that both a *longitudinal arch* and a *transverse arch* are created. Inasmuch as the longitudinal arch involves two columns of bones and is much higher on the medial side of the foot, it is convenient to regard it as consisting of a medial portion and a lateral portion. The posterior part of the calcaneus is the posterior pillar of both. In the "medial arch," the posterior pillar continues upward into the talus; the anterior pillar consists of the navicular, the three cuneiform bones, and the three medial metatarsals; the summit or keystone is the head of the talus. The "lateral arch" continues through the anterior part of the calcaneus, the cuboid bone, and the lat-

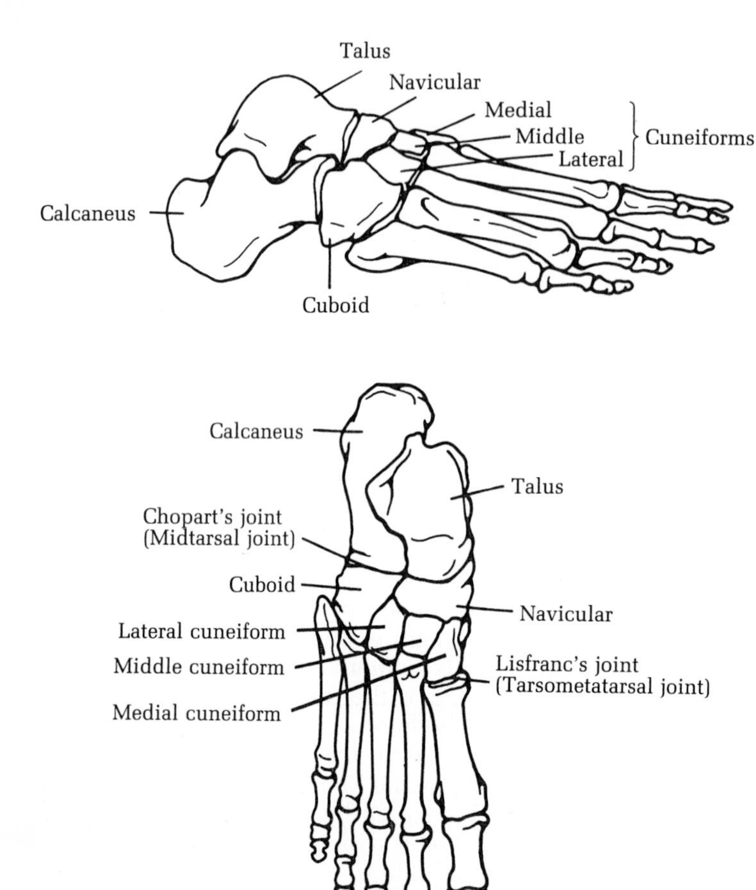

Fig. 4-12. The bones of the foot.

eral two metatarsals. The transverse arch is most evident along the line of the tarsometatarsal joints, and disappears as the metatarsals are traced toward their distal ends.

The joints between bones in the foot are synovial joints supported by collateral ligaments that are much stronger on the plantar side, where several of them cross more than one joint. The more notable of these ligaments are the *long plantar ligament* extending from the calcaneus as far as the base of the medial three metatarsals, completing a canal for the tendon of the peroneus longus muscle, and the *plantar calcaneonavicular ("spring") ligament,* passing from the calcaneus to the navicular and supporting the head of the talus. These and other longitudinally disposed ligaments are involved in creating and maintaining the longitudinal arch. In this function they appear to be assisted by the longitudinally coursing muscles of the foot and their tendons and by the tendons of muscles situated in the leg.

Dorsiflexion and plantar flexion occur primarily at the *talocrural (ankle) joint.* Inversion and eversion of the foot occur at the *subtalar joint* (between the talus and the calcaneus) and the transverse tarsal joints (talonavicular and calcaneocuboid). The forepart of the foot can be flexed and extended on the hind part at the transverse tarsal joint, flexion increasing the height of the arch (*pes cavus*) and extension decreasing it, an exaggeration of which results in a flat foot (*pes planus*).

With certain modifications and exceptions, the muscles and fasciae of the foot are comparable to those of the hand. With no counterpart in the upper limb, the extensor digitorum brevis on the dorsum sends a tendon to each of the four medial toes. On the plantar side, the *plantar aponeurosis* is comparable to the palmar aponeurosis. Immediately deep to the plantar aponeurosis, arising from the calcaneus, and sending a tendon to each of the lateral four toes is the *flexor digitorum brevis,* the equivalent of the flexor digitorum superficialis of the upper limb. Deep to the flexor digitorum brevis, the *quadratus plantae,* unique to the foot, arises from the calcaneus and inserts on the lateral side of the tendon of the flexor digitorum longus passing obliquely across the foot in the same plane. The other muscles of the foot are counterparts of comparable muscles of the hand, with two differences to be noted: in the foot there is no opponens hallucis, and the interosseous muscles are arranged about the second digit as the midline, whereas in the hand the middle finger serves as the midline.

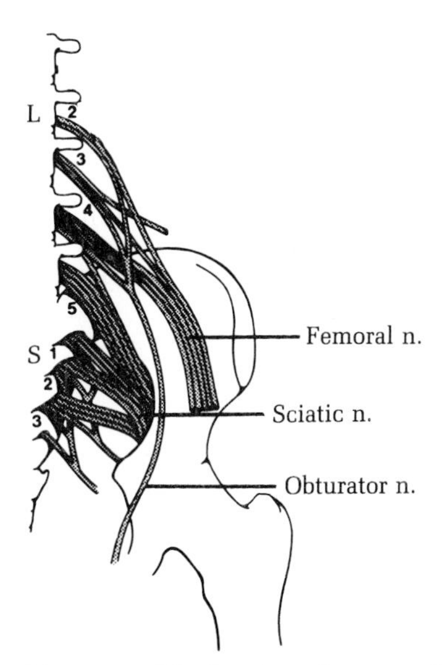

Fig. 4-13. The lumbar plexus and the lumbosacral plexus, and their chief branches.

THE NERVES

In thinking of the nerves of the lower limb, it is convenient to imagine the thigh flexed on the trunk as in a quadruped. In this posture, one set of nerves leaves the trunk cranial to the hip joint and another set caudal to the hip joint to enter the gluteal region.

Primary ventral rami of the five lumbar nerves and of the first four sacral nerves combine to form the *lumbar (L1-4) and lumbosacral (L4-S4) plexuses,* each giving rise to anterior and posterior branches (Fig. 4-13). The anterior branches supply flexor muscles of the limb, and the posterior branches supply extensor and adductor muscles, muscles that before rotation of the limb in the embryo were, respectively, anterior and posterior to the skeleton of the limb.

The derivatives of the lumbar plexus, the more cranial of the two plexuses, enter the limb anterior to the plane of the femur and the hip joint. The largest of these derivatives are the femoral nerve and the obturator nerve. The *fermoral nerve* (posterior branches of L2-4) enters the thigh after passing behind the inguinal ligament and, after giving branches to each of the components of the quadriceps muscle and cutaneous branches to the anterior thigh, it continues as the saphenous nerve, a cutaneous nerve to the tibial side of the leg. The *obturator nerve* (anterior branches of L2-4) enters the medial side of the thigh and supplies the adductor muscles and a variable extent of skin on the medial side of the thigh. Other derivatives of the lumbar plexus, which contribute to the cutaneous innervation of the anterior and lateral thigh, are the ilioinguinal nerve (L1), supplying a small area of the upper, medial part of the thigh; the genitofemoral nerve (L1, 2), supplying a small area inferior to the middle of the inguinal ligament; and the *lateral cutaneous nerve of the thigh* (L2-3), supplying the lateral and anterolateral thigh. Above the distribution of the lateral cutaneous nerve of the thigh, a variable area of skin on the lateral side of the thigh is supplied by the lateral cutaneous branch of the *iliohypogastric nerve* (L1).

The nerves arising from the lumbosacral plexus leave the pelvis posterior to the plane of the femur and hip joint. The *superior gluteal nerve* (chiefly L4 and 5) supplies the glutei medius and minimus and the tensor fasciae latae, and the *inferior gluteal nerve* (chiefly L5-S2) supplies the gluteus maximus. Small nerves derived from L4-S3 supply the lateral rotators of the thigh except the obturator externus, which is supplied by the obturator nerve. Much the largest derivative of the lumbosacral plexus is the *sciatic nerve,* which supplies the muscles of the posterior thigh and all of the muscles of the leg and foot. The sciatic nerve is composed of two portions, the *common peroneal nerve* and the *tibial nerve,* that usually separate in the upper part of the popliteal space, a space behind the knee bounded above by the tendons of the hamstring muscles and below by the two heads of the gastrocnemius muscle (Fig. 4-14).

The common peroneal nerve (L4-S2), the posterior component, supplies the short head of the biceps femoris in the thigh, crosses the lateral head of the gastrocnemius, and becomes subcutaneous behind the head of the fibula, where it is liable to injury. After penetrating the posterior intermuscular septum, it divides into the superficial and deep peroneal nerves. The *superficial peroneal nerve* is the nerve of the lateral compartment of the leg, lying first between the peroneus longus and the fibula and then between the peronei longus and brevis, supplying both muscles. The *deep peroneal nerve* courses forward around the fibula to enter the anterior compartment of the leg; it supplies the muscles of the anterior compartment and continues to the dorsum of the foot where it supplies the extensor hallucis longus and the extensor digitorum brevis.

The tibial nerve (L4-S3), the anterior component, supplies the muscles of the posterior thigh (except the short head of the biceps) and, after passing through the popliteal space posterior to the popliteal artery and vein, it enters the posterior compartment of the leg to lie deep to the transverse crural septum. In the popliteal space it gives off branches that supply the popliteus muscle, the two heads of the gastrocnemius, the soleus, and the plantaris muscles. In the posterior compartment it supplies the remaining muscles, the tibialis posterior, flexor hallucis longus, and flexor digitorum longus. The tibial nerve then passes behind the medial malleolus toward the plantar side of the foot. Under the flexor retinaculum it divides into the *medial plantar nerve* and the *lateral plantar nerve*. It will suffice to say that, speaking generally, the medial branch is the counterpart of the median nerve in the hand and the lateral branch is the counterpart of the ulnar nerve in the hand.

The skin of the gluteal region is supplied by four sets of nerves. In the lateral portion, the cutaneous nerves are *lateral cutaneous branches* of the 12th thoracic and the *iliohypogastric (L1) nerves*. The superior area receives *superior clunial nerves,* lateral branches of dorsal rami of L1-3. The medial area is supplied by *middle clunial nerves,* lateral branches of dorsal rami of S1-3. The inferior area receives *inferior clunial nerves,* branches of the posterior femoral cutaneous nerve.

The *posterior femoral cutaneous nerve* (S1-3) is derived from the lumbosacral plexus and accompanies the sciatic nerve in the gluteal region. Under cover of the gluteus maximus muscle, it gives off one or more perineal branches as well as the inferior clunial nerves, and continues downward in the midline deep to the fascia lata, giving off branches that supply the skin of the posterior thigh.

The skin of the leg is innervated by the *saphenous nerve*, the terminal portion of the femoral nerve, on the medial side; by the *lateral sural cutaneous nerve,* a branch of the common peroneal nerve, on the lateral side;

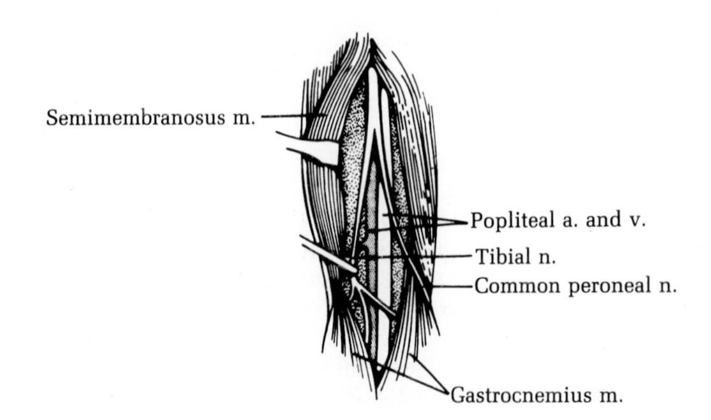

Fig. 4-14. The popliteal fossa.

and by the *posterior femoral cutaneous nerve,* above, and the medial sural nerve, a branch of the tibial nerve, below, on the posterior side. The *medial sural cutaneous nerve* is usually joined by a branch from the common perioneal nerve to form the *sural nerve* distributed to the lower part of the posterolateral side of the leg and, as the lateral dorsal cutaneous nerve, to the dorsal portion of the lateral side of the foot.

On the dorsum of the foot, the saphenous nerve supplies skin on the medial side and the sural nerve on the lateral side. A continuation of the superficial peroneal nerve supplies the middle portion, except the skin between the great toe and the next toe and the immediately adjacent area of the dorsum, which are innervated by the deep peroneal nerve. On the plantar surface, the cutaneous innervation resembles that of the hand, with the lateral plantar nerve supplying the lateral one fourth and the medial plantar nerve the medial three fourths. The skin over the calcaneus is supplied by the medial calcaneal nerve, a branch arising from the tibial nerve, just before its termination as the plantar nerves.

A schema of the dermatomes of the limb is shown in Figure 4-15.

THE BLOOD VESSELS

The arteries, like the nerves, leave the trunk to enter the lower limb both cranial to the plane of the femur and caudal to it.

The gluteal region is supplied chiefly by the *superior* and *inferior gluteal arteries,* both arising as branches of the internal iliac artery that leave the pelvis caudal to the plane of the femur.

The remainder of the limb is supplied largely by the *femoral artery* (Fig. 4-16), a continuation of the external iliac artery that leaves the trunk cranial to the plane of the femur, passing immediately behind the inguinal ligament. In the upper thigh, this artery lies between the femoral vein and femoral nerve in the femoral triangle, a space roofed by the fascia lata and bounded by the inguinal ligament above, the sartorius muscle laterally, and the adductor longus medially. It may be palpated in this region and used as a guide in aspirating the hip joint; a needle inserted one inch lateral to a point on the artery one inch below the inguinal ligament should enter the joint cavity.

The largest branch of the femoral artery in the femoral triangle is the *profunda femoris,* which arises on the lateral side of the femoral artery, arches posteriorly, and continues downward near the middle of the thigh. In addition to numerous branches to the adductor and hamstring muscles, it has two larger branches, the *lateral* and *medial circumflex femoral arteries* that supply the upper end of the femur. Branches of both arteries reach the bone at the level of attachment of the capsular ligament of the hip joint, and course along the neck as retinacular arteries to reach the head of the femur. The *retinacular arteries,* derivatives chiefly of the medial circumflex femoral artery, are liable to damage in fracture of the neck of the femur, resulting in ischemia and possibly necrosis of the head of the femur.

The main trunk of the *femoral artery* continues downward in the thigh deep to the sartorius muscle, accompanied by the saphenous nerve. Its general position is indicated by a line from the midpoint of the inguinal ligament to the adductor tubercle of the femur when the thigh is flexed, abducted, and laterally rotated. A bit above the knee, it reaches the posterior side of the thigh by passing through an opening in the adductor magnus muscle to enter the popliteal space as the *popliteal artery,* where it may be palpated if the subject is not obese. It sends paired sural arteries to the gastrocnemius and soleus muscles and ends by dividing into the anterior and posterior tibial arteries.

The *anterior tibial artery* passes through the gap above the interosseus membrane to enter the anterior compartment of the leg and supply its muscles. It continues on the dorsum of the foot as the *dorsalis pedis artery,* which gives off medial and lateral tarsal branches, and ends by dividing into the *arcuate artery* and the larger *deep plantar artery.* The arcuate artery has three *metatarsal branches* that, in turn, divide into dorsal digital arteries. The deep plantar artery sends *digital branches* to the great toe and the second toe and passes between the heads of the first dorsal interosseous muscle to the plantar surface.

The *posterior tibial artery* accompanies the tibial nerve in the posterior compartment

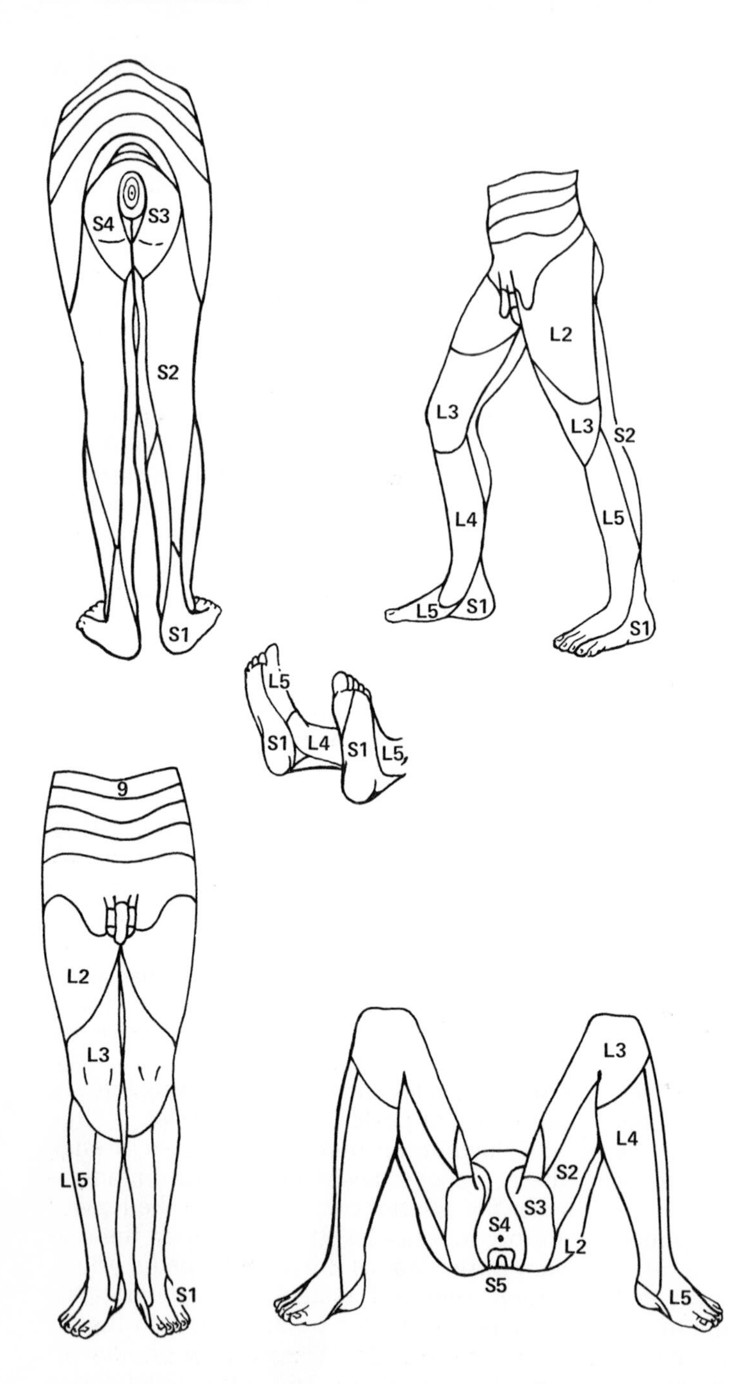

Fig. 4-15. Dermatomes of the lower limb.

of the leg, lying immediately deep to the transverse crural septum, and enters the plantar foot after passing behind the medial malleolus. The largest branch is the *peroneal artery* arising high in the leg and coursing downward in the posterior compartment lateral to and deeper than the posterior tibial artery. Both arteries have numerous branches to adjacent muscles and, in addition, the peroneal artery sends branches through the interosseous membrane to muscles in the anterior compartment and a nutrient artery to the fibula; the nutrient artery of the tibia is a large branch of the posterior tibial artery. The lateral compartment of the leg has no artery proper to it.

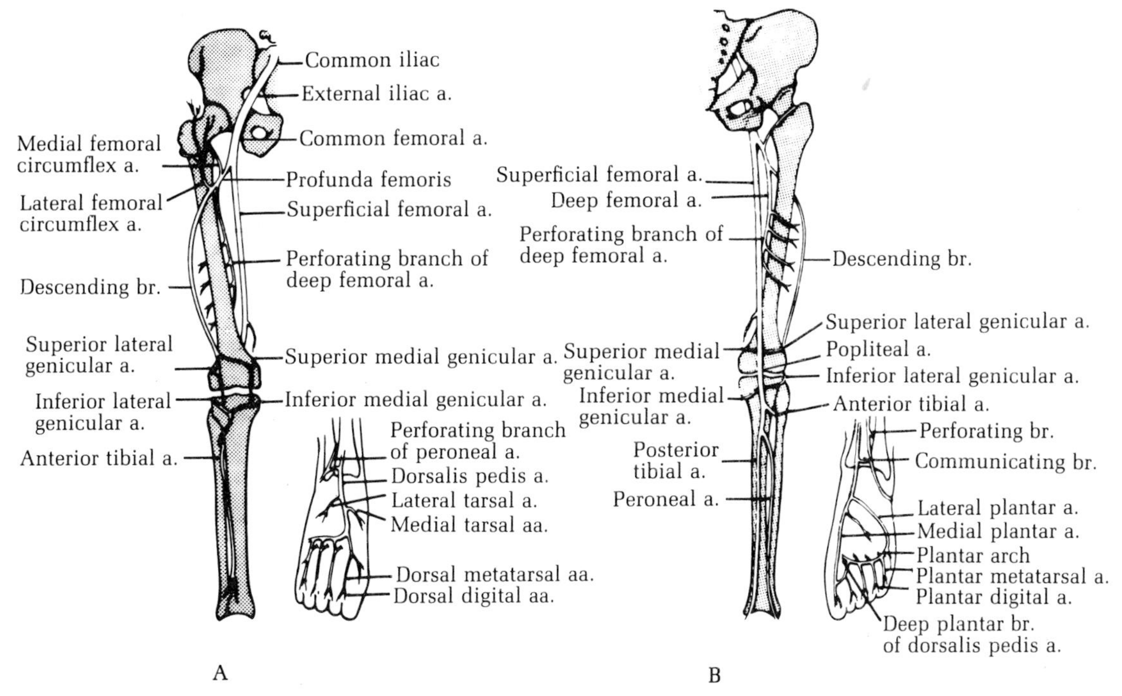

Fig. 4-16. The femoral artery and its derivatives. (*A*) Anterior aspect. (*B*) Posterior aspect.

Under the flexor retinaculum the posterior tibial artery divides into the *lateral and medial plantar arteries.* The medial plantar artery accompanies the medial plantar nerve and supplies the medial portion of the plantar foot. The larger lateral plantar artery accompanies the lateral plantar nerve to the base of the fifth metatarsal, where it arches across the foot to form the *plantar arch,* which is completed by the deep plantar artery from the dorsalis pedis. Five *plantar metatarsal arteries* arise from the plantar arch, and each divides into two *proper plantar digital arteries.* The three medial metatarsal arteries usually receive branches from the medial plantar artery.

Anastomoses between the superior and inferior gluteal arteries and the two femoral circumflex branches of the deep femoral artery, and between the deep circumflex artery (from the external iliac) and the ascending branch of the lateral circumflex femoral can provide *collateral circulation* when the femoral artery is occluded above the origin of the profunda femoris. Despite numerous arterial communications about the knee joint between branches of the femoral artery, the lateral femoral circumflex artery, the anterior tibial artery, and the popliteal artery, the collateral circulation here is usually inadequate when the femoral or the popliteal artery is suddently occluded. Numerous anastomoses between the anterior and posterior tibial arteries maintain viability when either is occluded.

Veins accompany the arteries of the lower limb, and those that accompany the three large arteries of the leg are paired, providing an important temperature-regulating mechanism. As in the upper limb, two superficial venous trunks have rich communication with the deep veins. The *small saphenous vein* begins along the lateral margin of the foot and courses upward along the posterior side of the leg; it ends in the popliteal vein. The *great saphenous vein* begins on the medial side of the foot and courses up the medial side of the leg, across the medial side of the knee, and upward to end in the femoral vein in the femoral triangle. Both are equipped with numerous valves.

GAIT

Normal *gait* consists of two phases: *stance phase* begins with heel-strike and ends with toe-off and, in terms of duration, constitutes two-thirds of the cycle of gait; *swing phase* begins with toe-off and ends with heel-strike, comprising one-third of the cycle. The duration of each phase is the same for both limbs, a circumstance, among others, that confers upon the normal gait an appearance of symmetry and rhythm. Abnormality of gait is usually a consequence of pain, weakness, or a difference in the lengths of the limbs.

Pain is a common cause of limp. Characteristic of such a limp is a shortened stance phase on the affected side. When the pain arises in the hip joint (coxalgia), there is also a lurch of the trunk toward the painful side during the stance phase. Moving the center of gravity of the body toward the painful hip decreases the moment arm of body weight to hip joint, reducing the total force on the hip.

A weak gluteus medius muscle allows the opposite side of the pelvis to tilt downward during stance on the weakened side. In an effort to compensate, the trunk lurches toward the weakened side *(abductor lurch)* during stance. This action moves the center of gravity nearer the fulcrum on the weak side, shortening the moment arm from the center of gravity to the hip joint and reducing the effort required of the abductors of the hip.

The gluteus maximus muscle begins to contract at the moment of heel-strike, slowing the forward motion of the trunk by arresting flexion of the hip and initiating extension. When the gluteus maximus is weak, the trunk lurches backward *(gluteus maximus lurch)* at heel-strike on the weakened side to interrupt the forward motion of the trunk.

When the quadriceps muscle is paralyzed, walking on a level surface may appear to be entirely normal. At a suitable speed the limb behaves as a pendulum, fully extending the knee joint preparatory to heel-strike. At full extension, action of the quadriceps is not necessary for stability of the knee joint; if the line of gravity is maintained anterior to the axis of motion of the knee joint, full extension persists through the stance phase. Such a patient, however, will be unable to run and may have difficulty walking on rough or inclined surfaces and stairs, because in those instances full extension is not attained and the knee tends to buckle into flexion. When this muscle is quite weak, a long leg brace may be needed to support the knee joint in full extension.

When the tendo calcaneus is divided or the gastrocnemius and soleus muscles paralyzed, ability to "push off" in the usual manner from the stance phase is lost. To compensate for this loss, extension of the hip by the gluteus maximus and the hamstring muscles is substituted. This is the disabling *calcaneus gait.*

A difference in the lengths of the limbs is termed *anisomelia.* A characteristic trait is lowering of the shoulder on the side of the shorter limb when that limb is in the stance phase. When the difference in lengths of the limbs is great, walking may be associated with a shift of the trunk to the short side during stance phase on that limb.

SELECTED REFERENCES

Daniels L et al: Muscle Testing Techniques of Manual Examination. Philadelphia, WB Saunders, 1952

Frankel V et al: The biomechanics of internal derangement of the knee. J Bone Joint Surg 53-A: 945, 1971

Grant JCB: An Atlas of Anatomy, 4th ed. Baltimore, Williams & Wilkins, 1958

Hollinshead WH: Anatomy for Surgeons, Vol 3. The Back and Limbs. New York, Hoeber Medical Division, Harper & Row, 1958

Kaufer H: Mechanical function of the patella. J Bone Joint Surg 53-A:1551, 1971

Last R J: Anatomy, Regional and Applied. Boston, Little, Brown & Co, 1954

Chapter 5

The Back

Charles W. Hooker

GOALS AND OBJECTIVES

Goals: To review the structure of the vertebral column as a whole; the structure of individual vertebrae at different levels; the structure of the intervertebral joints; the relationship of the spinal cord and spinal nerves to the vertebral column and to individual vertebrae; the blood supply of the column and of individual vertebrae; the relationship of structure to function of the vertebral column; and the organization of the muscles acting upon the vertebral column and their actions

Objectives: On completion of this unit, and using the text as a standard reference, one should be able to evaluate, describe, list, or recognize the following:

1. Representative individual vertebrae
2. Intervertebral joints and their ligaments
3. The spinal cord, meninges, and other contents of the vertebral canal
4. The manner of exit of spinal nerves and other spinal structures, their relationship to vertebral levels, and the significance of these relationships
5. The arterial supply and venous drainage of the vertebral column at the several levels
6. The relationship of structure to weight-bearing and movements
7. The groups of muscles acting on the vertebral column

OUTLINE

1. The vertebral column
   A. Structure of the vertebrae
   B. Intervertebral discs
   C. Spinal cord and meninges
   D. Joints and ligaments
   E. Blood supply

II. The muscles
   A. The splenius muscles
   B. The erector spinae
   C. The transversospinalis muscles
   D. The segmental muscles
   E. Innervation

III. Mechanical considerations
   A. Curvatures of the vertebral column
   B. Weight bearing
   C. Movements
   D. Actions of muscles

The bones, ligaments, muscles, and fasciae of the posterior portion of the trunk collectively constitute the back, an area of the first order of importance in support of body weight, in posture, and in locomotion.

THE VERTEBRAL COLUMN

The bones of the back are assembled to form the vertebral column, which serves as the axis of the body and, aided by its joints and muscles, is capable of both flexibility and rigidity. The head pivots on it; the limbs are attached to it; it transmits the weight of the body to the lower limbs; and it houses the spinal cord.

In the adult the vertebral column is typically composed of 33 osseous units, the *vertebrae*. Five vertebrae are fused to form the sacrum; 4 vertebrae usually comprise the coccyx, the first usually being separate and the succeeding three fused. The 24 remaining vertebrae persist as separate bones: 7 in the neck, 12 in the thoracic region, and 5 in the lumbar region. In keeping with their function of weight-bearing, the separate vertebrae become progressively larger, taller, and more massively constructed from above downward. Except between the first and second cervical vertebrae and in the sacrum and coccyx, the vertebrae are separated from each other by intervertebral discs that collectively account for roughly one fourth of the length of the vertebral column above the sacrum.

Structure of the Vertebrae

The vertebrae are constructed in accordance with a common plan; each consists of a body and an arch (Fig. 5-1). The body is the anterior and massive part of the vertebra, has the shape of a short cylinder, and is composed of spongy bone covered by a thin layer of compact bone. The arch projects posteriorly from the body and, together with the body, encloses the vertebral foramen through which passes the dural sac and the spinal cord or cauda equina, depending upon the level. The arch is composed of four portions, two pedicles and two laminae. Each pedicle projects posteriorly from the posterolateral surface of the vertebral body. From the posterior end of each pedicle, a lamina projects posteromedially to fuse with the other lamina.

From the area of fusion of the two laminae, the spinous process projects posteriorly. From the junction of pedicle with lamina on each side of the arch, a transverse process projects laterally. A superior articular process and an inferior articular process, projecting from the junction of pedicle and lamina on each side, provide for articulation of the vertebra with the vertebrae above and below. The pedicle has notches on its upper and lower borders. When the vertebrae are in place, these notches become portions of intervertebral foramina through which spinal nerves leave the vertebral canal.

Thoracic vertebrae (Fig. 5-1) have somewhat heart-shaped bodies, eight of them with two costal facets on each side, one along the upper and the other along the lower edge at the junction of the body with the arch. Each facet is in reality a demifacet that, together with a demifacet of the adjacent vertebra, forms a cup-shaped depression for articulation with the head of a rib. The 10th, 11th, and 12th vertebrae have single complete facets near the upper end of the body for artic-

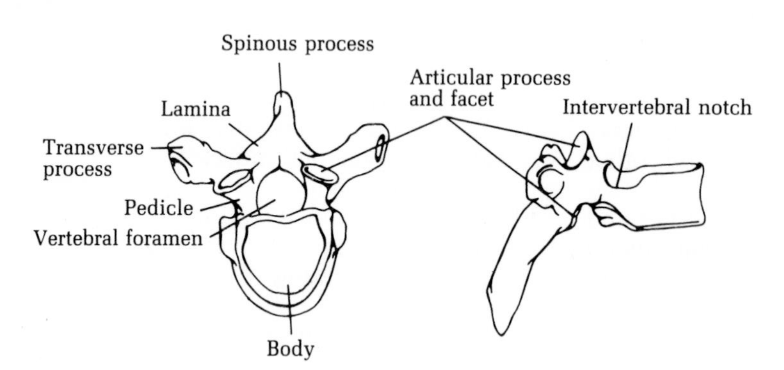

Fig. 5-1. A thoracic vertebra.

ulation with the head of the corresponding rib. The 1st vertebra has a complete facet near its upper end for the first rib, and a demifacet at its lower border that helps provide a facet for the second rib. The spinous processes of the 2nd to the 12th vertebrae are long and slope sharply downward; that of the 1st vertebra is particularly long and projects almost horizontally.

The laminae are broad and sloping and overlap like the shingles of a roof. The transverse processes extend posteriorly as well as laterally, and each ends in a clubbed extremity whose anterior surface has a small facet for articulation with the tubercle of the corresponding rib. The articular processes are thin, more or less triangular, and have flat articular surfaces somewhat oriented in a frontal plane. The superior articular facets face backward, upward, and medially; the inferior articular facets face forward and laterally. The movement most obviously permitted is lateral flexion (abduction and adduction).

Lumbar vertebrae (Fig. 5-2) have bodies that are somewhat kidney-shaped in cross section, with the concavity facing a triangular vertebral foramen; their heights are less than their horizontal diameters. The pedicles are relatively short and project from the upper half of the body. The laminae are thick and droop below the level of the pedicles but do not overlap. The spinous process is hatchet-shaped and projects horizontally, with its upper border well below the level of the upper end of the body, and its lower border at about the level of the upper end of the body of the next lower vertebra. Accordingly, there is an interval between the spinous processes and laminae of two adjacent vertebrae, through which an instrument can be passed into the vertebral canal. The transverse processes are long and thin, and they slant slightly backward and upward. The articular processes are heavy; in the main, the superior facets face almost medially and the inferior facets face almost laterally, placing the line of the interarticular joints in a nearly sagittal plane. The movement most obviously permitted is flexion and extension.

The region between the superior articular process and the remainder of the lamina is often called the pars interarticularis; failure of ossification in this area may be responsible for the condition known as *spondylolysis*. The superior articular processes of lumbar vertebrae and of the 12th thoracic vertebra have smooth, rounded enlargements on their posterior borders. These are the mammillary processes, to which are attached the larger slips of the multifidus muscle. It has been suggested that the mammillary process, the accessory process (a tubercle on the posterior side of the root of the transverse process), and the posterior part of the root of the transverse process together correspond to the transverse process of a thoracic vertebra, and that almost the entire transverse process of a lumbar vertebra is the homologue of a rib.

Cervical vertebrae (Fig. 5-3) form the most flexible portion of the vertebral column. In addition to their small size, these vertebrae are characterized by large vertebral foramina (providing for the cervical enlargement of the spinal cord), and by the presence of foramina in the transverse processes; the upper six of these transmit the vertebral artery, an important conduit for arterial blood to the brain. Their other attributes make provision for mobility and provide attachments for the muscles that provoke movement and confer

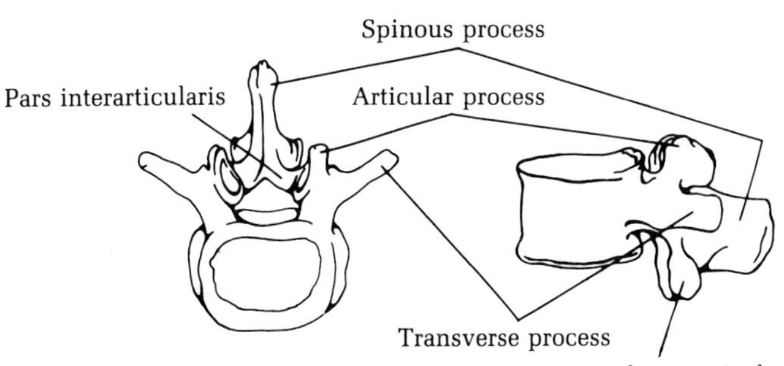

Fig. 5-2. A lumbar vertebra.

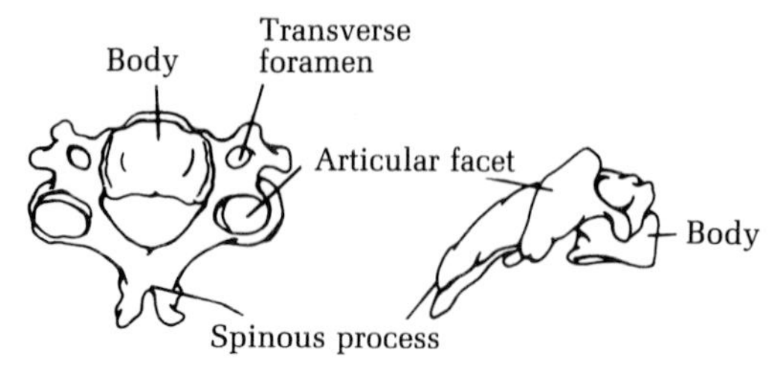

Fig. 5-3. A typical cervical vertebra.

stability. For the most part, the upper surfaces of the bodies are concave from side to side, and have lips that project upward to overlap the lateral portions of the inferior surface of the vertebra above. The lower surfaces of the bodies are convex from side to side, with the lateral portions beveled. The pedicles are short and rounded, and their projecting laterally as well as posteriorly contributes to the width of the vertebral foramen.

The laminae are relatively thinner, longer, and narrower from above downward than in other vertebrae. The spinous process is short and bifid to provide attachment for muscles, and it overlaps the spinous process below. The transverse processes are short, and each has two roots: the anterior root corresponds to a rib, and the posterior root corresponds to a true transverse process. Near their ends, the two roots are united by a bar of bone that completes the enclosure of the transverse foramen and is grooved on its upper surface to accommodate an emerging spinal nerve. The nerve lies posterior to the vertebral artery. Each root ends in a rounded tubercle for the attachment of muscles.

At the union of pedicle and lamina, the bone is much thickened as an articular mass forming a rounded pillar behind the transverse process. The upper and lower parts of the articular mass form the articular processes; their surfaces are sloping and nearly flat. The upper pair face backward and upward; the lower pair face forward and downward, the orientation of the joint approaching a nearly horizontal plane. Considerable movement in several directions is thus permitted.

The first and second cervical vertebrae are different in several respects from the other cervical vertebrae; the differences are related to articulation with the skull and to movements of the head. The first vertebra (the atlas), having lost much of its body, is essentially an oval ring of bone that also lacks a spinous process (Fig. 5-4). The lateral portions of the ring are thickened, and a transverse process longer than those of other cervical vertebrae projects from each portion. The upper surface of each lateral mass articulates with an occipital condyle. The articular surface, or fovea, is concave, kidney shaped, and faces medially, anteriorly, and upward. The movement permitted here is a "rocking" of the occipital condyle in the concave articular mass, as in nodding the head. The lower surface of each lateral mass is an articular surface that is almost flat and faces inferiorly, anteriorly, and slightly medially.

The second cervical vertebra (the axis) is distinguished by a heavy, toothlike protuberance projecting upward from the body (the dens; Fig. 5-5). The laminae are thick, and the spinous process is heavy and long compared with those of other cervical vertebrae. The articular processes arise from the body and pedicles rather than at the junction of pedicle and lamina. The superior articular facets are large, nearly flat, and face upward, posteriorly, and laterally. The dens provides a pivot on which the head and atlas can rotate, using the flat articular facets. The inferior articular facets are similar to those of other vertebrae.

The seventh vertebra is different from other cervical vertebrae, having a longer spinous process that often is not bifid. This vertebra usually has small transverse foramina that rarely transmit the vertebral arteries. As a variation, the usually small costal root of the transverse process sometimes becomes a cervical rib, more often on the right side than on the left.

The *sacrum* (Fig. 5-6), consisting of five fused vertebrae, is broadened by incorpora-

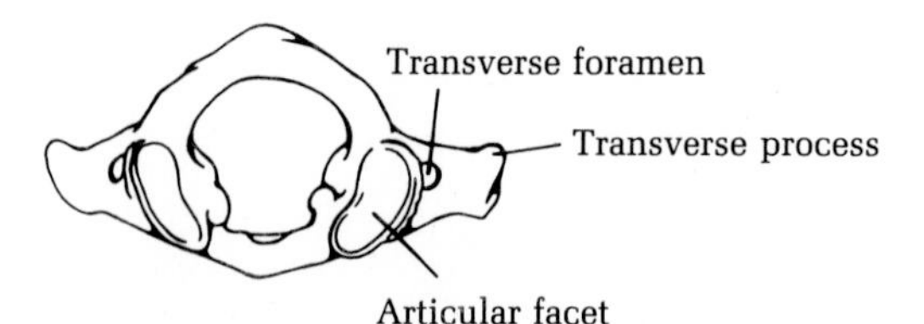

Fig. 5-4. The first cervical vertebra.

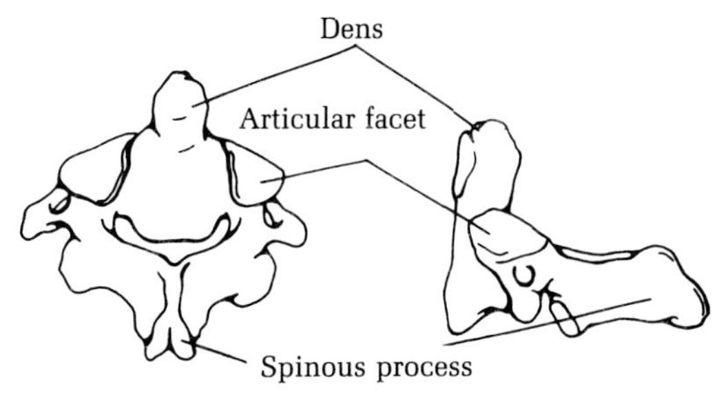

Fig. 5-5. The second cervical vertebra.

tion of large costal elements and transverse processes into a heavy pars lateralis on each side. It is triangular in shape, with the base upward when viewed from in front or behind; it is concave and fairly smooth on its pelvic surface, and convex and irregular on its dorsal surface. The pelvic surface has four transverse ridges marking the lines of fusion of the vertebrae. At the ends of the ridges are large pelvic sacral foramina through which the ventral rami of sacral nerves emerge. Extending laterally from the pelvic sacral foramina are conspicuous, converging grooves for these nerves.

On the dorsal surface, four spinous processes are more or less united to form the median sacral crest. About an inch lateral to the sacral crest are four dorsal sacral foramina, through which emerge the dorsal rami of sacral nerves. Just medial to the dorsal foramina is the intermediate sacral crest, a series of tubercles representing fused articular processes. Lateral to the sacral foramina are the lateral sacral crests representing transverse processes. The sacral canal is roofed by fused laminae, except for the fifth and sometimes the fourth vertebrae, where the laminae sometimes fail to meet, producing the sacral hiatus, an inferior entrance to the vertebral canal. The bone forming the lateral walls of the sacral hiatus ends above the apex of the sacrum as two sacral cornua.

The upper end of the sacrum, the base of the triangle, is directed forward and upward. In the middle is the upper surface of the body of the first sacral vertebra; its anterior border forms the sacral promontory. Behind the body is the large vertebral foramen leading into the sacral canal. The superior articular processes of the sacrum are supported by short heavy pedicles. The articular facets face medially and posteriorly.

The sacrum is situated between the two hip bones; the upper, wider part of the pars lateralis articulates with the ilium on each side. The sacrum is wider dorsally than ventrally; the weight of the body in forcing the sacrum down and forward wedges it between the two ilia.

The *coccyx* consists essentially of four fused vertebral bodies. As vertebrae they are rudimentary, possessing no laminae and few processes. The first, and much the largest, segment articulates with the apex of the sacrum. Projecting upward from its dorsal surface are paired cornua representing pedicles and superior articular processes; the first

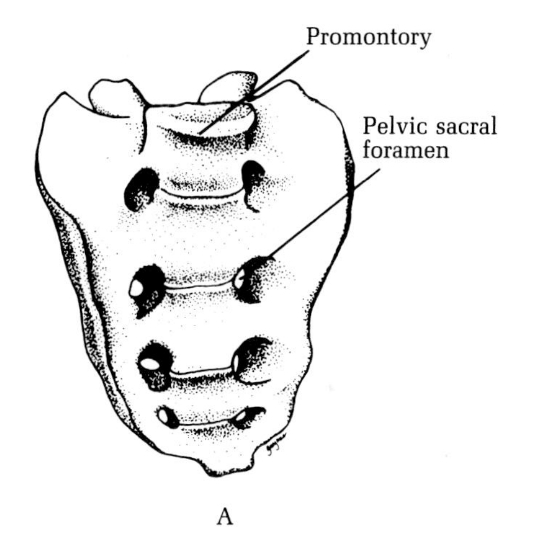

A

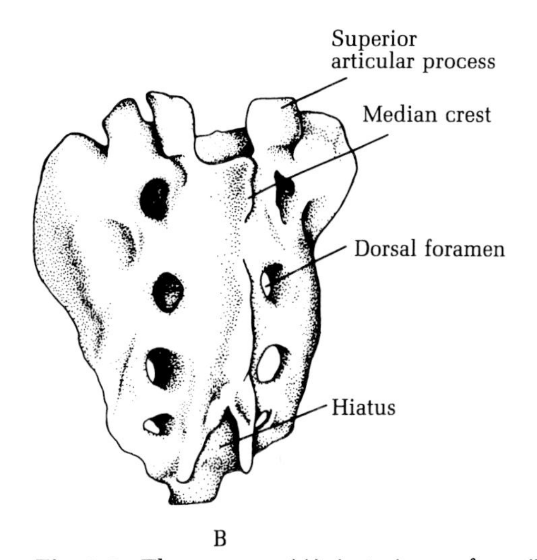

B

Fig. 5-6. The sacrum. (*A*) Anterior surface. (*B*) Posterior surface.

segment also has short transverse processes. Usually a fibrocartilaginous disc between the first and second segments permits movement at this joint. In advanced age, the mass may be fused to the sacrum.

Intervertebral Discs

From the lower surface of the second cervical vertebra through the junction between the lowest vertebra and the sacrum, the vertebral bodies have interposed between them intervertebral discs. In the cervical region, the discs are thicker anteriorly than posteriorly, a circumstance contributing to the usual cervical curvature. Their transverse diameter is slightly less than that of their associated vertebral bodies; consequently, the lower edge of one vertebra almost overlaps the upper edge of the next, especially posterolaterally. In the thoracic region, each disc is almost uniform in height, and thoracic curvature is due primarily to shapes of the vertebral bodies. The discs in the lower thoracic region are distinctly thicker than those in the upper region, a circumstance that could account for the greater mobility of the lower thoracic vertebral column. In the lumbar region, the discs are thicker anteriorly than posteriorly, maximally so in the fifth disc, which contributes much to the lumbosacral angle. The normal curvature of the lumbar column is due in part to the uneven thickness of discs, and in part to the shapes of the vertebral bodies.

Each intervertebral disc consists of two portions, the anulus fibrosus and the nucleus pulposus. The anulus fibrosus makes up the peripheral portion and is composed of fibrocartilage. The fibers of the anulus run obliquely between the vertebrae and are arranged primarily in concentric layers. The direction of the fibers in successive layers alternates, and the fibers of one layer cross those of adjacent layers at an angle between 30° and 60°, depending upon circumstances. Some of the peripheral fibers extend past the edge of the cartilage on the end of the vertebra to enter the bone of the body as Sharpey's fibers; the deeper fibers insert into the cartilage at each end of the disc. The anulus also blends with the nucleus pulposus. The anulus is wider anteriorly than posteriorly (*i.e.*, the nucleus pulposus is situated eccentrically).

The nucleus pulposus consists of a network of delicate collagenous fibers in a mucoprotein gel rich in polysaccharide. The nucleus has a high water content, apparently the result of imbibition by the gel. The water content declines with advancing age and is reduced by pressure borne by the disc, accounting for loss in the height of a person during an active day.

It is reported that, beginning during the later part of the third decade, there is gradual loss of fluid and concomitant fibrous replacement of the nucleus, so that by the sixth or seventh decade the nucleus has become fibrocartilage. Paralleling these changes in the nucleus, the anulus often shows coarsened and hyalinized fibers and fissuring of the lamellae.

A common problem involving the intervertebral disc is its protrusion or herniation, most often in the lumbar or cervical regions where motion and stress are greatest. This condition may involve a simple bulging of the disc or complete herniation of a portion of the nucleus pulposus through the anulus fibrosus. The protrusion is usually posterolateral into the vertebral canal, where it may compress the spinal cord or interfere with its blood supply (above the second lumbar vertebra); much more often, it may compress the roots of a spinal nerve (Fig. 5-7).

Spinal Cord and Meninges

When the vertebrae and intervertebral discs are assembled to form a vertebral column, the several vertebral foramina together become the vertebral canal, continuous from the foramen magnum through the sacral canal; the intervertebral notches become the intervertebral foramina.

The vertebral canal houses the spinal cord and its meningeal coverings. The medulla oblongata becomes continuous with the spinal cord at the foramen magnum, and the spinal cord usually ends inferiorly at the level of the first or second lumbar vertebra. From the tapered inferior end of the spinal cord, a cord of tissue, the filum terminale, continues inferiorly to merge with the periosteum on the dorsum of the coccyx as the coccygeal ligament.

Unlike the arrangement in the cranial cavity, the spinal dura is separated from the inner surface of the bones forming the ver-

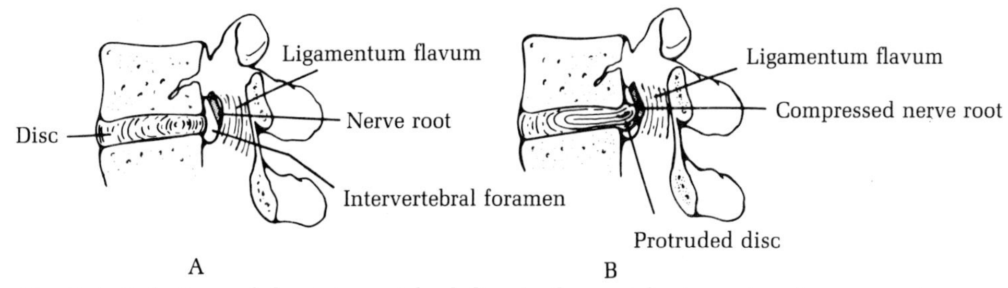

Fig. 5-7. Relations of the intervertebral disc to the vertebral canal and an emerging nerve in a hemisected lumbar vertebral column. (*A*) Normal relations. (*B*) The disc is protruded.

tebral canal by an epidural space containing fat and a rich plexus of veins. The dural sac continues inferiorly to about the middle of the second sacral vertebra. The pia mater is closely attached to the spinal cord, and the subarachnoid space, containing cerebrospinal fluid, is the space between it and the arachnoid which lies on the inner surface of the dura.

The *spinal nerves* leave the vertebral canal through the intervertebral foramina. Each nerve is formed by the union of a dorsal root and a ventral root, usually at the intervertebral foramen. The subarachnoid space is prolonged in a duralarachnoid sheath around each dorsal and ventral root, roughly to the level of union of the roots. Because the cord is shorter than the vertebral column, the nerves slope inferiorly from their levels of origin to the appropriate intervertebral foramina, and the angle becomes more acute from above downward. Below the inferior end of the cord, the duralarachnoid sac contains a leash of nerve roots and the filum terminale. This complex constitutes the cauda equina.

Except in the cervical region, spinal nerves are numbered relative to the vertebra *below* which they emerge; thus, the fifth thoracic nerve emerges through the intervertebral foramen below the fifth thoracic vertebra. Because there are eight pairs of cervical nerves and seven cervical vertebrae, cervical nerves are numbered according to the vertebra *above* which they emerge, the third cervical nerve emerging *above* the third vertebra. The eighth cervical nerve emerges between the seventh cervical and first thoracic vertebrae.

Because the spinal cord is shorter than the vertebral column, the level of emergence of a spinal nerve is below the level of the segment of the spinal cord from which it arises; the difference in these levels becomes greater from above downward. As a rule of thumb, the spinous process of the first lumbar vertebra overlies the five sacral segments of the spinal cord, and the spinous processes of the 11th and 12th thoracic vertebrae overlie the five lumbar segments. Between the 2nd cervical and 10th thoracic vertebrae, the number of the cord segment is the number of the spinous process, plus two. Thus, the spine of the 6th thoracic vertebra overlies the 8th thoracic segment of the spinal cord.

These generalizations concerning the emergence of spinal nerves are significant practically, as illustrated by the identity of the nerve root compressed by a protruded intervertebral disc. Because cervical nerves are numbered according to the vertebra *above* which they emerge, protrusion of the disc between the fifth and sixth cervical vertebrae would compress the roots of the sixth cervical nerve. Since the thoracic nerves are numbered according to the vertebra *below* which they emerge, protrusion of the disc between the fifth and sixth thoracic vertebrae would compress the roots of the fifth thoracic nerve.

The presence of the cauda equina and its many nerve roots below the second lumbar vertebra presents a different problem: although massive protrusion of a lumbar disc may compress much of the cauda equina, it is much more usual for only one or, less often, two nerves to be affected. The intervertebral foramina in the lumbar region are much larger than the lumbar nerves; each nerve emerges through the upper part of the foramen and lies against the body of the vertebra above (Fig. 5-7). Accordingly, protrusion of a lumbar disc would not be expected to affect the nerve corresponding in number to that disc; that nerve emerges above the disc. Instead, the protruded disc usually compresses the next lower nerve as that nerve crosses the level of the disc in its path to its foramen. As an example, protrusion of the fifth lumbar disc usually affects the first sacral nerve; it rarely affects the fifth lumbar nerve.

Joints and Ligaments

If a joint is taken to be the joining together of two bones, the vertebrae are related to each other by joints between body and body, between articular process and articular process, between lamina and lamina, and between spinous process and spinous process (Fig. 5-8).

The joints between adjacent bodies are symphyses, similar in principle to the symphysis pubis, with the intervertebral disc being the uniting fibrocartilage. The bodies of the vertebrae are bound together by two ligaments in addition to the intervertebral disc. The *anterior longitudinal ligament* is a broad collection of fibers extending along the anterior surfaces of the bodies. It begins above in a pointed attachment to the anterior tubercle of the atlas, and widens as it descends to end on the pelvic surface of the sacrum. The superficial fibers are long, but the deeper fibers extend over only one or two vertebrae. The *posterior longitudinal ligament* is in the vertebral canal on the posterior surfaces of the bodies. It is wider at its superior end and attaches to the occipital bone; its narrow lower end lies in the anterior wall of the sacral canal and continues into the ligamentous tissue on the dorsum of the lower coccyx. In thoracic and lumbar levels it has serrate margins, being broad over intervertebral discs and narrow over the vertebral bodies. The lateral extensions over the discs are much thinner than the central part of the ligament, a circumstance that may account for the fact that most protrusions of intervertebral discs are posterolateral rather than midline. The deeper fibers of this ligament attach to each vertebra, and its superficial fibers span three or four vertebrae.

Joints between articular processes are synovial joints surrounded by thin and somewhat lax articular capsules.

Joints between laminae are formed by the *ligamenta flava,* heavy bands composed primarily of elastic fibers connecting the laminae of adjacent vertebrae. Each is attached above to the front of the lower border of lamina and below to the back of the upper border of the succeeding lamina. They extend laterally as far as the articular capsules. Ligaments of each pair meet at the root of the spinous process, except for a slit in the midline for the passage of veins.

Joints between spinous processes are formed by the supraspinous ligament and the interspinous ligaments. The *supraspinous ligament* is a bundle of fibers running over the tips of the spinous processes, shorter fibers connecting adjacent spines and longer fibers connecting several in succession. According to some accounts, this ligament extends downward from the spine of the seventh cervical vertebra to the lumbar vertebrae. In the neck, the ligamentum nuchae is considered to be the equivalent of the supraspinous ligament. *Interspinous ligaments* are thin bands joining adjacent spinous processes. They occupy a position between the supraspinous ligament and the ligamenta flava. They are longer and stronger in the lumbar region, and may be relatively insignificant in the cervical region.

Intertransverse ligaments occur in the thoracic region, but they appear to have little significance.

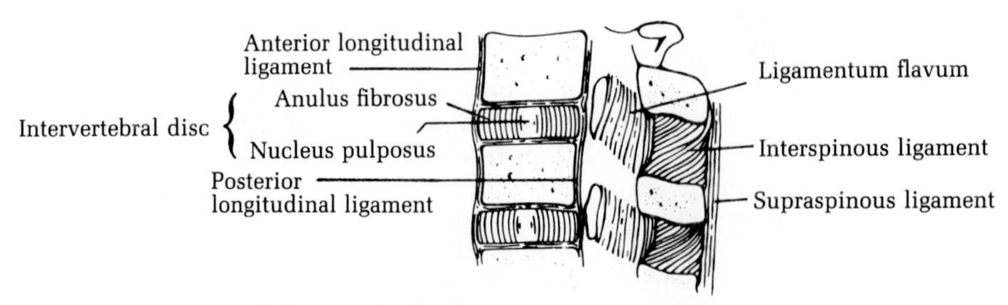

Fig. 5-8. Ligaments of the vertebral column.

Blood Supply

Blood is supplied to the vertebral column by way of segmental arteries that arise near it from the aorta, or from adjacent arteries in areas beyond the extent of the aorta. Thus, the sources are the vertebral and ascending cervical arteries in the neck; costocervical and intercostal arteries in the thorax; lumbar and iliolumbar arteries in the lumbar region; and lateral sacral arteries in the pelvis.

Typically, a segmental artery gives off branches to the body of a vertebra as it courses backward along the lateral surface of that body (Fig. 5-9). The segmental artery divides near an intervertebral foramen into a lateral branch, which constitutes its ventral continuation, and a spinal branch. The spinal branch enters the intervertebral foramen, where it divides into three terminal branches: dorsal, intermediate, and ventral. The dorsal branch helps supply the dura and the tissue in the epidural space, and anastomoses with similar branches above and below form small longitudinal arteries. The chief distribution of each dorsal branch is to a lateral half of the vertebral arch. The intermediate branch supplies the dura of the regional nerve roots. Additionally, this branch has a radicular branch that, when sufficiently large, contributes significantly to the arterial supply of the spinal cord.

The ventral branch divides into ascending and descending terminal vessels that course obliquely upward or downward toward the midlines of the two adjacent vertebrae. A portion of their course is between the posterior longitudinal ligament and the posterior surface of vertebral bodies, where they enter the vertebral body toward its middle. In the adult, the arteries in a vertebral body do not reach the disc; in the child, they penetrate the cartilage on the ends of the bodies to supply the discs.

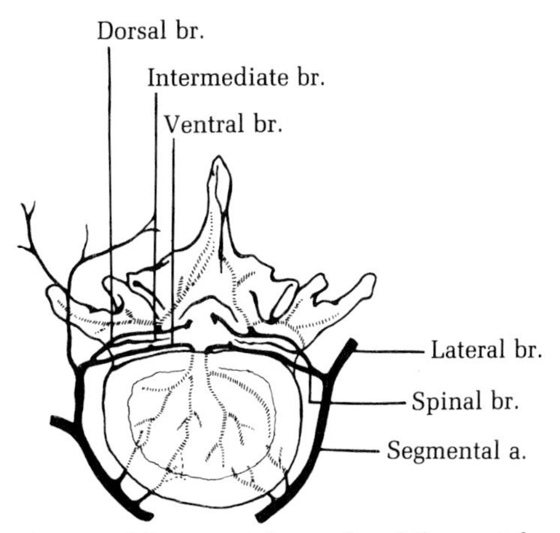

Fig. 5-9. The arterial supply of the vertebra.

The *veins* of the vertebral column make up rich plexuses that extend the length of the column, both inside and outside the vertebral canal. These veins communicate freely with the veins of the body wall, and have relatively few valves. Accordingly, they may provide collateral circulation in obstruction of the inferior vena cava as well as a pathway for dissemination of tumors in the pelvis to the vertebral column and cranium.

THE MUSCLES

The muscles of the back are arranged in three functional layers. Those of the superficial group are directly related to the upper limb. The intermediate layer is made up of two muscles of respiration, the serratus posterior superior and the serratus posterior inferior. The third group, the muscles of the vertebral column, is covered by the thoracolumbar fascia and consists of many muscles, in the main oriented longitudinally. These muscles occupy parasaggital gutters whose medial walls are the spinous processes of the vertebrae and whose lateral walls are, from below upward, the angles of the ribs, the ends of the transverse processes of cervical vertebrae, and the mastoid processes of the temporal bones. Their position suggests that the muscles of this group are for the most part extensors and lateral flexors of the vertebral column, and that they should also be stabilizers of the vertebral column. The group may be subdivided into several fairly distinct subgroups of muscles on the basis of origin and insertion, length, and direction.

The *splenius muscles* occupy the most superficial plane, originate in the midline, and run upward and laterally to their insertions. The splenius capitis is a flat muscle that arises from the lower half of the ligamentum nuchae and the spinous processes of the seventh cervical and upper three or four thoracic vertebrae; it inserts on the occipital bone and mastoid process of the temporal bone. The splenius cervicis is narrower; it arises from the spinous processes of about the third to the sixth thoracic vertebrae and runs upward and laterally to insert on the transverse processes of the upper two to four cervical vertebrae. These muscles extend the neck and head and, acting unilaterally, turn the face to that side in cooperation with the sternocleidomastoid muscle of the other side.

The *erector spinae* is the bulkiest and, except for the splenii, the most superficial subgroup of these muscles. It may be considered to arise as a single muscle from the dorsum of the sacrum and the adjacent portion of the iliac crest. As it ascends along the vertebral column, this muscle subdivides into three parallel columns of muscle: the *iliocostalis muscle* laterally, the *spinalis muscle* medially, and the *longissimus muscle* in an intermediate location. The iliocostalis inserts on the angles of the lower six or seven ribs, then, by overlapping relays of bundles of muscle, reaches the ends of the transverse processes of cervical vertebrae. The longissimus inserts on the ends of the transverse processes of the lower nine or more thoracic vertebrae and the ribs associated with them, then by relays of muscle to cervical trans-

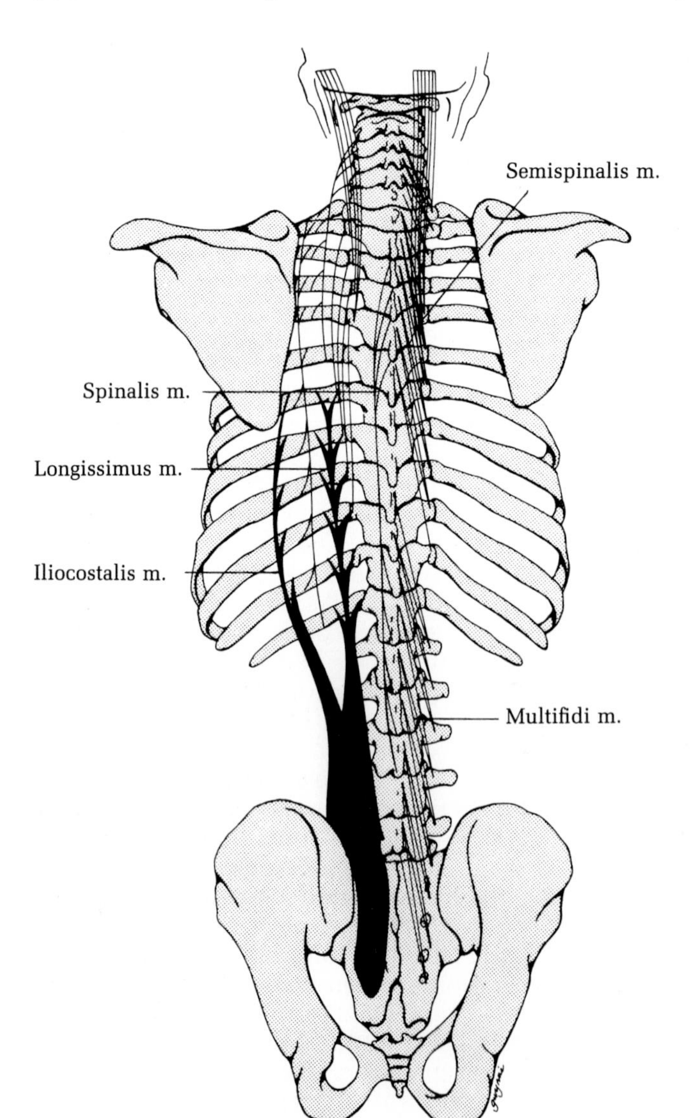

Fig. 5-10. The major deep muscles of the back. *Left:* The erector spinae. *Right:* The multifidi and semispinalis muscles.

verse processes, and finally to the mastoid process. The spinalis is often confined to the thoracic region, where it attaches below and above to spinous processes.

This group acting as a unit serves as an extensor of the vertebral column when acting bilaterally; acting unilaterally, the group acts as a lateral flexor. The action of small units of this group provokes the same movements in a local portion of the vertebral column. The *transversospinalis muscles* are deep to the erector spinae. This group consists of great numbers of small muscles whose fibers slant obliquely upward from transverse processes to spinous processes, and have a shorter span than the erector spinae. The most superficial layer of this group is the *semispinalis*, whose bundles span some three to six vertebrae. Its bundles do not extend below the thoracic region, and its upper fibers reach the occipital bone. More deeply situated are the *multifidus muscles* that span two to four vertebrae from the sacrum to the first cervical vertebra. Still more deeply situated and shorter are the *long and short rotator muscles*. Both arise from transverse processes; the short rotators extend to the spinous process of the next higher vertebra, and the long rotators extend to the spinous process of the second higher vertebra. The muscles of this group are extensors and lateral flexors of the vertebral column and, in addition, are rotators of the vertebral column. In all three actions, the span of movement is determined by the members of the group actively contracting (Fig. 5-10).

The *segmental muscles* are short muscles extending vertically from one vertebra to the next. The *interspinales* are paired muscles extending along the sides of the interspinous ligament from a spinous process to the next spinous process above. Six such pairs are present in the cervical region from the axis to the first thoracic vertebra. They are often absent in the thoracic region, but are well developed in the lumbar region. The *intertransversarii* are paired medial and lateral muscles between adjacent transverse processes in the cervical and lumbar regions, but are often absent in the thoracic region.

Belonging to none of these groups, the *levatores costarum* must be mentioned. Twelve short levatores costarum arise from transverse processes of the 7th cervical and upper 11 thoracic vertebrae, and insert on the rib below just medial to the angle. Long levatores costarum arise from transverse processes of usually the 7th to the 10th vertebrae and insert, along with the short levatores, on the 2nd rib below.

Innervation. All of the deep muscles of the back, with the possible exception of the lateral transversarii of the lumbar region, are supplied by primary dorsal rami of spinal nerves. Except in the first two cervical nerves, the primary dorsal rami divide into lateral and medial branches. In general, both branches run obliquely downward to supply muscles at their level of emergence and a segment or two below. The medial branches supply the more medial muscles and the lateral branches supply the lateral musculature. The lower multifidi are supplied by medial branches of the dorsal rami of the first three sacral nerves and by small branches from the posterior sacral plexus. The fourth and fifth sacral nerves usually do not innervate any muscle.

MECHANICAL CONSIDERATIONS

Only a few of the more obvious mechanical considerations can be mentioned here.

Curvatures of the Vertebral Column. In the early months of the fetus, the vertebral column has the shape of a C with the convexity backward (kyphosis). At birth, the cervical curve has begun to reverse itself and the lumbar portion has become nearly straight, but the thoracic and sacral portions have retained much of their earlier curvatures. When the infant begins to hold up its head, a cervical curvature with its convexity forward (lordosis) develops, presumably a result of the pull of muscles, and provides for a better balance for the head. When the child begins to stand and walk, an anterior convexity of the lumbar column develops, allowing balance of the body upon the sacrum.

Weight-bearing and the pull of muscles are factors of significance in establishing adult curvatures, but the intervertebral discs are also important by reason of their compressibility. Moreover, the shapes of both the discs and the vertebral bodies serve to preserve the curvatures. The curvatures contribute much to the ability of the vertebral column to withstand and absorb shock, such as that delivered by a jump from a height, or the jolts of ordinary walking. The compressible discs also serve as shock absorbers. As a consequence of anterior compression of osteoporotic vertebral bodies by weight-bearing forces, the vertebral column in the elderly may assume a C shape resembling that of the fetus.

Weight-Bearing. The most obvious adaptation to weight-bearing is the progressive increase in massiveness of the vertebrae from above downward, as the weight borne by each vertebra is greater than that of the one above it. The line of gravity along which the weight of the body is projected to the lower limbs is considered to pass in succession through the dens of the axis, the bodies of the 2nd and 12th thoracic vertebrae, and the promontory of the sacrum.

Movements. A consideration of movements of the back is complicated by the fact that the mechanisms employed in movement are also used to produce stability, a problem of no less significance. This circumstance is shared by many other joints but is magnified in the back by a succession of joints. Much of the information regarding movement has been obtained by roentgenographic studies.

The range of movement between any two successive vertebrae is slight, but the sum total of these movements is of considerable magnitude in the vertebral column as a whole. Flexion, extension, lateral flexion, and rotation occur at the interarticular joints, and the orientation of these joints is a factor in the magnitude of these movements. By virtue of their sagittal orientation, the joints between the upper lumbar vertebrae are best adapted to flexion and extension. In the thoracic region, the orientation of these joints in a frontal plane permits only limited flexion and extension. The roughly horizontal orientation of the joints in the cervical region leads to free extension and flexion, accomplished by a sliding and rocking motion of the joint surfaces on one another.

Rotation is a rather more complex movement, and is accomplished by sliding movements in these joints in the cervical and thoracic regions; in the lumbar region rotation is restricted. Provision for lateral flexion is best in the frontally oriented synovial joints of thoracic vertebrae, somewhat less favorable in the horizontally oriented joints of cervical vertebrae, and least favorable in the sagittally oriented lumbar joints. In the cervical and thoracic regions, lateral flexion is accompanied by some degree of rotation, and rotation is associated with some degree of lateral flexion.

A factor of significance in the range of mobility at the synovial joints is the laxness of the capsular ligaments, permitting excursions that would be restricted by taut ligaments. The thinness of these ligaments also constitutes a hazard.

Because of their compressibility, the intervertebral discs are factors in the degree of extension, flexion, and lateral flexion. Their relative thickness in the cervical region allows fairly extensive movements; their relative thinness in the thoracic region restricts these movements; and their thickness in the lumbar region allows such movements to occur fairly freely.

Several structural entities clearly serve to restrain movements. Each of the ligaments located posterior to the centers of vertebrae acts as a check ligament in flexion. The posterior longitudinal ligament, ligamenta flava, the supraspinous ligament, the interspinous ligaments, and the ligamentum nuchae replacing the supraspinous ligament in the neck are such ligaments. The presence of elastic fibers in the ligamenta flava and in the ligamentum nuchae presumably snub flexion gradually rather than abruptly. The ribs and sternum limit flexion of the trunk. Extension is restrained by the anterior longitudinal ligament and limited by the spinous processes of vertebrae. Lateral flexion is restricted by ligaments on the side opposite the direction of the flexion, by transverse processes, and, in the thoracic region, by the ribs and sternum. Rotation is limited by intervertebral ligaments and by intervertebral discs, a significant consideration here probably being the obliquity of the laminae of the anulus fibrosus. All the restraining ligaments are obviously subject to injury if excessively stressed, especially when the forces act perpendicularly to the direction of the fibers in the ligament (shear).

Actions of Muscles. The erector spinae are extensors of the vertebral column. Flexion is produced by contractions of muscles anterior to the vertebral column—psoas major, rectus abdominis, external oblique, internal oblique, sternocleidomastoid, scaleni, and probably the longus colli and longus cervicis muscles. Lateral flexion is produced by unilateral contraction of the erector spinae and transversospinales, aided by unilateral contraction of the psoas major, quadratus lumborum, external and internal obliques, scaleni, sternocleidomastoid, and other flexor muscles. Rotation is produced by unilateral action of transversospinales, external or internal oblique (depending upon the direction of rotation), splenii, and sternocleidomastoid. Stability results from simultaneous contractions of extensors and flexors, bilateral contraction of lateral flexors, and bilateral contraction of rotators.

Electromyographic study of the erector spinae indicates that these muscles are quiet when the subject is standing or sitting erect; that the muscles are active during partial flexion of the back, possibly exerting some regulation of this movement; and that they are quiet when the back is fully flexed.

The erector spinae also contribute to limitation or prevention of tilting of the pelvis when the weight is borne by the contralateral foot in standing and walking. In this action, the erector spinae are assisted by the gluteus medius on the weight-bearing side.

It should also be noted that extension of the trunk involves the hamstring muscles and the gluteus maximus in addition to the erector spinae.

SELECTED REFERENCES

Basmajian JV: Muscles Alive: Their Functions Revealed by Electromyography. Baltimore, Williams & Wilkins, 1962

Batson OV: The function of the vertebral veins and their role in the spread of metastases. Ann Surg *112*:138, 1940

Bick EM, Copel JW: The senescent human vertebra: Contributions to human osteogeny. J bone Joint Surg *34-A*:110, 1952

Coventry MB et al: The intervertebral disc: Its microscopic anatomy and pathology. Part II. Changes in the intervertebral disc concomitant with age. J Bone Joint Surg *27*:233, 1945

Davis PR et al: Movements of the thoracic and lumbar spine when lifting: A chronocyclophotographic study. J Anat *99*:13, 1965

Fielding JW: Normal and selected abnormal motion of the cervical spine from the second cervical vertebra to the seventh cervical vertebra based on cineroentgenography. J Bone Joint Surg *46-A*:1779, 1964

Gregerson GG, Lucas DB: An *in vivo* study of the axial rotation of the human thoracolumbar spine. J Bone Joint Surg *49-A*:247, 1967

Harris RS, Jones DM: The arterial supply to the adult cervical vertebral bodies. J Bone Joint Surg *38-B*:922, 1956

Hohl M: Normal motions in the upper portion of the cervical spine. J Bone Joint Surg *46-A*:1777, 1964

Hollinshead WH: Anatomy for Surgeons, Vol 3, pp. 79–206. New York, Harper & Row, 1969

Horton WG: Further observations on the elastic mechanism of the intervertebral disc. J Bone Joint Surg *40-B*:552, 1958

Miles M, Sullivan WE: Lateral bending at the lumbar and lumbosacral joints. Anat Rec *139*:387, 1961

Mitchell GAG: The lumbosacral junction. J Bone Joint Surg *16*:233, 1934

Morris JM et al: An electromyographic study of the intrinsic muscles of the back in man. J Anat *96*:509, 1962

Morris JM et al: Role of the trunk in stability of the spine. J Bone Surg *43-A*:327, 1961

Pauly JE: An electromyographic analysis of certain movements and exercises. I. Some deep muscles of the back. Anat Rec *155*:233, 1966

Peacock A: Observations on the postnatal structure of the intervertebral disc in man. J Anat *86*:162, 1952

Sub TH, Alexander L: Vascular system of the human spinal cord. Archives of Neurology and Psychiatry *41*:569, 1939

Willis TA: Nutrient arteries of the vertebral bodies. J Bone Joint Surg *31-A*:538, 1949

Part 3

BASIC PROCESSES IN BONE

Chapter 6

Histology and Growth of Bone

H. Robert Brashear
and Carole J. VanderWiel

GOALS AND OBJECTIVES

Goals: To familiarize the reader with the gross and microscopic structure of bone and how it attains its adult configuration; to relate the gross and microscopic structure of bone to its mechanical function; and to consider the mechanisms by which the shape of bone is altered in response to a change in function

Objectives: On completion of this unit, and using the text as a standard reference, one should be able to evaluate, describe, list, or identify the following:

1. Four functions of bone
2. Haversian systems, lamellar bone, cancellous bone, and immature bone
3. Two methods of formation of Haversian systems
4. The histologic properties and significance of immature bone
5. The processes by which bone grows and remodels and the importance of these mechanisms
6. Changes in the epiphyseal plate caused by rickets
7. The meaning of Wolff's law and an example of this law in action

OUTLINE

I. Gross structure
   A. Relationship of structure to function
   B. Types of bones
   C. Structure of long bones
II. Microscopic structure
   A. Haversian systems
   B. Lamellar bone
   C. Immature bone
   D. Osteocytes, lacunae, canaliculi
III. Cancellous bone
   A. Structure
   B. Location
IV. Circumferential growth
V. Longitudinal growth
   A. Mechanisms
   B. Epiphyseal plate
   C. Enchondral ossification

VI. Development of bone from a cartilage model
   A. Prenatal development
      1. Periosteal shell
      2. Primary ossification center
      3. Epiphyseal ossification centers
   B. Postnatal development
      1. Growth of the ossification center
      2. Epiphyseal plate
      3. Disturbances of the epiphyseal plate
         a. Injury
         b. Rickets
         c. Pituitary dwarfism
   C. Remodeling of bone

Bone is a living tissue characterized physically by hardness and rigidity of structure, and microscopically by a high ratio of extracellular substance to a relatively sparse cell population. The extracellular material or bone matrix consists of an inorganic portion, crystals of hydroxyapatite, and an organic part that is largely collagen. Thus, the extracellular part of bone is a two-phase system that might be compared to reinforced concrete, the collagen fibrils representing the steel rods, and the calcium phosphate crystals the cement. Entrapped within this hard tissue are small living cells, the *osteocytes*, whose only communication with the outside world is by means of thin cellular processes that lie in minute tubules, the *canaliculi*.

Bone has several functions. The most obvious is its mechanical function as a rigid supporting structure for the origin and insertion of muscles, and a lever arm through which muscles can act. Without this rigid tissue, our movements would be like those of the jellyfish. A second important function of bone is as a storehouse for minerals, particularly calcium and phosphorus. The tremendous surface area of bone makes available a vast supply of minerals whenever the body is in need of them. The mechanisms by which these minerals are made available to other tissues of the body are discussed in subsequent sections. A third role of bone is its function as a storehouse of the marrow elements for the formation of new blood cells. Bone also serves as a protective covering for the nervous system and other vital organs. It is the mechanical function of bone that will be emphasized at this time.

GROSS STRUCTURE

The gross structure of bone is very closely related to its function (Fig. 6-1). Its strength is greatest where greatest stress is applied. It is angulated or presents external prominences where such deviations from symmetry can best serve muscle function. There are three general categories of bone: *flat bones*, for example, the skull and pelvis; *cuboidal bones*, represented by vertebrae and tarsals; and *long bones*, such as the tibia and femur.

The typical long bone is broader at either end and narrower in its midportion. As a rule, the ends of the long bone are covered with articular cartilage and are broad in order to distribute weight-bearing loads over a wide area. The cartilage is supported by a bony plate, the subchondral bone, which is the visible margin of the joint seen on the roent-

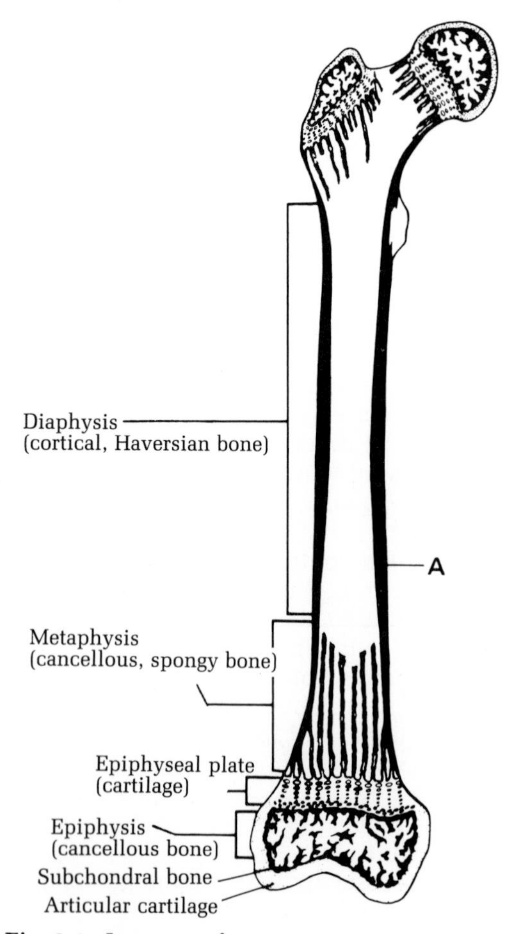

Fig. 6-1. Immature femur.

genograph and on the smooth end of the bone of a dried skeleton. This subchondral plate or surface is supported by a gridwork of cancellous or spongy bone, much as joists support the flooring of a house. Such an arrangement provides the most efficient structural means of supporting the articular surface against weight-bearing loads.

The upper and lower one fourth of a long bone, consisting of the joined epiphysis and metaphysis in an adult, are, for the most part, made up of cancellous bone surrounded by a thin covering of cortex on the surface. In the child, the epiphysis is separated from the metaphysis by the cartilaginous growth plate (Fig. 6-4*A*); after puberty, this epiphyseal plate is obliterated, and the two merge. The demarcation between the metaphysis and the shaft, or diaphysis, is not well defined. The diaphysis is composed of thick cortical bone; only a few spicules of cancellous bone are present in the marrow cavity. This thick, rigid, tubular part of the bone is structurally designed to withstand bending forces. Toward the metaphysis, the cortex becomes thinner, and there is a gradual increase in the amount of cancellous bone in the marrow area.

MICROSCOPIC STRUCTURE

It is in the compact cortical bone of the diaphysis that the Haversian systems are found (Fig. 6-2). If a transverse cut through the diaphysis is examined with the naked eye, the bone appears to be solid and ivorylike in texture. Under the low-power microscope, many small channels running in the direction of the long axis of the bone may be seen. Nutrients pass through these *Haversian canals* to the bone cells that lie buried in the thick cortex. Medium-powered microscopy will reveal that these canals are surrounded by concentric rings, each about 4 μ thick. These rings stand out strikingly under polarized light; they are layers of bone that contrast with one another under polarized light because of the different orientations of the collagen fibers in each layer.

Such layering is the hallmark of *mature* or *lamellar bone,* and may be contrasted with *immature, woven,* or *fiber bone* produced as a reaction to injury or disease. Immature bone is present normally only in the very young and does not have lamellae, and its coarse collagen fibers are randomly oriented. Within

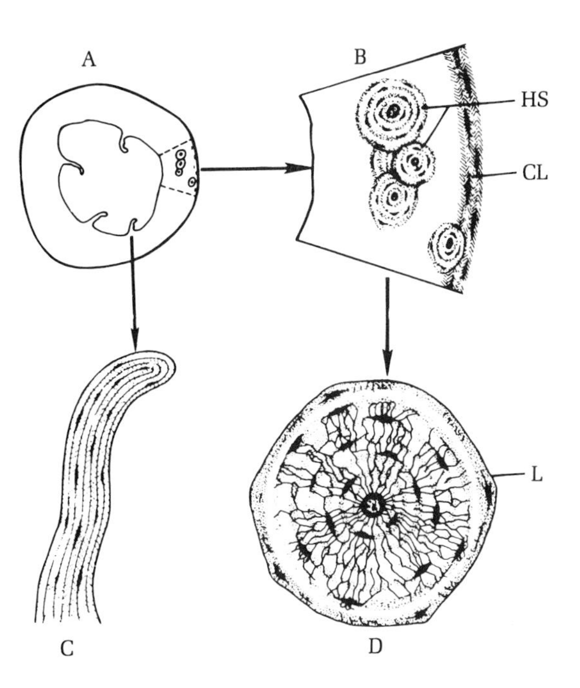

Fig. 6-2. (*A*) Cross section of diaphysis (at level A in Fig. 6-1) showing cortical bone with a few trabeculae of cancellous bone extending into the marrow cavity. Four Haversian systems are illustrated. (*B*) Enlargement of the wedge-shaped section seen in *A*; HS = Haversian systems; CL = circumferential lamellae laid down by periosteal osteoblasts on the surface. (*C*) Trabecula of cancellous or spongy bone. Note that cancellous bone is also lamellar bone. (*D*) A single Haversian system (osteon) showing concentric lamellae. Osteocytes in their lacunae are connected by fine canaliculi that communicate with the central canal with its contained vessel. L = the cement line that marks the outer border of the system.

the concentric lamellae of mature bone are small lacunae containing the osteocytes. From the lacunae extend fine *canaliculi* that contain the cell processes of the osteocytes. These processes connect the osteocytes to one another and to the Haversian canal, and are the pathways of nutrition from the canal to the bone cells. Canaliculi connect osteocytes within one Haversian system only; they do not cross cement lines to other systems. Since canaliculi are much too small to permit the passage of red blood cells, osteocytes must depend on diffusion and cell pumping mechanisms for their supply of oxygen and nutrients.

There are three types of cells intimately associated with bone: osteocytes, osteoblasts, and osteoclasts. *Osteocytes,* as noted above, dwell in small lacunae within the bone matrix. They are oval in cross section, their longest diameter being roughly parallel to the lamellae of mature bone.

Osteoblasts are found on the surfaces where bone is being formed. They vary in size and shape, most being 20 μ to 30 μ in diameter. They are usually arranged in a single layer of cells covering the bone surface, but where bone formation is very active, there may be several layers of cells. When mature bone is being formed slowly, the lining osteoblasts tend to be thin, flat, and elongated; when rapid osteogenesis occurs, the cells are usually quite plump and cuboidal. Osteoblasts have cytoplasmic processes that extend to adjacent osteoblasts and into the bone substance by way of canaliculi to join the processes of the osteocytes. Both the cytoplasm and the nucleus of osteoblasts contain the enzyme alkaline phosphatase.

The *osteoclast* is a large multinucleated cell that plays an active role in bone resorption. It is found in notches or indentations of bone surfaces called Howship's lacunae. These lacunae are 100 or more microns in length, just a bit larger than the associated cell, and appear to have been excavated by the osteoclast. Osteoclasts contain substantial amounts of the enzyme acid phosphatase. The surface of the osteoclast adjacent to bone has a striated or brush border. This ruffled border apparently plays an important role in the resorption of the underlying bone.

CANCELLOUS BONE

Cancellous or spongy bone is found at the ends of long bones and makes up the greater part of cuboidal bones. Its chemical composition and ultrastructure are identical to that of cortical bone. Cancellous bone is also formed in layers and is, therefore, lamellar bone. One difference between cancellous and cortical bone is the absence of Haversian systems in the former. Since cancellous bone is in the form of thin plates, its cells are never very far from the surface, and their canalicular systems are therefore adequate to supply nutrition; thus, there is no need for the complicated Haversian systems. Cancellous bone, like all other bone, is formed by osteoblasts that line the surface of the small trabeculae. The cancellous bone of the body presents a tremendously large surface area that responds readily to physical and metabolic demands of the body. It is more active metabolically than compact bone and its remodeling rate is higher.

CIRCUMFERENTIAL GROWTH

To understand the functions of and the reasons for the Haversian systems, one must consider the manner in which the diaphysis grows circumferentially. Since bone is a hard substance, it can grow only by adding new material to its surface. At birth, the diaphyseal portion of the human femur is a tube about 6 mm in diameter, with walls less than 1 mm thick. By adulthood, it attains a diameter of some 30 mm, with walls 5 or 6 mm thick. Such growth requires the addition of bone to the outer surface and resorption of bone from the inner surface. Osteoblasts are prominent on the outer surface of bone during the growing period. They produce the organic matrix of bone, which subsequently becomes calcified. The cells become incorporated in the matrix as osteocytes. This surface bone, being lamellar mature bone, is laid down in layers a few microns thick.

If the long bone were perfectly tubular, it would appear to be a series of hundreds of concentric, ever-enlarging rings of bone surrounding the marrow cavity, much like the rings of a tree trunk. The osteocytes buried within these rings would become separated by considerable distances from their nutritional supply at the surface, and would depend for survival on a very elongated canalicular system. Unfortunately, this system is not efficient and can support bone cells only for a limited distance—perhaps a few hundred microns. As the cortex of bone thickens with growth, it becomes impossible for the canalicular system to supply the deep-seated osteocytes. Blood vessels must be provided within the cortex for the nutrition of its osteocytes—thus, the need for Haversian canals.

Haversian systems are of two types, primary and secondary. Primary systems are formed on the growing surface of bone. Periosteal vessels running in the long axis of the bone become surrounded by bone, first in a trough, then completely buried in a canal. This canal is at first much larger than the vessels. Osteoblasts line the canal, and, by producing new concentric rings of bone at its periphery, gradually narrow the lumen until the vessels, now in a much smaller canal, come to lie within the concentric lamellae of bone that characterize an Haversian system. It should be noted that these systems are formed from the periphery of the canal toward the center.

Secondary Haversian systems are formed in newly eroded channels within the depths of the cortex. Constant internal remodeling of the cortex of bone takes place throughout life. Osteoclasts from the surface or from adjacent canals resorb bone to form new channels within the cortex. These channels are referred to as resorption canals or cutting cones. Vessels follow the osteoclasts into these resorption canals; later, the canal walls become lined with osteoblasts, and a new Haversian system is formed. This continuous alteration of the internal architecture of bone enables it to adapt to the changes in stress and metabolic demands throughout life.

LONGITUDINAL GROWTH

The longitudinal growth of bone is complicated by the physical limitations of bone tissue and by the need to maintain function during the growth process. As noted above, growth of bone tissue is limited to appositional growth, that is, the application of new bone on the surface of existing bone. This process is relatively simple in the instance of circumferential growth, but even this is complicated by the requirement of Haversian systems to maintain the viability of the osteocytes. Longitudinal growth might be accomplished by merely adding osseous tissue to the ends of the long bones, but this is prevented because of the presence of articular cartilage at each end. This cartilage must retain its specific shape and strength to permit proper joint function during growth.

Lengthwise growth of small bones, such as cuboidal bones, is accomplished through cell division and growth of the deeper layers of the articular cartilage, which is subsequently replaced by bone on its deep surface. The articular cartilage is thus constantly being pushed forward by the newly formed cartilage, which in turn is replaced by bone. This method of enlargement appears to be adequate for the cuboidal bones and for the epiphyses, which enlarge at a rate of only 1 mm to 2 mm per year. The long bones, however, lengthen at a much greater rate; a specialized structure, the epiphyseal growth plate, is required to permit their rapid growth.

The epiphyseal plate functions in much the same manner as do the deeper layers of articular cartilage in cuboidal bones; the deeper layers of cartilage cells multiply and enlarge, pushing the epiphysis and its overlying articular cartilage away from the metaphysis and diaphysis. Multiplication and growth of the epiphyseal cartilage cells tend to thicken the growth plate, but as rapidly as new cartilage cells are formed at the base of the plate, cartilage cells are destroyed and replaced by bone on the metaphyseal side of the plate. The plate, therefore, maintains a relatively constant thickness during the growing period. This process of exchanging cartilage for bone is called *enchondral ossification*. It is to be found in all growing bones of cartilaginous origin and is seen pathologically in the healing of fractures and in certain bone tumors.

DEVELOPMENT OF BONE FROM A CARTILAGE MODEL

The cartilaginous model of the long bones in the fetus undergoes a series of changes occurring in definite sequence that will ultimately transform this minute structure into an adult bone many times its size. The covering cells of the cartilage model, the *perichondrium*, change from cartilage-producing cells to bone-forming cells, osteoblasts, in the middle portion of the shaft. The newly created *periosteum* forms a thin shell of bone about the middle of the cartilage model. The cells within the center of the model hypertrophy, and vessels grow into the shaft from the surface. As the vessels come into contact with the cartilage cells, these cells are destroyed and replaced by bone. This bone nucleus spreads lengthwise in both directions from the middle of the model, until the bone reaches the level of the future epiphyseal plate. Thereafter, growth in length of the cartilage keeps pace with the growth in length of the bone. What remains at this point is a shaft of bone covered on either end by a large mass of cartilage cells, which is the status of most long bones at the time of birth.

This mass of cartilage represents the articular cartilage, the future epiphysis, and the epiphyseal plate. At a time that varies in each epiphysis, the cartilage cells in the center of the mass hypertrophy, there is an ingrowth of blood vessels, and bone replaces cartilage just as it did in the shaft at an earlier stage. This process gives rise to the *epiphyseal ossification centers.* These centers make their appearance in a specific order: the center at the distal end of the femur is always present at birth; the center at the proximal end in the head of the femur appears between 2 and 8 months following birth; the center in the proximal end of the radius is not present until after 3 years of age. As the ossification center enlarges, it does so at first in all directions at the expense of the surrounding cartilage, until it becomes bounded on the metaphyseal side by the epiphyseal plate and on all other sides by articular cartilage. From this time on, the bony epiphysis grows only on the sides adjacent to the articular cartilage. Its method of growth, therefore, is similar to that of the cuboidal bones.

The *epiphyseal plate,* which is responsible for the length growth of the shaft, is a complex structure (Fig. 6-3). It consists of four indistinct zones of cells that merge into one another without clear demarcations. Immediately adjacent to the epiphysis are irregularly scattered cartilage cells, called the *resting cell zone.* On the metaphyseal side of this zone, the cartilage cells become aligned into well-defined columns, the second zone (also called the *zone of cellular proliferation*). It is at the base of these columns that mitotic activity is found. In this small area, two or three cells thick, occurs the cell di-

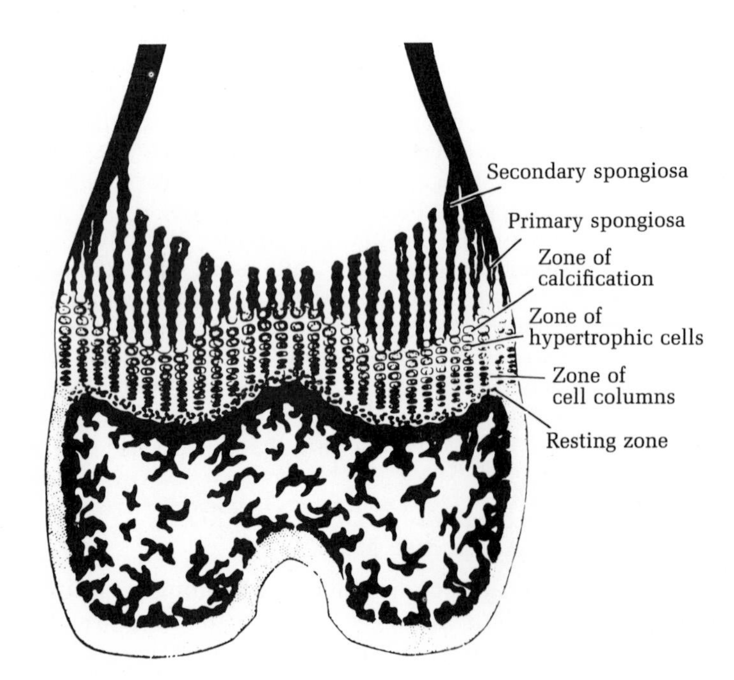

Fig. 6-3. Distal end of the femur showing the four layers of the cartilaginous growth plate and the primary and secondary spongiosa of the metaphysis.

vision upon which the entire growth in length of the bone depends. Failure of these cells to thrive results in cessation of growth at that end of the bone.

The columns of cartilage cells extend toward the metaphysis, being constantly lengthened by cell division occurring at the base. The cells nearer the metaphysis begin to undergo changes that ultimately lead to their destruction. They hypertrophy at the expense of extracellular matrix, and these enlarged cartilage cells constitute the third zone, or *hypertrophic zone*. The last two or three cells in the column of cartilage cells are in the fourth zone, the *zone of provisional calcification*. It is in this area that the extracellular chondroid matrix becomes impregnated with calcium salt. This calcification of matrix seems to be necessary for the next steps, which are the invasion of the cartilage cells by blood vessels from the metaphysis, the destruction of the cartilage cells, and the formation of bone along the remaining walls of calcified cartilage matrix. The juncture between epiphyseal plate and the metaphysis is secured by the welding of metaphyseal bone to calcified cartilage matrix.

The bone at this point has a very characteristic microscopic appearance as seen in hematoxylin and eosin sections. Trabecular pink bone, aligned perpendicularly to the epiphyseal growth plate and parallel to the shaft of the bone, contains central cores of blue-staining cartilage; this *enchondral bone* is found only in bone of cartilaginous origin. In this area, it is also referred to as the *primary spongiosa*, and it extends into the metaphysis for only a few millimeters. This primary spongiosa, or enchondral bone, is destroyed little by little at its metaphyseal end as the epiphyseal plate grows away from it. It is replaced by new trabeculae of bone with similar longitudinal orientation but without a central core of cartilage matrix. Thus, true enchondral bone exists for only a short time, and the adult skeleton contains little, if any, of this type of bone.

Bone formed without a preceding cartilaginous base is termed *membranous bone*. Circumferential growth of the diaphysis of long bones and most of the growth of the skull is by intramembranous bone formation.

The dividing cartilage cells at the base of the zone of cell columns determine the rate and the amount of growth that take place at the end of any given bone. Just what regulates this process so precisely is not known. It may be that a given set of cartilage cells in a certain location is allotted a specific number of mitoses or a specific rate of mitotic activity. The ultimate fate of these cells is under hormonal influence, since they stop dividing at puberty. When new cartilage cells are not provided to the growth plate, the continuing process of enchondral ossification on the metaphyseal side destroys the remaining cartilage cells, and the plate is obliterated. During their growth period, however, the activity of these cartilage cells cannot be explained entirely on a hormonal basis, for cells at the distal end of the femur grow more rapidly (1.3 cm per year) than those of the proximal tibia (0.9 cm per year). Cells at the proximal end of the humerus and distal end of the radius divide about four times as fast as the corresponding epiphyseal cartilage cells at the elbow. Each epiphyseal plate contributes a specific percentage of growth in length to a bone.

As might be expected where such mitotic activity is present in one localized area, many things can go wrong. Injury in the form of fracture through the growth plate can result in cessation or retardation of growth in length and a shortened limb. The amount of shortening will depend upon the age when the injury occurs. For example, should the distal femoral epiphysis be damaged in a 6-year-old boy, shortening that would develop in the remaining 10 years of growth would roughly amount to 10×1.3 cm or 13 cm. If only one side of an epiphyseal plate is injured, the opposite side may continue to grow, producing angulation.

The growth plate is sensitive to nutritional and metabolic changes. In *rickets*, the zone of provisional calcification is deprived of calcium salts; as a result, enchondral ossification is disrupted. Cartilage continues to accumulate in the form of hypertrophic cells, but failure of a zone of provisional calcification to form prevents the ingrowth of blood vessels and the replacement of cartilage by bone. The result is a grossly enlarged epiphyseal plate (Fig. 6-4). The rachitic rosary of the costochondral junctions and the swollen wrists seen in children with rickets are

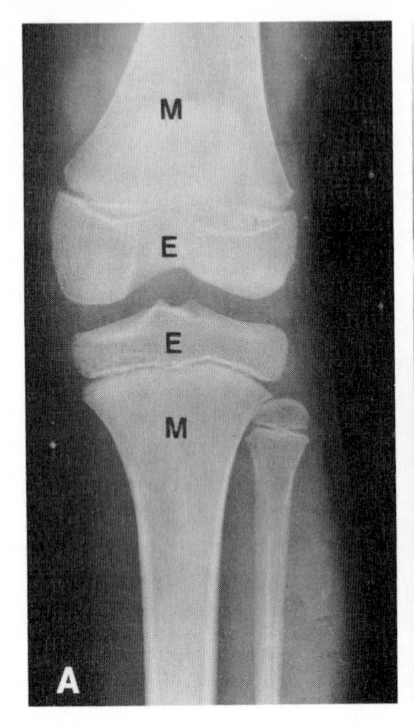

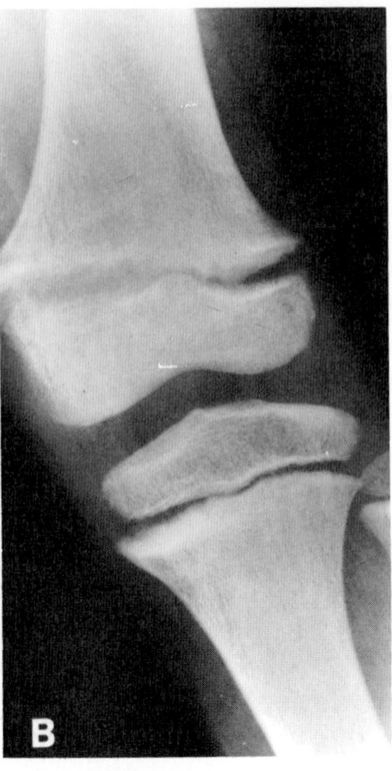

Fig. 6-4. (*A*) Normal distal femur and proximal tibia in a growing child. M-metaphysis, E-epiphysis. (*B*) Distal femur and proximal tibia in child with vitamin D-resistant rickets. Note the wide and irregular epiphyseal plate which is caused by the accumulation of cartilage cells. Note also the valgus or knock knee deformity.

produced by these accumulations of cartilage.

In certain hereditary disorders such as achondroplasia, a severe disruption of the growth plate occurs, resulting in *dwarfism*. In the *pituitary dwarf*, an insufficiency of somatotropic hormone leads to a slowing of mitotic activity in the epiphyseal plate, thereby retarding overall growth.

During normal growth, the epiphysis and epiphyseal plate constantly enlarge in a transverse direction. Thus, the number of columns of cartilage cells increases, and the width of the metaphysis increases as growth in length occurs. If the addition of new cartilage and bone at the epiphyseal plate were the only process involved in growth, the adult bone would have the appearance of two inverted cones with their apices at the point of origin of the embryonic bone, and their bases at the joints. This structure, however, is considerably modified by the constant remodeling of bone during growth, and even after growth stops. The periphery of bone in the metaphyseal area is undercut by osteoclasts, a process that has been referred to as *funnelization*, while the diaphysis is enlarged transversely by the periosteal growth described earlier. As the external diameter increases, there is also an enlargement of the marrow cavity within. This change is the result of osteoclastic activity on the endosteal surface of the diaphysis, a process of diaphyseal remodeling called *tubulation*.

Muscle attachments influence the shape of bone, as do functional demands. Bone responds to changes in function and to stress put upon it by remodeling, bone being added where needed and removed where it is not required. The general principle of this remodeling process was described by Julius Wolff in 1868. Wolff's law holds that every change in the form or function of a bone is followed by certain definite changes in its internal architecture and its external shape. An active, athletic person has dense, heavy bones. If that same person is rendered inactive for a prolonged period, his bones become thinner and less dense. With age, the shafts of long bones increase in external diameter but decrease in cortical thickness and density.

SELECTED REFERENCES

Bloom W, Faucett A: Textbook of Histology, 10th ed. Philadelphia, WB Saunders, 1975

Ham AW, Cormack DH: Histology, 8th ed. Philadelphia, J B Lippincott, 1979

Urist MR: Fundamental and Clinical Bone Physiology. Philadelphia, JB Lippincott, 1980

Chapter 7

Chemistry and Biochemistry of Bone

Carole J. VanderWiel

GOALS AND OBJECTIVES

Goals: To describe the chemistry of bone along with the biochemical and cellular processes that support bone formation and resorption

Objectives: On completion of this unit, and using the text as a standard reference, one should be able to evaluate, describe, list, or recognize the following:

1. The gross composition of dry bone in terms of mineral, proteinpolysaccharide, collagen, noncollagen protein, and lipid, along with the probable functions of each
2. The physical state of collagen in bone with respect to its relationship to other organic fractions and the mineral
3. Cellular participation during the formation and resorption of bone
4. Current concepts concerning the mechanism of bone mineralization and resorption

OUTLINE

I. The chemistry of bone
   A. Organic constituents of bone
      1. Collagen
      2. Proteinpolysaccharides
      3. Noncollagenous protein
      4. Lipids
   B. Inorganic constituents of bone
      1. Hydroxyapatite crystals
      2. Amorphous calcium phosphate
   C. Arrangement of organic and inorganic matrix
II. Bone formation
   A. The osteoblast
   B. Collagen biosynthesis
   C. Collagen disorders
   D. Mechanisms of mineralization
III. Bone resorption
   A. The osteoclast
   B. Mechanisms of bone resorption
   C. The osteocyte

Bone is a unique connective tissue because

of its high content of inorganic material. The orderly deposition of bone mineral confers on this tissue a rigidity that is necessary for the attachment of muscles and the protection of vital organs. This chapter describes the basic chemical nature of bone along with the novel arrangement of its organic and inorganic constituents that provide for its inflexibility. The two major physiologic processes in bone, formation and resorption, are also discussed along with their respective biochemical and cellular processes.

THE CHEMISTRY OF BONE

Organic Constituents of Bone

On a dry weight basis, the organic matrix of bone comprises approximately 35% of its total weight, of which about 95% is collagen. Other constituents are the proteinpolysaccharides (mucoproteins or glycoproteins) and lipids, including phospholipids.

Collagen. The protein collagen is the predominant component of the organic phase of bone as well as of other connective tissue, and is widely distributed as a highly organized system of fibers. Collagen can be found in all connective tissues—bone, dentin, skin, tendon, cartilage, kidney, liver, and lung. There are at least five different genetic types of collagen, each made up of three alpha chains. Type I is the major collagen of tendon and bone, but it is also predominant in lung, skin, dentin, heart valves, fascia, scar tissue, cornea, and liver. Type I collagen is essential for the tensile strength of bone; it is the final amount and distribution of these collagen fibers that will determine the size, shape, and ultimate density of the bone.

Collagen fibers are characterized by an axial periodicity of 640 angstroms (Å) to approximately 700 Å depending upon the source of collagen. The presence of high and low protein densities give it distinctive light and dark bands. Collagen is a unique protein in that it contains about one third glycine residues. It is also rich in hydroxyproline and hydroxylysine residues, contains many alanine residues and very few aromatic amino acids. A single collagen fibril is composed of three polypeptides called alpha chains. Variations in the alpha chains exist in their sequence of amino acids, their extent of hydroxylation of lysine and proline, and their glycosylation of hydroxylysine residues.

The sequence of amino acids in collagen is basically very simple and can be used to determine the collagen type, since all four types have similar x-ray diffraction patterns. Every third amino acid residue is glycine, which is usually followed by proline and then by hydroxyproline. There are approximately 333 glycine residues, 100 proline residues, and 100 hydroxyproline residues in the alpha chain. Hydroxyproline is an interesting residue in that when collagen is broken down, hydroxyproline is excreted in the urine and can be measured colorimetrically as an indicator of collagen turnover.

The alpha chain is also rich in lysine and hydroxylysine residues, which are the ultimate determinants of the nature and number of crosslinks. Type I collagen is composed of two $\alpha 1$ chains and one $\alpha 2$ chain. These three peptide chains are each coiled into a left-handed helix, and the three adjacent helices are bound by intermolecular and intramolecular cross-linkages. All Type I collagen has the same amino acid sequence, but the tissue it was extracted from is distinguished from other tissues by the pattern of cross-links. The first cross-link type is formed by the condensation of two aldehydes to form an aldol or an intramolecular cross-link. The second type is the Schiff base or intermolecular cross-link formed by an aldehyde reacting with an amino group. The most important type is the intermolecular cross-link that is formed from amino and aldehyde groups of lysine and hydroxy lysine residues.

The three peptide chains held into the left-handed helices by their cross-links are twisted around a common axis or right-handed super helix to form a three-stranded coil. This unique helical formation gives the molecule its highly stable, rigid, rodlike shape. These fibrils become more soluble as the salt concentration of the extracting fluid increases; the general thesis is that the more insoluble the collagen, the older it is. When salt-extractable (newly synthesized) collagen is denatured, it separates into the collagen polymers ($\alpha 1$, $\alpha 1$, $\alpha 2$), each with a molecular weight of about 94,000 daltons. Each chain has approximately 1030 residues with each residue 2.9 Å long and weighing 91 daltons.

The newly synthesized chains twisted into a super helical conformation have a molecular weight of 282,000 daltons. Older collagen gives rise to two double and one triple chain (β11, β12, and γ112) whose molecular weights are 200,000 and 300,000 respectively.

Protein Polysaccharides. Protein polysaccharides account for approximately 4.4% of the organic components of bone and may be defined as compounds of carbohydrate and protein in which the carbohydrate is a polysaccharide attached to a protein by covalent bonds. The principle polysaccharide (mucopolysaccharide) of bone is chondroitin-4-sulfate (chondroitin sulfate A). The chondroitin sulfates are found in particularly high concentrations in the proliferative zone of epiphyseal cartilage where they may play an inhibitory role in calcification. (For a discussion of the physical and chemical properties of the protein polysaccharides, please refer to Chap. 17, Chemisty and Biochemistry of Cartilage and Synovial Fluid). In certain genetic diseases known as mucopolysaccharidoses, there is a mutation-produced deficiency in the lysosomal enzyme activity needed to degrade certain mucopolysaccharides, which results in an accumulation of the mucopolysaccharides within cells of various organs and increased excretion of the polysaccharides into the urine. Loss of these polysaccharides from bone and cartilage causes specific skeletal defects such as stiff joints, flattened vertebrae, generalized osteoporosis, and hip and thoracic deformities.

Noncollagenous Protein. The noncollagenous protein of bone amounts to about 0.5% of the organic fraction. Most of these proteins are probably bound to polysaccharides. One such compound is gamma-carboxyglutamate, which acts as a strong calcium-binding site. Although its function is obscure, there is evidence suggesting its involvement in regulating mineralization and calcium movement.

Lipids. The lipids of bone comprise less than 0.1% of the organic fraction and consist of triglycerides, free fatty acids, phospholipids, and cholesterol. Although some of the lipids are probably structural parts of the cell membrane, evidence suggests that lipids may also be involved in calcification and ossification. It has been observed that phospholipids disappear just before calcification occurs. Further, the absence of lipid-staining material in the epiphyseal cartilage of rachitic animals and its return after treatment with vitamin D suggests a correlation between the vitamin, lipids, and ossification. Other physiologic substances that influence skeletal metabolism (e.g., parathyroid hormone, vitamin A, and glucocorticoids) also affect the biosynthesis of bone lipids. Thus, although the role of the lipids in skeletal metabolism is unknown, there is no doubt that in some manner they are involved in ossification and maintenance of a normal skeleton.

Inorganic Constituents of Bone

The inorganic phase of bone accounts for about 65% of its dry weight. The bulk of the mineral in bone is composed of calcium and phosphate, which in the adult is primarily crystalline in structure and resembles synthetic hydroxyapatite crystals. The minor mineral constituents of bone are magnesium, sodium, potassium, and a number of trace elements (zinc, manganese, fluoride, and molybdenum) considered to be adsorbed on the bone surface. It is not known whether these trace elements have a role in skeletal metabolism or merely represent adsorption resulting from their presence in foodstuffs. Carbonate forms 3.5% of dry, fat-free human bone, but whether it is an integral part of the hydroxyapatite crystal or only a surface-limited ion has not been completely resolved. *In vivo*, carbonate may exchange for phosphate, and fluoride for an hydroxyl ion. Citrate ion is also found to an appreciable extent in dry, fat-free bone. Although the amounts of calcium and phosphate do not vary significantly in different species, those of magnesium and citrate do.

In addition to the high content of inorganic material, bone also contains a large amount of water. Approximately 15 percent of the total water volume is located in bone spaces occupied by the canaliculi, Haversian canals and osteocytic lacunae. The major volume of water is found in the organic matrix, around the collagen fibers and ground substance, and in the hydration shells of the bone crystals. The water content of bone varies with its age, being high in young, rapidly growing bones and low in older bones. As bone ages, the lost water is replaced by mineral; however, the actual percentage of mineral also varies with the specific bone.

Hydroxyapatite crystals. Most investigators believe that calcium and phosphate are present in the form of an apatite, because on x-ray diffraction analysis, bone gives patterns very similar to hydroxyapatite $[Ca_{10}(PO_4)]_6(OH)_2$. However, some believe that octacalcium phosphate $[Ca_8H_2(PO_4)]_6 5H_2O$ may be either the major crystalline fraction of bone or a precursor. The exact nature of the crystalline form is still not known because it is involved in a complex biologic system that is affected by the presence of other ions as well as by an organic matrix.

Some of the differences between crystalline hydroxyapatite and bone mineral are as follows:

1. The theoretic calcium-to-phosphate ratio of apatite is 1.66 on a molar basis, but it rarely equals this value in bone and may range from 1.33 to 1.66
2. The heating of bone crystals from 200° to 600° C causes formation of pyrophosphate; this reaction does not occur with synthetic hydroxyapatite
3. Extraneous ions (e.g., sodium, potassium, carbonate, magnesium, citrate, and fluoride) are associated with the mineral phase of bone, whereas none are present in synthetic hydroxyapatite
4. Bone crystals have a considerable amount of bound water that can be removed by heating, which differs from synthetic hydroxyapatite that has no water of crystallization

In general, synthetic hydroxyapatite and bone crystals are very small; their x-ray diffraction patterns are diffuse and poor, but they are similar. X-ray diffraction will distinguish hydroxyapatite from other structures but cannot positively distinguish "pure" and "impure" apatite. Basically, bone crystal may be considered to be a "modified" hydroxyapatite. Even though there is divergence of opinion about the size of hydroxyapatite crystals, most investigators agree that the smallest dimension is about 25 Å to 50 Å; the other dimensions are on the order of 400 Å × 200 to 350 Å. There is good evidence, based on x-ray diffraction and electron microscopic studies, that the direction of the long axis (C axis) of the crystal is parallel to the collagen fibers.

Although the surface area of the crystals is tremendous, only about 0.65% of human bone calcium is part of the readily exchangeable pool. Since the vast bulk of bone calcium is not rapidly exchangeable, only certain areas in bone contain calcium that is rapidly exchanged. In living bone, these areas have been identified by autoradiography as the lining of Haversian canals or resorption cavities. The sites of new bone deposition, for example, subperiosteal or newly mineralizing osteons, do not appear to participate to any great extent in these exchange reactions. Also, as bone ages, expulsion of water during calcification prevents significant chemical diffusion into the interior of fully mineralized bone tissue.

All crystals in a liquid are surrounded by a layer of water that is called a hydration shell (Fig. 7-1). Theoretically, ions pass readily to and from the aqueous phase and can exchange with each other rapidly. At the crystalline surface, ions are held by electrostatic charges, and only those of similar chemical properties can actually enter into the crystals. Strontium, sodium, radium, and lead can replace calcium on the surface of the crystal lattice and thus become entrapped and buried within bone. Fluoride is known to replace the hydroxyl ion on the crystal surface, and it can also form a fluoroapatite crystal. These substitutions are less rapid than exchange in the water layer. Sometimes ions enter defects in the crystal lattice. Exchange within the crystal itself is a very slow process. Other ions, such as potassium and magnesium, are believed to be adsorbed on the surface. However, bone behaves differently from pure hydroxyapatite crystals, perhaps because it contains a variety of macromolecules in an intimate association with the crystals, and, as a living tissue, it also contains cells that are capable of taking in and expelling ions.

Autoradiographic studies show that monovalent ions diffuse freely through skeletal tissue, unlike divalent ions which vary with respect to their diffusibility. Thus, the

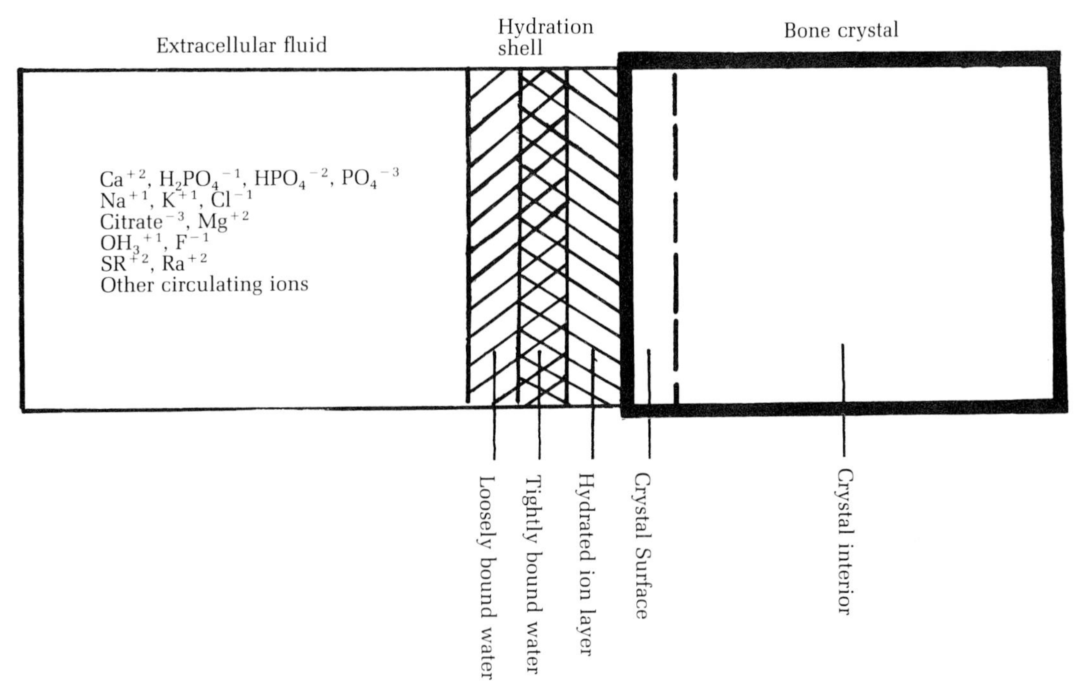

Fig. 7-1. Schematic representation of a hydration shell that is bound to the bone crystal surface. The crystal is comprised of three zones: (1) hydration shell, (2) crystal surface, and (3) crystal interior. The first two zones represent the surfaces for ion exchange. (Modified from Neuman WF, Neuman MW: The Chemical dynamics of the Bone Mineral. Chicago, University of Chicago Press, 1958)

concept of "available" bone mineral is dependent on the type of mineral, the age of the animal, and the site of bone chosen for analysis. To account for gradients in mineral content in bone and extracellular fluid, one must assume some sort of "membrane" separation of fluid compartments in cortical bone.

Amorphous Calcium Phosphate. In addition to the crystalline form of calcium and phosphate in bone, there is also an amorphous, or noncrystalline, mineral phase. X-ray diffraction studies have shown this fraction to be a major component of bone mineral; approximately 40% of the mineral in the adult human femur is noncrystalline. This component decreases with age and is replaced by crystalline apatite as bone matures. The amorphous calcium phosphates, like the apatites, do not have a strictly defined chemical composition. The molar calcium-to-phosphate ratio varies from 1.44:1 to 1.55:1, depending on the conditions of preparation of the bone samples. These amorphous calcium phosphates are not stable in an aqueous medium and hydrolyze into crystalline apatite. The rate of conversion *in vivo* is controlled by the apatite product and not by the amorphous precursor.

Arrangement of Organic and Inorganic Matrix

The arrangement of collagen fibrils allows for packing of inorganic crystals around and within the collagen fibrils without changing their volume. Linear polymers of collagen molecules in fibrils overlap by about 9%. The fibrils are arranged so that adjacent macromolecules are staggered by a fourth of their length. This arrangement gives the so-called native type (640–700 Å axial repeat) collagen fibril appearance. The net effect is the appearance of holes that may be continuous or that may occur as broken channels throughout the fibrils (Fig. 7-2). These holes occur once each axial period and can accommodate the mineral crystals without altering the basic structure of the fibrils.

The actual bone salt is made up of atoms

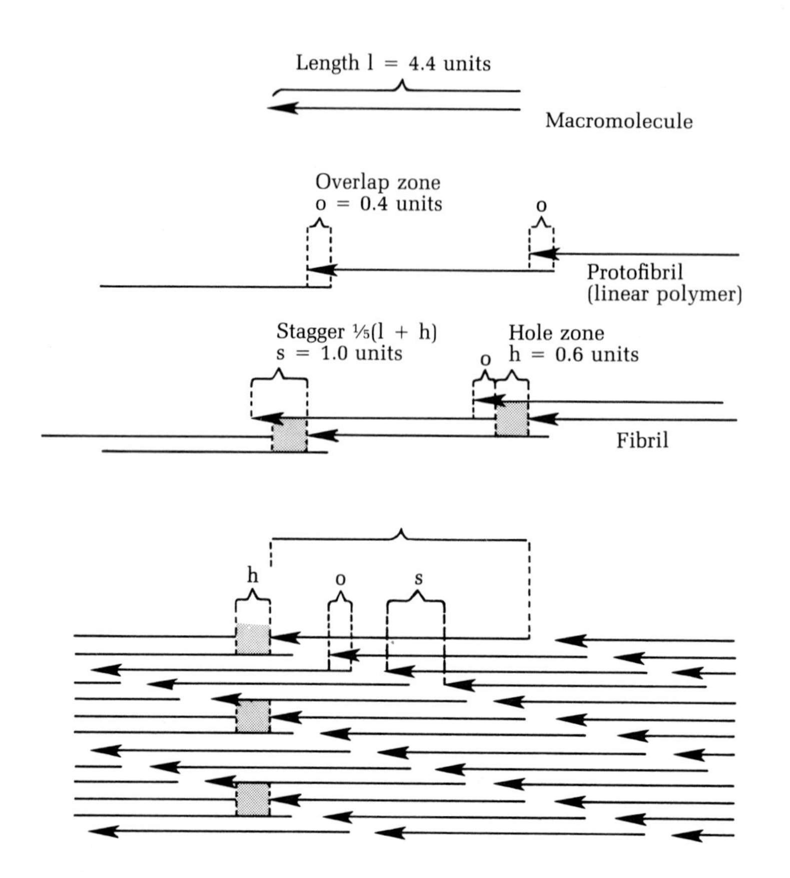

Fig. 7-2. Suggested model for alignment of collagen fibrils to account for deposition of hydroxyapatite. (Glimcher MJ, Krane SM: Treatise on collagen. New York, Academic Press, 1968)

organized into a regularly repeating three-dimensional array forming a crystal lattice. The smallest repeating unit of the lattice is referred to as a unit cell that is in the shape of a right-handed rhomboid. The dimensions of the unit cell in bone salt, as revealed by x-ray diffraction, are 9.4 × 9.4 × 6.9 Å. The crystal lattice, made up of eight or more unit cells, is visible under the electron microscope as an electron density seen at regular intervals along the longitudinal axis of the collagen fibers. These intervals are between 600 and 700 Å apart and correspond to the normal axial repeat of the collagen fibril. This finding establishes that bone mineral is deposited along specific regions of the collagen fiber, but the actual relationship of bone mineral to the collagen structure is still uncertain. It is believed that the channels, or "holes," within the collagen alignment may hold as much as 50% of the mineral phase of bone. Also, the microfibrillar arrangement can account for 40% more of the total crystal volume.

After the initial formation of the extracellular collagen fibrils and prior to their mineralization, there is a lag time of 8 to 10 days, which accounts for the layer of uncalcified collagen or osteoid between osteoblasts synthesizing collagen and the underlying calcified bone. In osteomalacia, the organic material fails to properly calcify, and patients develop wider osteoid seams. The collagen appears normal, but there is an abnormal arrangement of the collagen fibrils, making calcification more difficult.

BONE FORMATION

The Osteoblast

Bone formation is a two-step process that involves matrix formation and mineralization. The cell responsible for this formation is the osteoblast, which has the capacity to synthesize collagen and to control its subsequent mineralization. The active osteoblast is cuboidal in shape and is in contact with the surface of bone. Each cell ranges from 20 to 30 μ in maximum diameter. The collagen-synthesizing osteoblast contains a large number of mitochondria, a wide Golgi zone, many free ribosomes, small vesicles, and a well-developed endoplasmic reticulum (Fig. 7-3). These osteoblasts exhibit polarity in that they normally only secrete collagen and protein polysaccharides into the matrix space adjacent to the osteoid, and they extend their cytoplasmic processes out into the osteoid seam.

Electron micrographs have shown that active osteoblasts contain granules with a high calcium and inorganic phosphate content. Whether or not these calcium–phosphate granules form during fixation, their presence supports the concept that mitochondria are involved in the storage and transport of intracellular calcium and may play a role in mineralization. In fact, at the growth plate, chondrocytes have been shown to accumulate calcium within their mitochondria in a region anterior to the zone of provisional calcification. These granules rapidly decrease in number after the initiation of matrix mineralization.

Collagen Biosynthesis

The biosynthesis of collagen is initiated within osteoblasts (Fig. 7-4). These intracellular events involve protein synthesis on endoplasmic reticulum to form three polypeptide chains, which make up protocollagen. Protocollagen is hydroxylated to form procollagen, which is glycosylated at the endoplasmic reticulum. The degree of hydroxylation of the lysine residue is important in that it will determine the number of cross-links and therefore the strength of the collagen. Procollagen is converted to a triple helix before secretion from the cell by microtubules. The procollagen helices are actually longer than the collagen molecule owing to an amino-acid terminal and a carboxy terminal endpiece that keep the collagen soluble while inside the cell. All the intracellular processes require more than eight enzymes, have over 150 modifications of each chain, and alter one-tenth of the amino acids. Recent pulse-chase experiments have shown that the synthesis of an alpha chain occurs sequentially from the amino terminal end to the carboxy terminal endpiece. Procollagen chains can be synthesized at a rate of 200 residues per minute, with approximately 6 to 7 minutes for the synthesis of a complete chain.

Once the osteoblast secretes procollagen, a procollagen peptidase splits off the terminal endpieces, and polymerization and

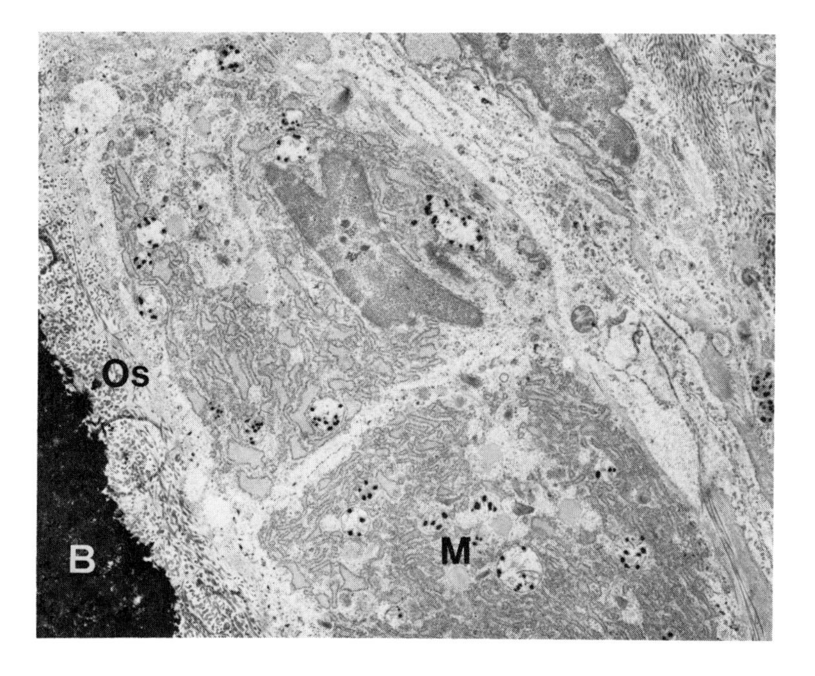

Fig. 7-3. An electron micrograph of two adjacent osteoblasts on the surface of bone. The cells are separated from the electron dense bone (B) by a collagenous matrix of osteoid (Os). With a special fixation technique using pyroantimonate, the mitochondria (M) are shown to contain many electron-dense granules. Original magnification × 4500.

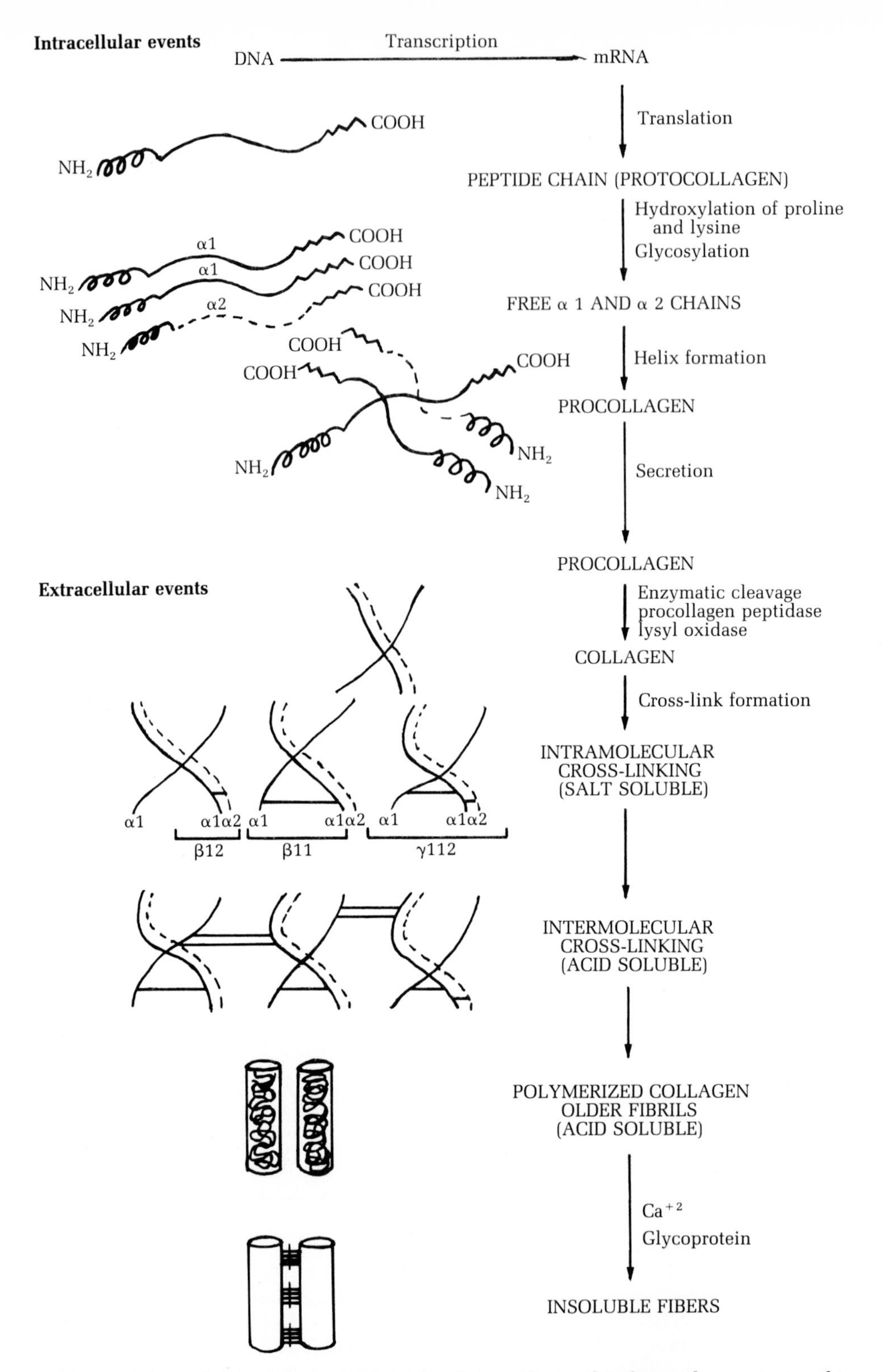

Fig. 7-4. Biosynthesis and maturation of collagen fibers. This figure demonstrates the probable sequence of events from peptide chains that are formed within cells to the formation of mature collagen fibrils that occur extracellularly. This "classical" scheme of collagen synthesis varies slightly for the collagen of bone, cartilage, and soft tissue, each of which possesses genetic heterogenity of its component alpha chains.

maturation naturally follow. Five collagen molecules will polymerize to form a microfibril, and these microfibrils will polymerize to form fibrils that are visible under the electron microscope. Covalent bonds are formed between the adjacent collagen molecules both within microfibrils and between adjacent microfibrils. These crosslinks will determine the maximal tensile strength of the tissue collagen and its subsequent solubility, and thus extractability.

Collagen Disorders

The biosynthesis of collagen involves many complex processes that are subject to biologic control. These processes can be disrupted at any point by metabolic disorders that may become manifest as diseases. For example, a disease that can affect the intracellular biosynthesis of collagen is scurvy, which is caused by vitamin C (ascorbic acid) deficiency. The specific defect appears to be an inability of the tissue to hydroxylate proline, and there is a decreased hydroxylation of lysine. Less collagen will be formed, and the collagen that is formed will be of a poor quality. In scurvy, the collagen fibrils appear swollen and contain increased amounts of polysaccharides. New bone formation is prevented, and the older bone becomes brittle. Old scars and wounds tend to rupture more easily when a patient lacks an adequate intake of this vitamin.

If the extracellular processes of cross-link formation are inhibited, the collagen will remain soluble, which is the case in a disease known as lathyrism. The ingestion of certain agents called lathyrogens, including β-aminopropionitrile, causes profound alterations in the collagen of connective tissue and bone. Most lathyrogens act by inhibiting the enzyme lysyl oxidase, which is responsible for the synthesis of aldehydes. These aldehydes are needed for the formation of the bonds that link two chains together. A copper deficiency also causes a disorder similar to lathyrism because lysyl oxidase is a copper-requiring enzyme. Recently, penicillamine and cystamine have been investigated for their ability to react with aldehydes in collagen and to break cross-linkages formed. If these intermolecular and intramolecular cross-linkages are inhibited or broken, the net effect is a marked increase in the amount of collagen that can be extracted under mild conditions from bone and other connective tissue. Lathyritic animals are known to have soft, deformed bones, many joint dislocations, and aortic aneurysms.

Many of the genetic collagen diseases have biochemical defects in the biosynthesis of collagen that are still unknown. An excellent example is Ehlers-Danlos syndrome (EDS). The inherited connective tissue disorders known as EDS have been categorized into seven different types based on clinical, genetic, and biochemical data. Each group can be defined by a subset of distinct clinical findings and, in some cases, by a known biochemical defect. The classic clinical picture is one of hyperextensible joints, hyperelastic fragile skin that tears and stretches easily, poor wound healing, and easy bruising owing to the delicate collagen fibers within the blood vessels. The collagen extracted from patients with Ehlers-Danlos syndrome is known to be deficient in hydroxylysine. Also, the Type VII Ehlers-Danlos syndrome is now known to be caused by a deficiency in procollagen peptidase. Once the osteoblast secretes procollagen, the patient either has no procollagen peptidase to remove the amino terminal endpiece or the patient does have procollagen peptidase, but it is inactive due to a defect located within the chain.

Mechanisms of Mineralization

Tissue mineralization is considered to be the last step in bone formation following cellular differentiation and matrix formation. The principal mineral salt of bone exists primarily in the form of crystalline hydroxyapatite, which is the thermodynamically stable phase at normal tissue *p*H. The first step in the precipitation of bone salts must involve some type of nucleation, that is, the formation of a mineral arrangement of calcium and phosphate ions capable of crystal growth. The phenomenon of nucleation or "seeding" is explained by the concept of the undersaturation of body fluids with calcium and phosphate until the first precipitate is formed. For example, the local phosphate concentration would have to be raised to three times the serum phosphate concentration before a spontaneous precipitation could occur. The body fluids would be undersaturated until the first precipitation of calcium phosphate, and then the body fluids would become supersaturated in respect to the solubility of the precipitate, and crystal growth would occur automatically. How nucleation occurs is an unsolved problem in skeletal metabolism. Several theories have been proposed to explain this phenomenon, but all have severe limitations:

Spontaneous Mechanisms. British chemist Robert Robison proposed that the alkaline phosphatase in bone hydrolyzed free phosphate esters to produce sufficient inorganic phosphate for the supersaturation necessary to precipitate apatite. The organic matrix was not involved, and there was no concomitant increase in calcium ions. It is doubtful that the local concentration of phosphate could be raised to three times its serum concentration as necessary for spontaneous precipitation. Also, alkaline phosphatase is present in a great number of other tissues that do not calcify. Robison's theory is therefore mainly of historic interest.

Local Mechanisms. Interest focused next on some component of the organic matrix as the initial event of mineralization. Since collagen appeared to be intimately connected to the mineral, many investigators have espoused this protein as the main component responsible for seeding of bone mineral. However, other than the fact that bone mineral is deposited for the most part along or within collagen fibers, there is insufficient evidence to support the idea that it initiates mineralization. Further, electron microscopy has demonstrated that bone crystals may be found in areas completely devoid of collagen.

Cellular Mechanisms. All cells are programmed during their embryonic development to synthesize specific products. In the case of skeletal cells, it is well established that certain cells (osteoblasts) are capable of synthesizing all components of the bone matrix. Further, these cells are also capable of taking in calcium and phosphate, and their mitochondria can bind large quantities of calcium liberated by hormonal action. Although osseous cells are the only ones designed to make bone, there may be intracellular calcification of cells in other tissues under pathologic conditions. Recent studies have indicated that calcification may originate in a cellularly derived globule or matrix vesicle originating in the Golgi apparatus. These vesicles contain apatite crystals and have a high level of alkaline phosphatase, pyrophosphatase, and ATPase activity to prepare the matrix for mineralization. Thus, the cell contains all the ingredients necessary for the ossification process.

It is unlikely that extracellular conditions are such that the levels of calcium and phosphate ions are high enough to produce spontaneous precipitation of amorphous calcium phosphate, the supposed precursor of hydroxyapatite. The problem of bone formation is even further complicated under the concepts of a separate bone fluid compartment with even lower concentrations of calcium. The most logical theory is that the cells, in addition to producing organic matrix, can concentrate calcium and phosphate and transport it to an extracellular location in an amorphous form along with associated lipids and proteins. This theory is attractive because it permits cellular control over the seeding process even in the embryo, in which, because of the adherence of the cellular layer and the osteocytes to the underlying matrix, the bone fluid compartment is not only very small but has little or no contact with the extracellular fluid. In any event, it would seem that a cellular mechanism for calcification is more plausible than other mechanisms that have been suggested.

BONE RESORPTION

The Osteoclast

The opposite of bone formation is bone resorption, which involves the hydrolysis of collagen and the dissolution of bone mineral. The cell primarily responsible for bone resorption is the osteoclast. The actual amount of bone resorbed is dependent upon the number of osteoclasts present and each osteoclast's activity. These large cells are multinucleated, with cytoplasm full of mitochondria, free ribosomes, vesicles, prominent Golgi apparatus and lysosomes (Fig. 7-5). Osteoclasts have three cellular organelles that are

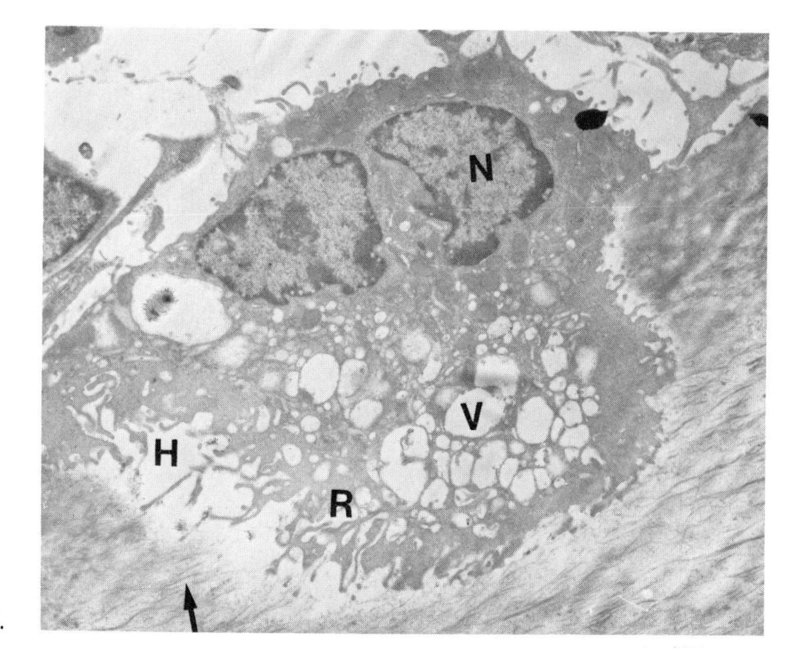

Fig. 7-5. An electron micrograph of a multinucleated (N) osteoclast that is occupying a resorptive cavity or Howship's lacunae (H). The mineralized bone surfaces are irregular, and the demineralized bone shows exposed fibrils within the lacunae (*arrow*). The osteoclast has a large, ruffled border (R) and many smooth vesicles (V) in the cytoplasm. Original magnification × 2800.

believed to be involved in resorption: mitochondria, lysosomes, and a ruffled or brush border. Evidence that mitochondria play a role in the osteoclasts' resorptive activity stems from microscopic data demonstrating that there is a significant increase in the number of electron-dense mitochondrial granules during states of active bone resorption.

Lysosomes are membrane-bound vesicles containing a wide spectrum of acid hydrolase enzymes. These organelles are found in almost all cells and are capable of absorbing, digesting, and breaking down material. Within the osteoclasts, lysosomes have two possible roles: to release enzymes from the cell onto the bone resorptive surface or to coalesce with intracellular vascular debris in order to allow the lysosomal enzymes to degrade their contents.

The ruffled border of the osteoclast is a series of membranous evaginations and invaginations at the resorptive site. This border is in immediate contact with the bone surface to allow the cellular processes to penetrate the bone matrix. Although the precise functional organization and structure of the ruffled border is yet unknown, it is of primary importance to the osteoclast during bone resorption. It is here that the osteoclast will secrete acid, collagenases, pyrophosphatases, and other enzymes to partially decalcify and hydrolyze the organic matrix. Thereafter, bone fragments could be ingested by the cell and incorporated into lysosomes for further digestion and decalcification.

Mechanisms of Bone Resorption

Bone resorption involves the dissolution of mineral crystals along with a breakdown of the bone matrix. The actual mechanisms and sequence of events have been under investigation for years, but the answers remain elusive. Calcium is probably removed before the matrix is degraded, yet these events are closely linked. Morphological data indicate free collagen fibers beneath the ruffled border, but a large amount of decalcified matrix never accumulates. Also, the enzymes involved in bone resorption are not capable of breaking down a fully calcified bone matrix. The mineral deposits must prevent the enzymes from reaching their substrate.

Once bone mineral dissolution has begun, collagenolytic enzymes may act on the insoluble collagen molecules and convert them to large, soluble fragments. Collagenase, cathepsin D, acid protease, acid phosphatase, deoxyribonuclease, and other acid hydrolases are believed to be involved in further degradation of the collagen fragments.

In tissue-culture experiments, it has been demonstrated that resorption is enhanced by acidosis and inhibited by alkalosis. It may be that a low pH is required as an initial step in the mobilization of calcium.

There is still a question as to whether collagen hydrolysis and mineral dissolution are entirely extracellular events. It appears more likely that matrix and mineral are incompletely degraded within the bone fluid compartment and then are taken up by osteoclasts, wherein dissolution and hydrolysis can be completed.

The Osteocyte

The osteocyte should be mentioned for possibly having some resorptive capabilities. It is the most numerous type of bone cell derived from an osteoblast that is no longer synthesizing collagen. These osteocytes were once considered to be dormant, metabolically inactive cells; now there is clear evidence that they can synthesize collagen, control bone mineralization within their lacunae, and possibly carry out bone resorption, referred to as osteocytic osteolysis. Although there is no direct evidence for the latter, in certain disease states, such as hyperparathyroidism, Pagets' disease, or disuse osteoporosis, there is excessive bone resorption. At the light microscopic level, the lacunae appear to be enlarged with ragged borders in many of these cases. Whether this appearance is due to an osteocytic resorptive capability is yet to be answered.

SELECTED REFERENCES

Bornstein P, Byers P: Current Concepts in Collagen Metabolism. Kalamazoo, MI, Upjohn & Co (A Scope Publication), 1980

Eanes ED, Posner AD: Structure and chemistry of bone mineral. In Schraer H (ed): Biological Calcification, pp. 1–26. New York, Appleton-Century-Crofts, 1970

Glimcher MJ, Krane SM: "Structure and Chemistry of Bone Mineral" In Ramachandran GN (ed): Treatise on Collagen, pp. 67–241. New York, Academic Press, 1968

Neuman WF, Neuman MW: The Chemical Dynamics of the Bone Mineral. Chicago, University of Chicago Press, 1958

Trifitt JT, Terepka AR, Neuman WF: A comparative study of the exchange *in vivo* of major constituents of bone mineral. Calcified Tissue Research 2:165, 1968

Vaughan J: The Physiology of Bone. Oxford, Clarendon Press, 1975

Chapter 8

Physiologic Processes in Bone

Roy V. Talmage, Stephen A. Grubb, and Carole J. VanderWiel

GOALS AND OBJECTIVES

Goals: To help the reader understand the process of bone remodeling and the control by bone of plasma calcium concentrations; to provide the background for the interrelationships between these two physiologic processes; and to demonstrate how malfunctions in these processes lead to metabolic bone disease

Objectives: On completion of this unit, and using the text as a standard reference, one should be able to evaluate, describe, list, or recognize the following:

1. The state of calcium in the body
2. Properties of calcium that influence its role in the control of metabolic processes
3. Maintenance of intracellular calcium homeostasis and current concepts of transcellular calcium transport
4. Maturation of bone cells to replenish osteoblasts, osteocytes, and osteoclasts, and how this process can be modified in pathologic situations
5. The process of bone remodeling in the adult, and the link between bone resorption and bone formation
6. Mechanisms for maintenance of constant plasma calcium levels
7. Roles of magnesium and phosphate in bone metabolism

OUTLINE

I. Important physical properties of calcium
   A. Low solubility of vital calcium salts
      1. Calcium carbonate
      2. Calcium phosphate salts and their solubilities
   B. Complexing of calcium by organic compounds

This chapter considers the process of bone remodeling and the role played by bone in calcium homeostasis. These processes, when functioning normally, aid in maintaining constant calcium concentrations in plasma; when altered, they lead to pathologic conditions of the skeleton.

One of the distinguishing characteristics of vertebrates is a living endoskeleton, which contains cells capable of specific metabolic processes that control the inert skeleton, permitting appropriate compensations for the growth of the individual. There are also special problems caused by salts of extremely low solubility within the body, and special adaptations that permit the skeleton to aid in the control of the ionic composition of the extracellular fluid while providing an ever-changing skeletal basis for the attachment of muscles and the support of soft tissues.

To understand the problems of the skeleton, it is necessary to understand the problems all cells have to contend with in regard to the element calcium. From the very origin of life, and millions of years before animals with internal skeletons appeared on earth, the calcium ion was a major factor in the metabolism of cells. It is quite probable that the cellular processes that control bone are merely adaptations of those that all cells use to protect themselves from calcium while making valuable use of this ion for metabolic processes.

IMPORTANT PHYSICAL PROPERTIES OF CALCIUM

The physiologic roles of calcium are well established. Calcium is a necessary component in the basic processes of blood clotting, cellular secretion, mitosis, enzyme activity, membrane structure, and nerve-impulse propagation. Clinically, calcium is important in controlling the strength of the heartbeat. Abnormally low concentrations of this ion permit spontaneous discharges of both sensory and motor fibers in peripheral nerves, leading to tetany; at elevated levels, nerve impulses are blocked, leading to coma. Calcium is also a necessary and important addition to cell membranes, giving strength to these structures and regulating permeability. Finally, calcium salts make up the major inorganic component of our skeletons. These aspects of calcium are based on two physical characteristics that make it both a dangerous ion and, at the same time, one of the most important keys in the regulation of intracellular processes.

Low Solubility of Vital Calcium Salts. The first characteristic of calcium is the insolubility of its primary salts, the anions (phosphates and carbonates), which play a significant biologic role. Although calcium carbonate is found in lower animal forms, including some vertebrates, the internal milieu of man and other mammals contains only the small amount of calcium carbonate associated with hydroxyapatite.

The calcium phosphates (secondary and tertiary) form the basis of the internal skeleton, and their ions circulate freely in controlled amounts within our body fluids. It is the compatibility of these two phases (solid versus liquid) that makes the story of bone physiology an intricate and interesting one. The least soluble of these salts is tertiary calcium phosphate, $Ca_3(PO_4)_2$. It is found in bone as apatite crystals and has a solubility in the order of 10^{-4}M. Another form, secondary calcium phosphate, $CaHPO_4$, has a solubility of greater than 10^{-3}M. The ions of this form circulate in the fluids of the body at approximately one-half saturation. These contrasting solubilities have led to the concept of plasma (and extracellular fluid) as undersaturated with calcium and phosphate ions but considerably supersaturated in respect to the solid phase of bone.

The questions that need to be addressed because of this situation of "undersaturation vs. supersaturation" are as follows: How can this apparent contradiction of physiochemical properties exist in the living mammal, and how is it possible to remodel bone and produce controlled growth under these conditions?

Complexing of Calcium by Organic Compounds. The second important characteristic of calcium is that it is complexed by many organic compounds, particularly proteins. The amount of complexing and its reversibility depends upon the structure of the individual protein and the availability of calcium. As calcium ions are attached to the protein, the three-dimensional conformation and the chemical characteristics of the protein are subject to change. This unique characteristic of calcium is the basis for its role in muscle contraction, for its importance in the structure and permeability of cell membranes, and for its influence on most intracellular metabolic processes.

Some of the important proteins that bind and release calcium in proportion to the ionic concentration of this mineral are (1) calmodulin, which is believed to be an important regulator of intracellular calcium in all cells; (2) troponin, which, on binding calcium onto the thin filament of muscle fibers, permits contraction; and (3) the plasma proteins, which bind calcium proportional to its ionic concentration. Also important is the fact that cell membrane proteins bind calcium in proportion to its concentration in extracellular fluid. Another unique calcium-binding protein is found primarily in the intestinal mucosa and is dependent upon the presence of Vitamin D metabolites.

So important is this relationship between calcium and proteins that it is doubtful if a cell could live if the intracellular calcium ion concentration exceeds 10^{-5}M for any length of time. Therefore, this characteristic of calcium is even more limiting than the insolubility of the calcium phosphate salts discussed above. Without an internal skeleton, animals could maintain an independence from problems of calcium phosphate precipitation by maintaining normal *p*H and concentrations of these ions in the range of 10^{-3}M. However, for normal functioning of the cells, intracellular calcium ion concentration has to be maintained in the range of 10^{-7}M.

A simplified model for intracellular calcium homeostasis is shown in Figure 8-1. This model demonstrates the major difference between the ionic calcium concentration of extracellular fluids and intracellular fluids. It also illustrates the relative impermeability of cell membranes to this divalent ion. Despite its relative impermeability, calcium is continuously entering cells owing to chemical gradients. Thus, cells must have mechanisms to allow precise control of internal ionic calcium concentrations. The uptake and release of calcium by mitochondria may play an important role; however, recent data suggest that the protein calmodulin is central to the control of intracellular calcium. The mechanism of action of calmodulin may relate to control of the calcium "pump." This pump represents a biomechanical mechanism located in the cell membrane for transferring calcium against a chemical gradient out of the cell. Calmodulin, it has been proposed, alters the calcium-dependent ATPase component of this "pump." Furthermore,

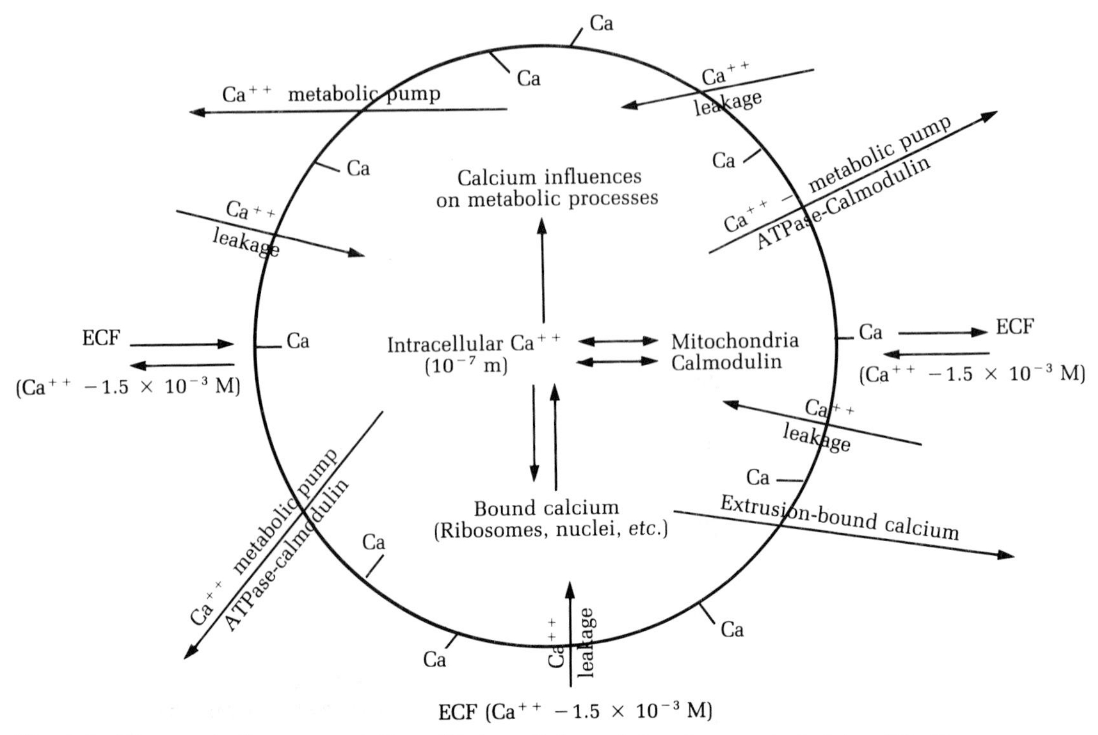

Fig. 8-1. Diagrammatic representation of intracellular calcium homeostasis (simplified).

other protective mechanisms may exist within the cell to provide for the sequestration and excretion of excess calcium.

Obviously, one of the first problems to face a large multicellular organism in regard to calcium is the need to transport this ion rapidly across one or more layers of cells without disturbing cellular processes. A probable solution, based on studies of intestinal absorption of calcium in man and other mammals, has been described as follows:

Calcium is rapidly transported across the mucosal layer of the small intestine, which entails its passage through cells. A similar situation exists in the renal tubule, where calcium is rapidly and almost completely reabsorbed after glomerular filtration (Fig. 8-2). This process involves a more permeable membrane on the lumen side of the cell and a greater concentration of calcium pump activity on the serosal side next to capillaries. Rapid entry, mitochondrial or calmodulin control, and rapid pumping permit transcellular transport without raising the intracellular concentration of this ion above permissible limits.

Some investigators have questioned the adequacy of the method described above for the high-rate transcellular movement of calcium. What would be the energy requirements if all calcium absorbed from food were moved by this procedure? No method for calculating this answer has been devised. An alternate method, supported by minimal evidence, is based on the immediate attachment of calcium ions to intracellular membranes. The non-ionized calcium would then be transferred into microtubules or along the membrane for excretion to the receiving compartment. It is unfortunate that even in the intestine, where the major work on transcellular calcium movement has been centered, the manner by which this process is actually accomplished is unknown.

THE STATE OF CALCIUM IN BODY FLUIDS

With these characteristics of calcium in mind, it is not surprising that the concentration of ionic calcium in the blood must be kept below the solubility product of the appropriate

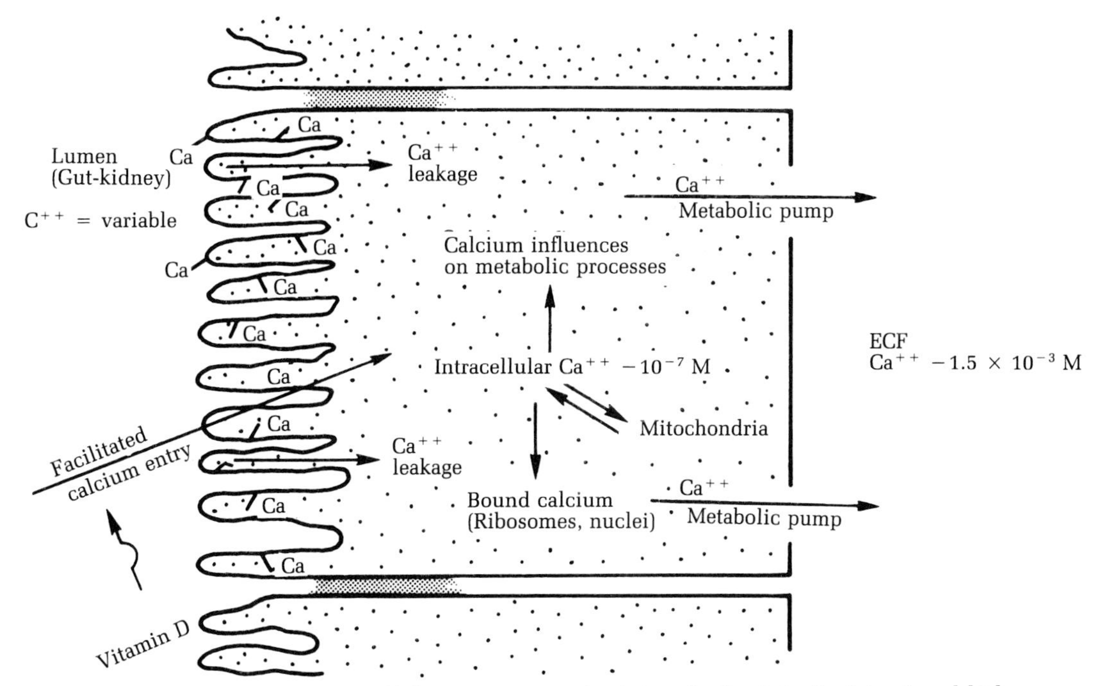

Fig. 8-2. One mechanism for transcellular movement of calcium in the intestinal tract and kidney. One side of the cell membrane is more permeable to calcium; the Ca^{++} metabolic pump is concentrated on the other sides of the cell. Calcium must be moved across the cell without significantly raising the intracellular ion concentration above 1×10^{-7}M.

calcium phosphate salt, and that additional calcium is reversibly complexed with plasma proteins. The total calcium concentration in plasma is approximately 10 mg/100 ml, whereas the ionized portion is slightly greater than 50% of this amount, that is, between 5 and 6 mg per 100 ml, or approximately 1.5×10^{-3}M. The distribution of calcium in plasma is given in Figure 8-3. In extracellular fluids other than blood in which the protein content is low, the calcium content varies between 6 and 7 mg per 100 ml; however, the ionized portion is similar to that in plasma.

A second process of equilibration occurs continuously between calcium ions in extracellular fluid and those complexed to cell membranes. In the final analysis, it is because these equilibrating processes occur that a relative constancy of extracellular calcium concentration is required to prevent major changes in the calcium content of cell membranes. Most clinical problems of either hypo- or hypercalcemia are the result of continued *net* movement of calcium in only one direction between cell membranes and extracellular fluid.

The calcium in blood is by no means stagnant. The normal calcium balance for an average 70-kg man is illustrated in Figure 8-4. These ions are absorbed from the digestive tract, are continuously reabsorbed by the renal tubule after glomerular filtration, enter into the equilibration processes described, and move into and out of the various compartments of bone.

THE APPLICATION OF PHYSICAL PROPERTIES OF CALCIUM TO BONE PHYSIOLOGY

Intracellular control of calcium is only one part of the problem. The extracellular fluids, while undersaturated with $CaHPO_4$, are supersaturated with respect to calcium phosphate salts making up the solid phase of bone [variations of $Ca_3(PO_4)_2$] with which this fluid comes in contact. There must be processes in bone that not only combat this problem of supersaturation, but also, at the same time,

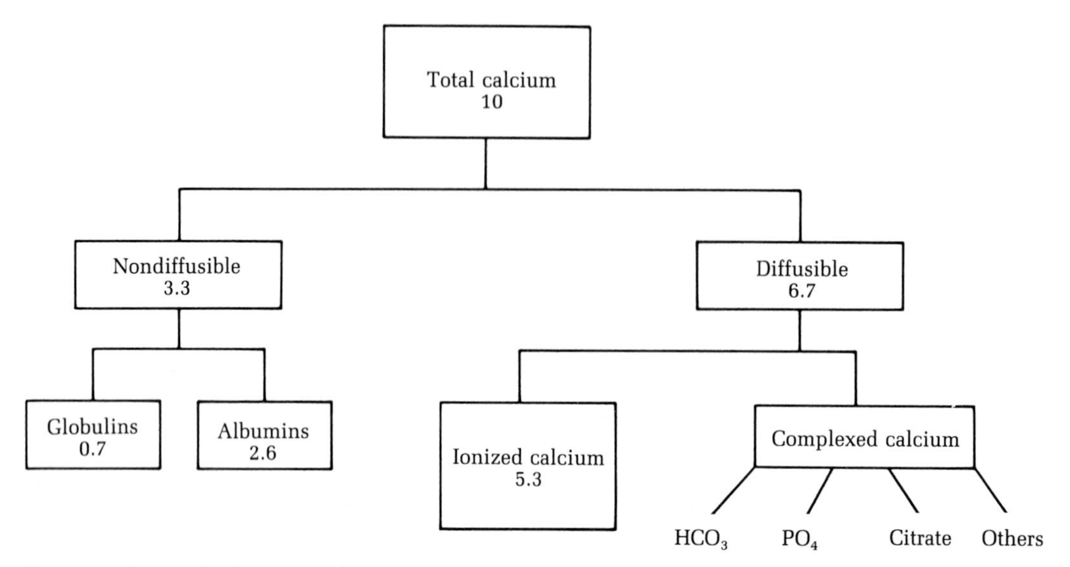

Fig. 8-3. State of calcium in the serum (given as mg/100 ml).

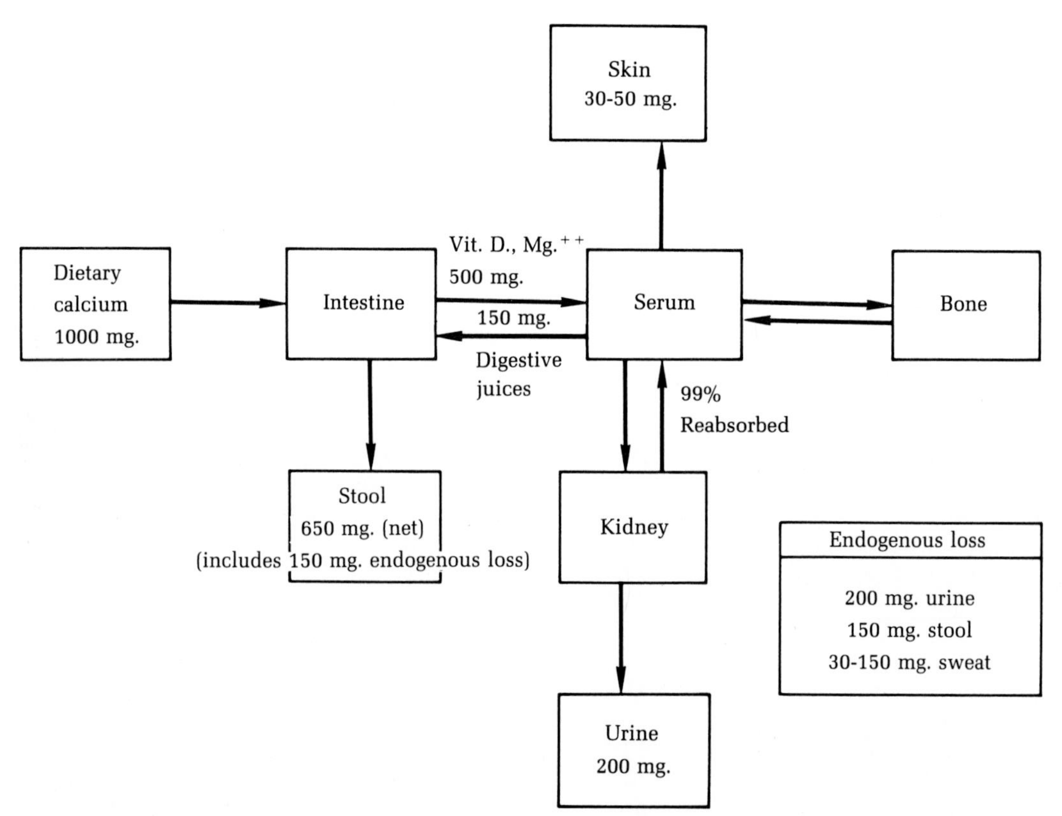

Fig. 8-4. Calcium transfer within body compartments. See Fig. 8-7 for details of calcium movement between serum and bone.

allow both the deposition of additional calcium phosphate salts where needed and the dissolution and transport of calcium phosphate already present. These processes are an integral part of the bone resorption and formation that occur during the modeling and remodeling of bone for growth and repair. Simultaneously, bone tissue must also play a major part in "calcium homeostasis," the maintenance of a constant plasma calcium concentration.

Our concern, therefore, will be how these two processes (bone remodeling and calcium homeostasis) are accomplished within the framework of the unique physical characteristics of calcium. For many years, it was generally accepted by physiologists that one process was merely a reflection of changes in rates in the other: plasma calcium concentrations were said to be controlled by changes in the rate of bone resorption. This concept, although still found in textbooks, is no longer held by most investigators. Therefore, the two processes are presented below as distinct entities with overlapping functions.

Bone Remodeling

The processes of bone remodeling function to replace preexisting bone. These processes permit the "modeling" or reshaping of bone during growth and the replacing of damaged or old bone. Since it is a replacement process, it is not surprising that bone remodeling starts with new loci of bone resorption, followed in place by bone formation. The bone remodeling process occurs as a preordained sequence of bone cell activity, the bone multicellular unit (BMU). This sequence is activated (A) by one of many stimuli, for example, parathyroid hormone. It proceeds through a period of osteoclastic resorption (R) of preexisting bone during which both organic and inorganic components are removed. The sequence then proceeds to formation (F) of new bone by osteoblasts, replacing the bone resorbed. The sequence can be written A→R→F (ARF). In the normal adult, the length (sigma) of one sequence is about 4 months. Theoretically, the replaced bone should exactly equal the amount resorbed. If this does not occur, there will be a net loss of bone. The failure to complete each BMU is now considered to be a primary cause of gradual bone loss with aging.

In the adult, over 95% of bone formation occurs in the BMU. Only in the periosteal envelope does any significant amount of bone formation occur outside of this bone remodeling sequence. However, the rate of periosteal bone formation decreases with age and is a minor component of total bone formation in the adult, so that in the aging person it is essentially impossible to stimulate bone formation without first stimulating bone resorption. In other words, bone formation rates fluctuate with bone resorption rates, allowing for the lag time between bone resorption and the start of formation to replace lost bone.

Hormones, drugs, and physical stresses may appear to affect only one step in the sequence, and they are transitory effects. The so-called transients occur because (1) there is a lag between changes in bone resorption rates and the subsequent parallel effects on formation, and (2) direct effects on preexisting osteoblasts do little other than speed up or slow down the completion of their preordained job. The failure to recognize effects as transients has been a major cause of misinterpretation of clinical tests of new modes of treatment for a variety of metabolic bone diseases.

These bone remodeling processes occur in the growing person as well as in the adult. However, there are two processes that permit increased bone mass during growth. The first of these is longitudinal growth through the activity of the epiphyseal plate and the formation of calcified cartilage. The second process is the far more active rate of bone formation in the periosteal envelope in the young. In the adult, the absence of the former and the reduction in the latter explain why it is essentially impossible to add bone mass after physical maturity. One exception to this generalization may be the effect of muscular exercise on the activity of the periosteal envelope.

Bone remodeling that occurs in compact bone is involved in the replacement of osteons, which is illustrated in Figure 8-5. When a BMU is activated, a cutting cone of osteoclasts forms that proceeds longitudinally, followed by osteoblastic activity, which fills the hole formed by the osteoclasts. Trabecular bone can also be remodeled. The acti-

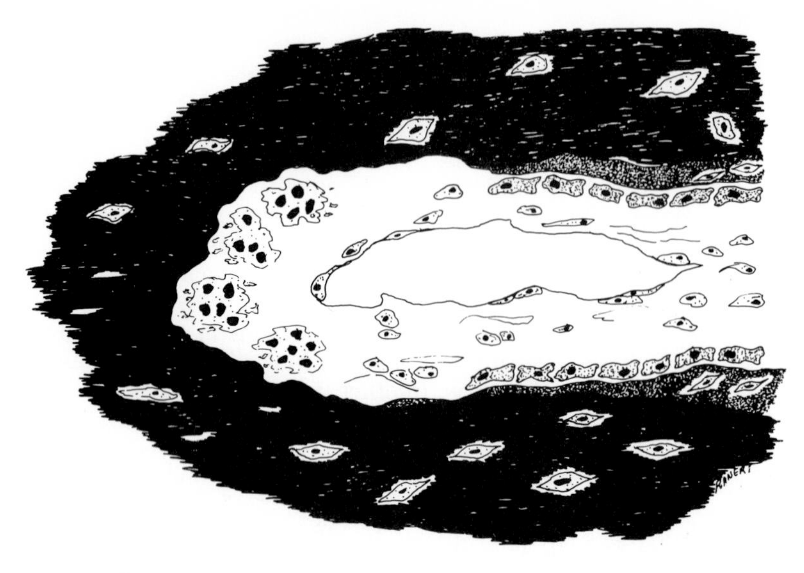

Fig. 8-5. Diagrammatic representation of the remodeling of compact bone. The cutting cone of osteoclasts is followed by a brief inactive phase and osteoblastic bone formation. The total process, one BMU, forms a new Haversian system, theoretically with no net loss of bone.

vation stimuli create loci of osteoclasts on the surface that soon form resorption cavities called Howship's lacunae. The osteoclasts are replaced by osteoblasts that fill in the cavity. This process is visualized diagrammatically in Figure 8-6. It is easy to see that if the BMU is not completed, compact bone will contain larger vascular channels; trabeculae will be reduced in size and, eventually, may even disappear.

The link between bone resorption and bone formation can only be broken to the detriment of the person because it results in "runaway resorption." In pathological situations, this process can occur if resorption loci (Rs) become so numerous that the cutting cones cross and destroy newly developing osteons. A more innocuous break in the sequence occurs when osteoclastic activity is stimulated to the extent that subsequent osteoblastic activity cannot keep up. In both examples, the net effect is bone loss.

The process of bone remodeling requires a continous supply of new cells throughout the life of the person, followed by their appropriate maturation into osteoclasts and osteoblasts. This activation portion of ARF is a major key to the eventual rate of bone resorption.

The primary, if not the only, source of osteoclasts is monocytes derived from the reticuloendothelial system. Not only does the vascular system supply the osteoclast progenitor cells, but agents secreted by the vascular system play a necessary role in the transformation of monocytes into osteoclasts. This area is now under intense experimental investigation as it bears on diseases caused by the lack of osteoclasts, such as osteopetrosis. While it is not yet clear whether these transformed monocytes are capable of multiplying to produce a large population of osteoclast stem cells, a single transfusion of specific blood products can, in experimental genetically induced animal models of osteopetrosis, permanently cure the disease.

Osteoblasts also appear to be derived from stroma cells of the vascular endothelium, although the actual transformation of vascular cells to osteoblast progenitors has yet to be identified owing to the large population of these preosteoblasts and the absence of a disease entity known to result from a failure of cell transformation. The ubiquitous mesenchymal population from which osteoblasts are derived provides a continuous source of new osteoblasts as needed.

The bone remodeling sequence can be influenced by such agents as hormones, vitamins, drugs, and physical stress. None of the above has, as yet, been shown to change the sigma in spite of the fact that the normal 4-month period is extended to more than 2 years

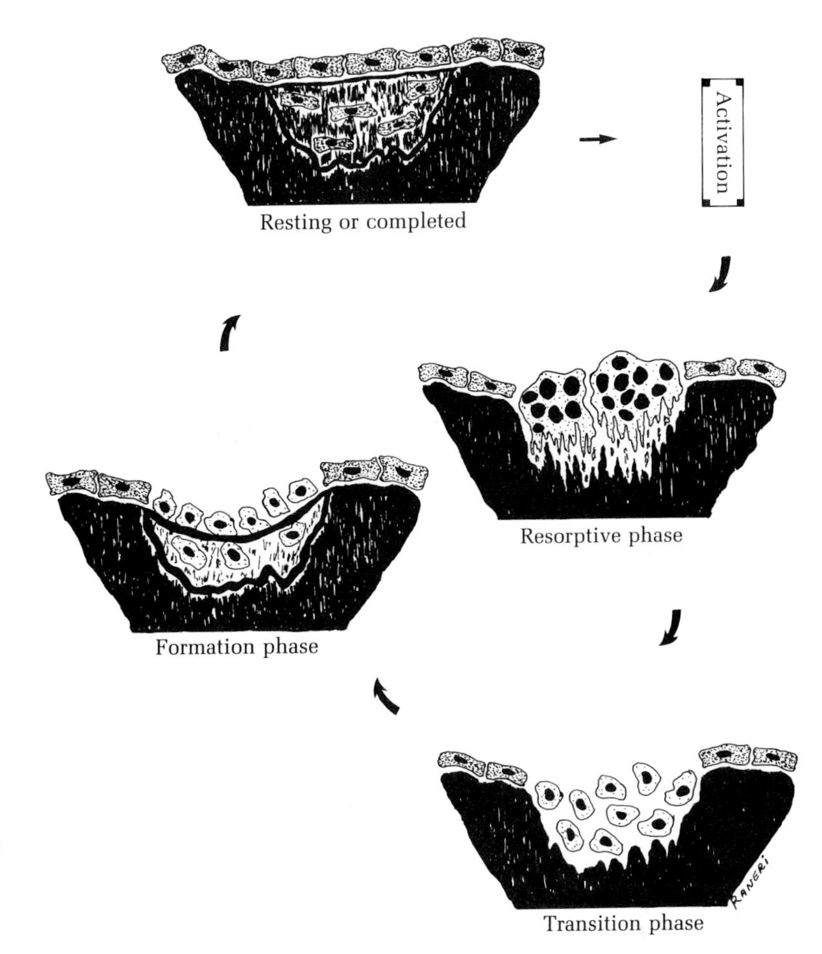

Fig. 8-6. Diagrammatic representation of the remodeling of trabecular bone. The process follows the same pattern as in compact bone except that the osteoclasts move along the surface of bone. Failure to complete the BMU leads to a net loss in size of the trabecula.

in such diseases as osteoporosis. These agents primarily effect the rate at which new sequences are initiated and, secondarily, the activity of individual osteoblasts and osteoclasts. A change in the "A" frequency can have a major long-range effect on bone morphology. The change in activity of cells can temporarily upset the balance between bone resorption and bone formation. In extreme cases, these two changes can break the link between resorption and formation to the detriment of the health of bone. Bone remodeling in disease is discussed in more detail in Chapter 10.

Calcium Homeostasis

For our purposes, calcium homeostasis is defined as the sum total of physiologic processes involved in the regulation of plasma calcium concentrations. Since bone contains approximately 99.9% of the calcium in the body, it would be expected that bone processes should play a major role in controlling the minute fraction of this amount found in body fluids. Despite this relatively small quantity, calcium is maintained in blood at a closely regulated concentration for reasons summarized earlier in this chapter.

In considering the control mechanisms for plasma calcium, it is important to recall that most of the calcium in bone is in the solid phase, consisting of a variety of calcium phosphate compounds, primarily hydroxyapatite. This solid phase, because of its physico-chemical properties, adsorbs calcium and phosphate from any fluid with which it comes into contact. The following section examines the interactions of the large mass of calcium with that in body fluids. Through these processes the concentration of plasma calcium is controlled, dietary calcium is processed, and bone metabolism is influenced.

Rates of Calcium Movement Into and Out of Bone. A general scheme for calcium addition to and loss from the body was provided in Figure 8-4. To complete the picture, estimates for rates of calcium movements between bone and blood are provided in Figure 8-7. For ease of comparison to Figure 8-4, these data are given in mg per day based on a 70-kg adult human. Comparison of these two figures will show that most of the units for calcium transfer are in the range of 200 to 300 mg per day. These values include net calcium absorption from the intestines, net renal calcium excretion, calcium derived from bone resorption, and that lost from blood through bone formation. Even the total amount of ionized calcium found at any one time in the vascular compartment is within this range. The only exception is the quantity of calcium transferred in both directions between blood and the so-called exchangeable fraction of bone that includes calcium in the bone fluid and calcium readily accessible on bone surfaces. It is between these two compartments that the major calcium fluxes occur; they are at least 15 times greater than those transferring calcium between other compartments. These fluxes involve the movement of a minimum of 6 g of calcium per day in each direction between these two compartments and represent a transfer of an amount of calcium equivalent to the total found in blood into and out of this bone compartment at least once every hour. Because of the relative magnitude of these fluxes, it would be naive to conclude that they are not involved in some way in the processes that establish plasma calcium concentrations.

A Postulate to Explain the Rapid Control of Plasma Calcium Concentrations. It is not surprising that the leading postulate states that the primary method of plasma calcium control is control of the rapid calcium fluxes existing between blood and bone. It is agreed by all investigators that calcium influx into

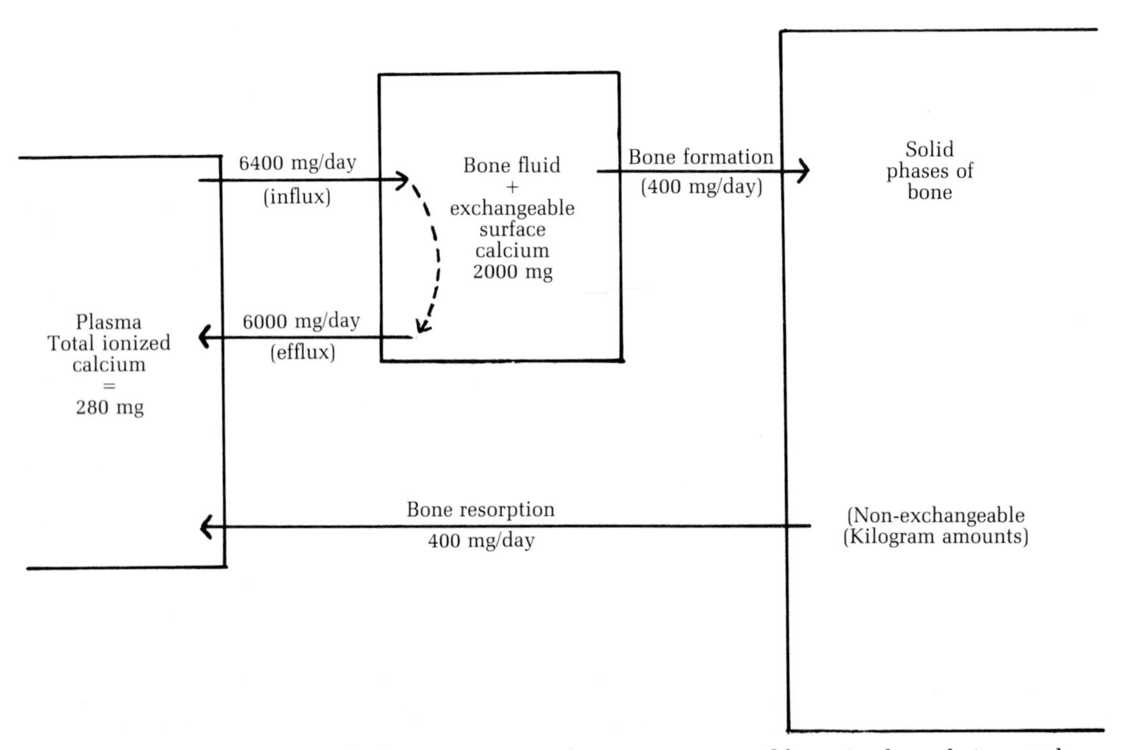

Fig. 8-7. Approximate rates of calcium movement between serum and bone (24-h totals in a 70 kg adult). By far the major calcium movement is the two-way flux between serum and bone fluid.

bone is not metabolically controlled. The rate of passive calcium influx is the result of laws of diffusion and pressure of gradients of calcium ions. The control of calcium fluxes must, therefore, lie in cellular processes that influence and regulate calcium efflux from bone. Small, rapid changes in calcium efflux would buffer plasma calcium against changes in bone remodeling rates, changes in calcium absorption from the intestinal tract, and the small changes that occur in renal tubular reabsorption of calcium. Persistent higher rates of efflux would maintain plasma calcium at elevated levels once calcium influx rates come into equilibrium with efflux rates.

To permit rapid small changes in calcium efflux, a sensitive feedback system between plasma, ionic calcium concentrations, and the controlling mechanism is required; this is accomplished by a negative feedback between plasma calcium ion levels and parathyroid hormone secretion. This hormone induces a rapid elevation of the rate of calcium efflux. Since the system involves bidirectional calcium fluxes tending toward equilibrium, no source of additional calcium is needed when the two fluxes are in equilibrium. The amount needed to make minor adjustments in efflux rates is small compared to the total amount of calcium found in the bone fluid compartment and exchangeable fraction (see Fig. 8-7).

The Bone Fluid Compartment. Physicochemical considerations, particularly the low solubility of calcium phosphate salts in bone, suggested the existence of a fluid compartment in bone in which the ion makeup was different from that of the primary extracellular fluid compartment. A variety of physiological experiments, particularly those involving rates of equilibration of ionized and non-ionized substances, have confirmed the existence of this separate fluid compartment, which is maintained distinct and apart from the extracellular fluid.

Separation of Bone Fluid from the Extracellular Fluid. Although evidence is accumulating to support the existence of a unique bone fluid compartment, determination of the actual site of the interface between it and the primary extracellular fluid compartment has been elusive. Ultrastructural studies of bone have established that active surfaces of bone tissue are covered by a layer of cells such as illustrated diagrammatically in Figure 8-8. These cells are packed tightly and are separated from adjacent cells by narrow, open channels permitting movement of solutions between them. An example of such a cell on the surface of human bone is shown in Figure 8-9. However, in the adult human, approximately 80% of bone surfaces are quiescent (inactive with respect to bone formation). In trabecular bone, and probably also in compact bone, these surfaces are also covered with a layer of cells. Such cells are shown in Figure 8-10; these are thin, fibroblastic-like cells separated from each other by gaps through which solutions can freely flow. Regardless of the type of bone surface, bone-lining cells send protoplasmic extensions into the solid phase of bone, where they make direct contact with similar extensions of buried osteocytes. Quiescent bone surfaces have one distinctive characteristic: the actual bone surface is modified into a rather unique structure called the lamina limitans, which may serve as an interface to slow the passage of water and ions into deeper bone.

The conclusion, although not yet proven, is that bone lining cells and their underlying osteocytes form a metabolic unit for the active transfer of calcium from bone to the extracellular fluid. It is the quiescent surface of bone that, by this theory, would control the rate of calcium efflux from bone, the lining cells serving as message centers while the osteocytes are the actual calcium transfer units. On active surfaces of bone where matrix formation and mineralization occur, the interface between bone fluid and the extracellular fluid is believed to be moved out to the lining cells themselves owing to the absence of the lamina limitans. Thus, active osteoblasts are capable of controlling the extracellular environment needed for the mineralization process while participating in the control of plasma calcium concentrations.

The osteocyte–lining cell units act as "calcium pumps," returning this ion to the extracellular fluid as fast as it filters into the bone fluid compartment. One might compare this situation to a "leaky dike" system separating two bodies of water maintained at different levels by a series of pumps return-

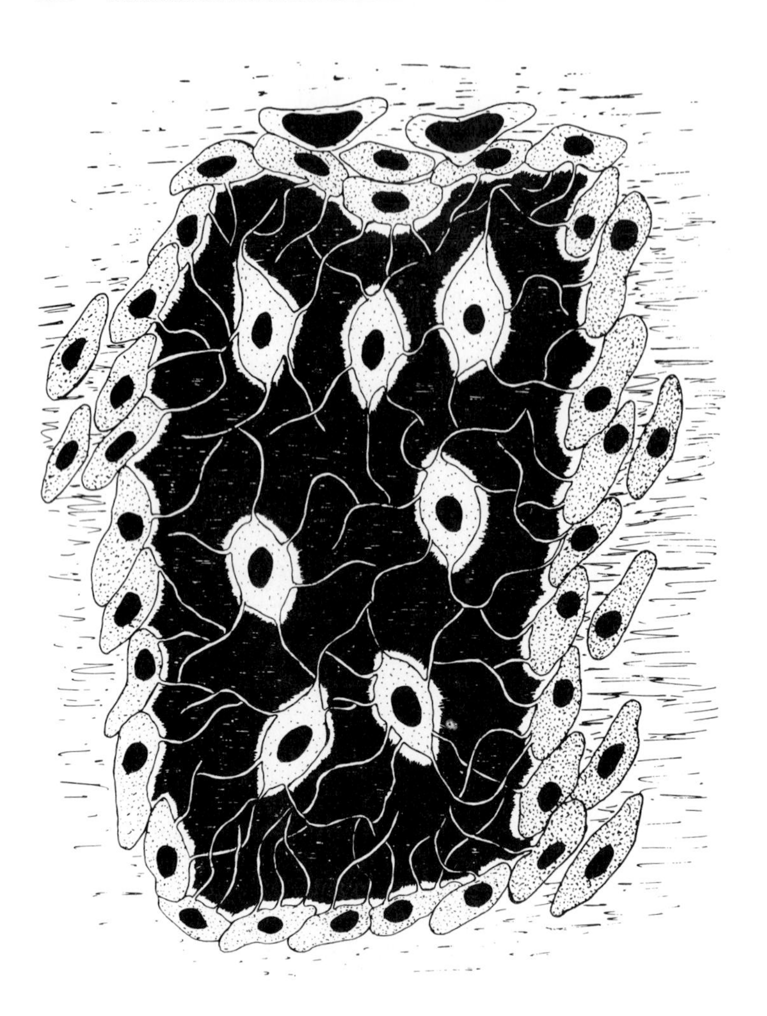

Fig. 8-8. Diagrammatic representation of the cell layer lining active bone surfaces. Narrow channels separate these cells, permitting intercellular diffusion from serum to bone fluid. On active bone surfaces, these cells are believed to form the interface between the bone fluid compartment and the primary extracellular fluid compartment of the body. (Talmage RV: Calcium homeostasis, calcium transport, parathyroid action. Clin Orthop 67:210, 1969)

ing the water to the upper level as fast as it leaks through the dike.

It is suggested that this transcellular calcium movement at the surface of bone is accomplished by metabolic energy, using the identical systems found in intestine and kidney. In all three situations, calcium ions are transported toward the extracellular fluid. The source of the ions for transport by the gut is, primarily, nutritional intake from food; those ions transported through the epithelial lining of the renal tubule come from the glomerular filtrate, and those transported by the lining cell–osteocyte complex of bone come primarily from the calcium entering the bone fluid by diffusion and ion gradients.

The situation in bone differs from that in kidney and intestine in one very important aspect. Intestinal absorption of calcium depends upon a dietary source; renal reabsorption of calcium can never exceed 100% of that filtered by the glomerulus. In bone fluid, however, bone can be called upon if the source from the extracellular fluid is limited. Bone fluid, being in physicochemical equilibrium with the bone crystals and other precipitated forms of calcium phosphate, has an essentially limitless supply of calcium that can be transported toward the extracellular fluid to keep the concentration of calcium at required levels in this fluid.

Contribution by Other Systems to Plasma Calcium Control. Because of the magnitude of the bidirectional calcium fluxes between blood and bone fluid (exchangeable fraction), control of calcium efflux from bone constitutes the primary method for control of plasma calcium concentrations. Three other systems also contribute to this control, either

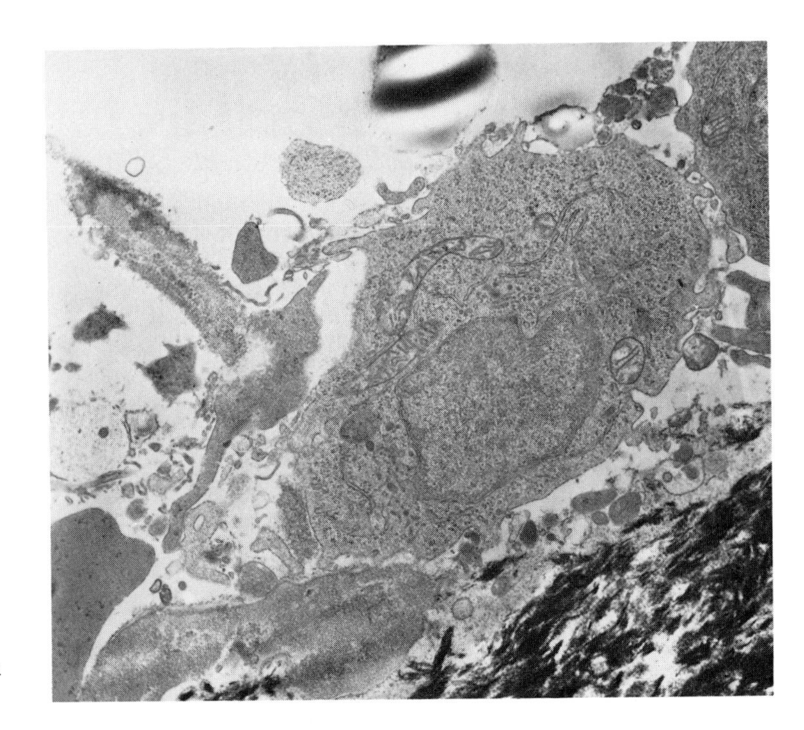

Fig. 8-9. An electron micrograph of an "active" lining cell (osteoblast) on the surface of human trabecular bone. This is an example of cells described in Fig. 8-8 (taken from the iliac crest of a 49-year-old male).

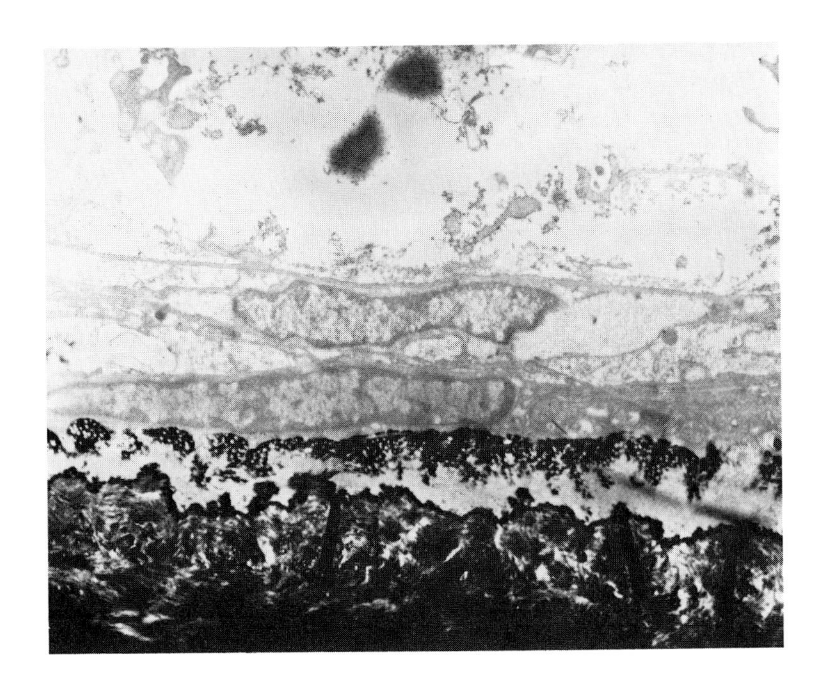

Fig. 8-10. An electron micrograph of lining cells on a quiescent surface (no bone formation in progress) of human trabecular bone. The bone fluid compartment between the lining cell and the bone surface contains a lanthanum staining precipitate (taken from iliac crest of a 28-yr-old female).

increasing or decreasing the metabolic work required in influencing calcium efflux. These three systems involve net calcium absorption from the intestinal tract, changes in rates of renal tubular reabsorption of calcium, and changes in rates of bone resorption. Figure 8-11 summarizes this coordinated activity.

The amount and timing of calcium absorption from the intestine is obviously directly related to the frequency of eating and

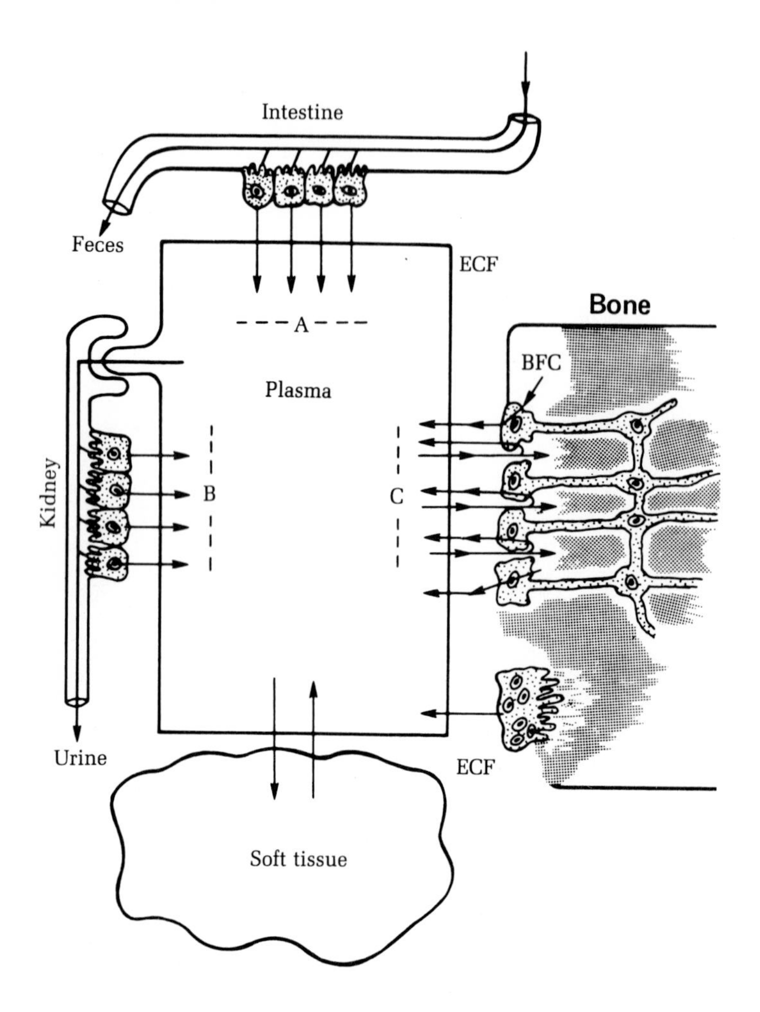

Fig. 8-11. Coordination of the roles played by bone, gut, and kidney in control of plasma calcium concentrations. Bone formation occurs within the primary flux system (C). Bone resorption, represented by the osteoclast, occurs outside of the calcium flux system (D). In the presence of ample dietary calcium, primary control is accomplished by the calcium flux system (C) with the aid of the kidney (B). In the absence of dietary calcium, the source of calcium is shifted from the intestine (A) to the osteoclast (D).

the calcium content of the meal. Because of its irregularity, the rate of intestinal absorption of calcium cannot be used as a method for regulating the level of plasma calcium; it will, however, influence the work of other systems.

The kidney plays a major role in conserving body stores of calcium by reabsorbing nearly 100% of the filtered load. Small increases in this reabsorption rate decrease renal calcium loss slightly but exert little or no influence on setting plasma calcium levels.

Bone resorptive processes transfer calcium directly into extracellular fluid. These rates are relatively low and are almost equaled by bone formation rates with which they are linked. However, in pathological situations in which this link is broken and bone resorption uncontrolled, the rates may become sufficiently high to produce lethal hypercalcemia.

The Calcium-Regulating Hormones. Although all the primary hormone systems in man are capable of indirectly influencing calcium homeostasis, there are only three hormones that are considered to have the control of calcium movements in the body as one of their major functions. These are parathyroid hormone, 1,25-dihydroxycholecalciferol (1,25-vitamin D_3), and calcitonin.

Parathyroid Hormone. Parathyroid hormone rates its importance because of the sensitive negative feedback system between the hormone and the ionized calcium of blood. This importance is magnified by the fact that it works against primary physicochemical pressures tending to lower plasma calcium concentrations. Although it has been demonstrated that the calcium efflux system from bone responds to very low doses of parathyroid hormone, its overall role is complicated by its ability to activate new sequences of bone remodeling, which commence with increased osteoclastic activity.

1,25-Vitamin D_3. The best-established action of 1,25-vitamin D_3, a vitamin D metabolite, is to increase absorption of calcium from the intestinal tract. It also has direct influence on bone processes, including the calcium efflux system, but this influence is not clearly understood and may include a primary effect on the lining cell–osteocyte complex. The amount of the metabolite in circulation is regulated primarily by parathyroid hormone. Because the feedback system for the formation of the metabolite is slow (relative to that for parathyroid hormone), this hormone cannot make rapid adjustments in plasma calcium concentrations and functions primarily to assure the entry of adequate supplies of calcium into the extracellular fluid compartment from the intestines. 1,25-vitamin D_3 is extremely important for the overall control of calcium homeostasis and for the health of bone. Malfunctions involving this metabolite are a major cause of metabolic bone disease.

Calcitonin. The role of this hormone in calcium homeostasis is unresolved. Calcitonin circulates in the blood of humans of all ages, but no pathology can be attributed to its absence or excess. Although it has a feedback system with ionized calcium in blood, it cannot play any significant role in the maintenance of plasma calcium concentrations. It obviously is able to act as an antihypercalcemic agent, but when hypercalcemia becomes a problem, its protective action is easily overridden. In reports from our own research group, we suggest that its physiologic action is related to postprandial handling and processing of dietary calcium. We have proposed that its presence postprandially maintains parathyroid secretion at a time when it would normally be reduced by calcium entering the blood from the digestive tract; through this action, it indirectly (by way of parathyroid hormone) reduces postprandial renal calcium excretion. Finally, it directs additional calcium into bone, possibly into temporary storage for return to blood during intermeal fasting periods. Calcitonin, in pharmacologic doses, reduces osteoclastic action and has proven effective for Paget's disease. Until the physiologic role of this hormone has been delineated, its role in the development and cure of bone diseases will remain in doubt.

The Physiologic Balance Between Bone Remodeling and Calcium Homeostasis

Because bone remodeling and calcium homeostasis are continuous in bone at all times, they must be in balance in the normal person and out of balance in certain disease states. The control of these two systems rests primarily with parathyroid hormone; this hormone and its action are discussed in Chapter 10. Both systems respond to parathyroid hormone because of the ability of the hormone to increase entry of calcium into cells. Since it is suggested that the remodeling process requires sufficient increase in intracellular calcium to stimulate the internal machinery of the cells, the remodeling process has a higher threshold for response and, once activated, it continues until completion of the BMU.

Transcellular transport of calcium, which is the key to calcium homeostasis, is also stimulated by increased calcium entry into those cells forming the cellular interface on the surface of bone. Because of the adequate calcium transfer system in these cells, calcium is pumped out of the vascular or marrow side with little or no effect on other metabolic processes in the cell.

The calcium transport system is therefore the most sensitive to changes in parathyroid hormone titer. In the normal person with adequate calcium intake, bone remodeling and calcium homeostasis are in balance, with primary control being exerted by small changes in the rates of calcium transport.

Sources of Calcium for Serum. In man and other mammals, the maintenance of plasma calcium levels has the highest physiologic priority, even if eventual damage is done to bone. There is an order in which calcium is removed from bone to reduce to a minimum the possibility of such damage. It is for this reason that metabolic bone disease occurs over extended periods and that repair is so difficult by the time damage can be detected.

As described above, the first means of control is the return of calcium to the extracellular fluid as it filters through the open channels between the cells lining bone. In a healthy person with sufficient calcium and a high calcium-to-phosphate ratio in his diet, the maintenance of plasma calcium levels requires little or no participation of bone other than the calcium transfer system at the interface between the extracellular fluid and the bone fluid compartment.

If adequate calcium sources are not available from the diet, the first source from the bone appears to be from the surfaces in contact with bone fluid. As the need for calcium continues, the titer of parathyroid hormone rises, and the rates of bone resorption are increased with a long-term emphasis on the production and activity of osteoclasts. These cells attack all components of bone and, in resorbing bone, add calcium to the extracellular fluid. Unfortunately, when this event occurs, the remodeling sequence is broken, causing eventual damage to bone itself.

OTHER MINERALS INVOLVED IN BONE METABOLISM

In discussing physiologic processes in bone, this chapter has dealt primarily with the relationship of calcium to these processes. However, a few comments should be included as to the role of magnesium and the importance of phosphate.

Magnesium. Magnesium, a divalent cation, belongs to the same family of elements as calcium. However, its salts, are more soluble, and it does not complex to the same degree with organic molecules, although a fractional amount is bound to plasma proteins. There are therefore marked contrasts in the effects of these two ions on metabolic processes.

The total magnesium content of the body is about one fiftieth of that of calcium. In contrast to bone containing 99% of all the calcium in the body, only two thirds the supply of magnesium is in the bone, and half the remainder is in muscle. Magnesium is not readily absorbed through the intestinal mucosa, and its concentration in body fluids is relatively low (0.75×10^{-4}M). In bone it is found only on the surface of crystals. Since ions in this location are in close equilibrium with those in solution, bone magnesium acts as a buffer for plasma concentrations of this ion.

Although diets deficient in magnesium are uncommon, such deficiencies may lead to muscle hyperactivity such as tetany and, in extreme cases, to delirium.

Magnesium is a cofactor for numerous intracellular enzymatic reactions, particularly in various steps of the glycolytic cycle. In many processes it acts as an antagonist to the action of calcium. However, in other reactions the two ions can be exchanged or are synergistic.

No direct hormonal control of magnesium metabolism is known, though it has been implicated in both the control and the action of parathyroid hormone. Although parathyroid hormone affects plasma magnesium concentrations, this effect is considered to be incidental to its control of calcium. It is not known whether there are active metabolic processes for transcellular transport of this ion or the control of its fluid concentration.

Phosphate. Phosphate is too important an ion to be treated lightly, primarily because of its relationship to energy delivery in biochemical processes. Since space does not allow a complete treatise on this ion, only its relationship to calcium will be covered. This relationship starts with the state of phosphate in plasma. Phosphate is one of blood's primary buffers; there are continuous shifts between HPO_4 and H_2PO_4 in plasma, whereas only minute amounts of the trivalent form, PO_4, are present. Most phosphate in plasma (85%) is in the divalent form, HPO_4, which has a relatively soluble calcium phosphate salt, accounting for the fact that plasma is only 50% saturated with calcium phosphate. The inorganic phosphate concentration of plasma averages 4 to 5 mg per 100 ml in humans.

Despite major differences in plasma concentration of phosphate in different species, it is not considered to be under any specific hormonal control. However, it is known to be influenced by most hormones, although these effects are believed to be indirect results of other primary actions of these agents. Examples of these indirect effects are the increased urinary excretion of phosphate following parathyroid hormone injection; its entry into cells after insulin administration; its increased absorption by the gut following vitamin D treatment; and the hypophosphatemic action of calcitonin. Most steroids also affect phosphate metabolism.

Recently, investigators interested in the vitamin D metabolites and in calcitonin action have been giving more attention to the relation of these hormones to phosphate. Reports are now suggesting that a primary concern of these hormones may be phosphate. It is also believed that there may be specific biochemical processes for transporting this ion into and through cells and tissues. It would not be surprising if, during the next few years, the concept of the passive nature of the supply and demand for this ion is replaced by evidence for a rather exact biochemical control.

Obviously, deficiencies in the supply of phosphate would lead to severe health problems; however, in man it is usually oversupplied in the diet. The clinical manifestations of oversupply are subtle and related primarily to the relationship of phosphate to calcium. High plasma phosphate-to-calcium ratios, for whatever reason (e.g., diet or renal damage), produce a low level hyperparathyroidism, the manifestations of which may not appear clinically for years. Hyperparathyroidism caused by renal diseases produces more acute shifts in these ratios. From a nutritional viewpoint, the average person would do well to either reduce his phosphate intake or increase his calcium intake in order to produce a calcium-to-phosphate ratio of 1 or greater.

SELECTED REFERENCES

Baud CA: Submicroscopic structure and functional aspects of the osteocyte. Clin Orthop 56:227, 1968

Canas F et al: Potassium and the milieu interieur of bone. Am J Physiol 2175:117, 1969

McLean FC, Urist MR: Bone, 2nd ed. Chicago, University of Chicago Press, 1967

Neuman WF et al: Cyclic concept in exchange in bone. Calcified Tissue Research 2:262, 1969

Parfitt AM: Integration of skeletal and mineral homeostasis. In DeLuca HF, Frost H (eds): Osteoporosis: Recent Advances in Pathogenesis and Treatment, pp 115–126. Baltimore, University Park Press, 1981.

Talmage RV et al: Evidence for an important physiological role for calcitonin. Proc Natl Acad Sci USA 77:609, 1980

Talmage RV, Meyer RA: Physiological role of parathyroid hormone. In Aurbach GD (ed): Handbook of Physiology, Vol 7, p 344. Washington, American Physiological Society, 1976

VanderWiel CJ, Talmage RV: Comparison of the effects of prostaglandin E_2 and parathyroid hormone on plasma calcium concentrations and osteoclast function. Endocrinology 105:588, 1979

Part Four

PATHOLOGIC PROCESSES IN BONE

Chapter 9

Vascular Disorders of Bone

H. Robert Brashear

GOALS AND OBJECTIVES

Goals: To familiarize the reader with the anatomy and physiology of the circulation of bone, and to introduce him to those clinical conditions associated with pathologic alteration of this blood supply

Objectives: On completion of this unit, and using the text as a standard reference, one should be able to evaluate, describe, list, or recognize the following:

1. Four sources of blood supply to the long bones
2. Three sources of blood supply to the head of the femur
3. Four clinical conditions associated with avascular necrosis of the head of the femur
4. The microscopic and roentgenographic features of avascular necrosis of the femoral head and the correlations between them
5. Four bones that are particularly subject to avascular necrosis
6. The causes and effects of increased circulation to the long bones of a growing child

OUTLINE

I. The anatomy of the circulation of bone
   A. Nutrient artery and its terminal branches
   B. Metaphyseal vessels
   C. Epiphyseal circulation
   D. Periosteal blood supply
   E. Circulation in growing bone versus adult bone
   F. Anatomy of circulation in special areas
      1. The femoral head
      2. The scaphoid
II. The physiology of the circulation of bone
   A. Blood flow
   B. Blood pressure gradients in diaphysis, metaphysis, epiphysis
   C. Effect of interruption of blood flow to bone
      1. Disruption of the periosteal blood supply

2. Disruption of the nutrient artery
3. Disruption of the epiphyseal blood flow

III. The clinical features associated with interruption of the circulation to bone
   A. Avascular necrosis of the femoral head
      1. Traumatic: fracture, dislocation, manipulation
      2. Idiopathic: adult and child
      3. Septic
      4. Hemoglobinopathies
      5. Decompression sickness
      6. Steroid therapy
      7. Collagen disease
   B. Treatment and prognosis in avascular necrosis of the femoral head
   C. Avascular necrosis of other bones
      1. Scaphoid
      2. Talus
   D. Bone infarction

IV. The clinical conditions associated with increased blood flow to bone
   A. Childhood
      1. Arteriovenous fistula
      2. Hemangioma
      3. Infection
   B. Adulthood
      1. Paget's disease
      2. Osteoarthritis

There is a tendency to look upon bone as we see it in the inert laboratory skeleton. Bone, however, is a dynamic living tissue constantly undergoing internal reorganization and remodeling as the result of changing physical and metabolic demands of the body. For this reason, bones are provided with an elaborate vascular system. The needs for a circulatory system within bone are several. The blood supply furnishes access to the great mineral reserves of bone, particularly calcium and phosphorus. The circulation provides nutrition and access to the blood-forming elements of the marrow. An active circulation is needed to maintain the bone-forming and bone-destroying cells that function in the remodeling of bone according to the needs of the body and in its repair when injured.

THE ANATOMY OF THE CIRCULATION OF BONE

There are four sources of blood vessels to a typical long bone: the *nutrient artery*, the *periosteal vessels*, vessels that enter through the many small openings in the *metaphysis*, and vessels that penetrate the bone of the *epiphysis*. The nutrient artery enters the long bone through an oblique canal. The direction of the canal is determined by the relative amount of growth that has occurred at the proximal and distal ends of the bone. Nutrient canals slope away from the knee in the femur, tibia, and fibula and towards the elbow in the radius, ulna, and humerus.

The nutrient artery divides when it reaches the medullary cavity, sending branches in proximal and distal directions. Some of these branches supply the marrow substances; others, coursing close to the endosteal surface, enter the cortex to supply the Haversian systems of the inner two thirds or more of the cortex. Several major branches of the ascending and descending portions of the nutrient artery continue in more or less parallel alignment to the metaphysis. In the growing child, these vessels terminate at the metaphyseal side of the epiphyseal plate, where they participate in enchondral ossification (Fig. 9-1).

Examination of the metaphyseal portions of the long bone of a dried skeleton will reveal numerous small foramina. Through

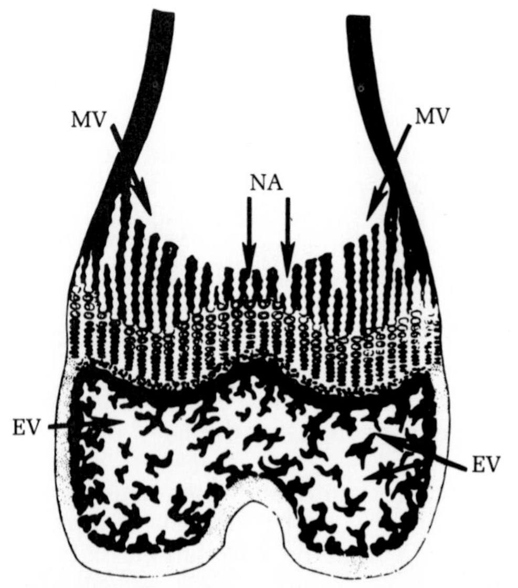

Fig. 9-1. The various sources of blood supply to the epiphyseal plate (*arrows*). NA = vessels derived from the nutrient artery. MV = vessels entering the metaphysis. EV = vessels entering the epiphysis.

these channels pass vessels that enter the marrow cavity to anastomose with vessels derived from the nutrient artery. Most of these metaphyseal channels, however, contain veins that permit egress of blood from the narrow cavity.

In the epiphysis are similar openings that permit the passage of a large number of vessels into and out of the ossification centers. In the growing child, these epiphyseal vessels are isolated from those of the rest of the bone, but with closure and obliteration of the cartilage growth plate there are extensive anastomoses between the epiphyseal vessels, the metaphyseal vessels, and the terminal branches of the nutrient artery. As will be seen later, the femoral head is an exception to this general arrangement.

The fourth source of blood to the long bones is the vasculature of the periosteum. This extensive network of vessels covers the entire length of the shaft. During youth, while the periosteum is actively engaged in circumferential bone growth, the blood supply in this area is much more abundant than it is in the adult. These periosteal vessels send small branches through minute channels in the cortex to supply no more, and possibly less, than the outer third of the cortex.

The circulation of bone in the child differs from that in the adult because of the requirements of growth and the presence of the epiphyseal plate. As the terminal branches of the nutrient artery, augmented peripherally by the metaphyseal vessels, approach the growth plate, they branch repeatedly, always keeping a parallel relationship. When the vessels reach the growth plate, branches are so numerous that there is almost one vessel for every column of cartilage cells. In the final few millimeters before the terminal arteriole reaches the cartilage, it is encased in a tube of enchondral bone. As the vessel extends to the last cartilage cell of the column, it makes an abrupt 180° turn to enter a larger venule. It is here that slowing of the circulation may permit the lodging and proliferation of bacteria to produce an early focus of hematogenous osteomyelitis. The function of this extensive vascular supply on the metaphyseal side of the growth plate is to supply nutrition for the active cells involved in enchondral ossification.

Vessels that enter the epiphyseal ossification center send branches to bone underlying the articular cartilage where, in the child, they participate in the slower-paced enchondral ossification by which the epiphysis enlarges. Other branches of these vessels reach the epiphyseal side of the growth plate and come to lie in small cavities among the resting cartilage cells of the plate. These vessels are extremely important, for they supply the dividing cells of the growth plate and hence are responsible for maintaining longitudinal bone growth.

The *venous drainage* of bone is complex and less well understood than the arterial supply. The arterioles on the metaphyseal side of the growth plate, after making their hairpin turn, enter venules, which in turn open into larger venous sinusoids. These sinusoids empty into a large central vein that has a much greater capacity than the nutrient vein. Much of the outflow from bone is through the many venous channels in the metaphyseal–epiphyseal system.

There are certain areas of bone in which the vascular supply is precarious. These areas are subject to infarction and *avascular necrosis*. Three such regions are the head of the femur, the body of the talus, and the scaphoid. They have the common feature that a very large portion of their total surface is covered with articular cartilage through which vessels do not penetrate. The blood supply for these bones enters through very restricted spaces, and there is limited collateral circulation. When the principal route of the circulation to these bones is interrupted by trauma or disease, necrosis ensues.

The head of the femur receives most of its blood supply from branches of the medial femoral circumflex artery (Fig. 9-2). Only a small and variable amount of the femoral head is nourished by the artery of the ligamentum teres. Branches of the medial circumflex artery enter the capsule of the hip joint near its distal insertion and are directly approximate to the femoral neck as they make their way toward the head. The most prominent vessels are on the posterosuperior aspect of the neck, where they enter the lateral edge of the epiphysis and extend across it to anastomose with the smaller vessels of the ligamentum teres. These large lateral epiphyseal vessels, derived from the medial femoral circumflex artery, are the principal blood supply to the weight-bearing dome of the femoral head. The nutrient artery of the femur

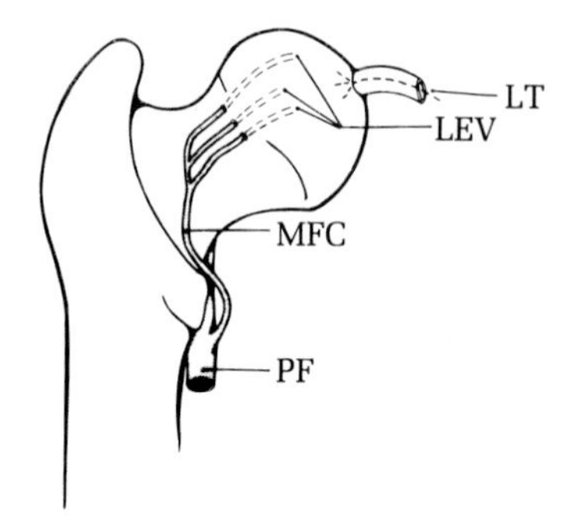

Fig. 9-2. Posterior view of the left hip. The principal blood supply is derived from the medial femoral circumflex artery (MFC) that takes origin from the profunda femoris artery (PF). The branches of the medial circumflex enter the head near the synovial reflection on the articular cartilage and become the lateral epiphyseal vessels (LEV). The vessels of the ligamentum teres (LT) supply only a small part of the femoral head.

sends branches to the metaphysis or neck but does not contribute significantly to the head.

Even after closure of the epiphyseal plate, there is little tendency for anastomosis between the epiphyseal and metaphyseal circulations, which remain essentially independent. Since the greatest portion of the blood supply to the head of the femur is derived from the vessels on the posterior superior surface of the femoral neck, disruption of these vessels, as might be caused by fracture or dislocation, can result in death of the head. Though the lateral epiphyseal vessels supply the bulk of the circulation to the femoral head at all ages, there are variations during the growth period in the relative amount contributed by various sources. For example, during the first 6 years of life, few, if any, vessels are provided by the ligamentum teres.

Much of the surface of the scaphoid bone is covered by articular cartilage, and only a narrow area of its neck, and an even smaller distal portion, are accessible to blood vessels. Fractures across the scaphoid may destroy the meager blood supply to its proximal part. The body of the talus is furnished with blood vessels derived from its inferior surface in the sinus tarsi and from its neck. These vessels are also vulnerable to injury, and necrosis of the body of the talus is a complication of fractures through its neck.

THE PHYSIOLOGY OF THE CIRCULATION OF BONE

Because of the numerous vascular channels in bone and the several sources of its blood supply, the study of the physiology of bone blood flow has been difficult. Attempts to isolate the arterial and venous circulation of a single bone have required such dissection that a true physiologic condition is not obtained. The use of radioisotopes in the study of bone circulation yields indirect information about the rate of flow but furnishes probably the most accurate data available. Such studies suggest that the rate of blood flow through bone is about 10 ml/min per 100 g of wet bone, including its marrow.

The pressure within the marrow cavity of the long bones varies with the systemic blood pressure. The pressure in the diaphysis is much higher than in the epiphysis and is one quarter to one half the systemic blood pressure. The pressure in the metaphysis is less than that in the diaphysis but greater than the epiphyseal pressure. There is a definite pulse pressure in bone and a rhythmical fluctuation in pressure that is synchronous with respiration. In general, a rise in systemic pressure produces elevation of the marrow pressure; however, the injection of epinephrine (Adrenaline), causing a rise in systemic blood pressure, will result in a distinct fall of the marrow pressure. This occurrence is probably due to vasoconstriction of the nutrient artery. A similar restriction of bone blood flow is seen in shock. Muscular activity, by compressing the veins of the periosteum, causes a rise in marrow pressure and exerts a pumping effect on bone circulation.

Disruption of the various components of the blood supply of bone causes changes in the areas served by these components. Obliteration of the periosteal circulation by stripping the periosteum from the shaft results in the death of osteocytes in the outer one quarter to one third of the cortex. This situation occurs in scurvy, in which excessive subperiosteal hemorrhage may lift the periosteum from the shaft. Acute pyogenic infection may do the same. Provided that the remaining circulation is intact, such periosteal stripping causes little harm. The periosteum is stimulated to form new bone, and the dead outer cortical bone is gradually replaced.

Disruption of the nutrient artery in growing bone results in necrosis of a large portion of the marrow and of the inner two thirds of the cortex. This cortical death does not occur in adult bone because the combined epiphyseal–metaphyseal collateral circulation is sufficient to maintain these areas. Loss of circulation in the terminal vessels of the nutrient artery of growing bone results in changes in the epiphyseal plate that interfere not with growth of the cartilage plate but with enchondral ossification. New cartilage continues to form, but it is not resorbed and replaced by bone. Thus, the growth plate becomes thicker until the metaphyseal circulation is restored, which usually occurs very quickly.

Obliteration of the epiphyseal blood supply results in necrosis of the epiphysis and deprives the deeper cartilage cells of the growth plate of their nutrition. Longitudinal growth ceases, and, if collateral circulation is not restored, permanent closure of the epiphyseal plate occurs.

There are a number of clinical conditions that result from alterations in bone circulation. The most common are those associated with avascular necrosis of the femoral head. As noted earlier, a fracture of the neck of the femur may tear the delicate retinacular vessels supplying the head and cause avascular necrosis. Distention of the hip joint capsule by fluid or pus may produce pressures that exceed the epiphyseal marrow pressure and thereby cut off its circulation. At times, usually in male children between the ages of 5 and 10, avascular necrosis of the femoral head develops for no apparent reason. This condition is known as Legg-Calvé-Perthes' disease. One theory of its cause is compression of capsular vessels from swelling due to unrecognized trauma. Other causes of avascular necrosis of the hip include the hemoglobinopathies, such as sickle cell anemia, steroid therapy, caisson disease (the bends), and several connective tissue diseases.

CLINICAL FEATURES ASSOCIATED WITH INTERRUPTION OF THE CIRCULATION TO BONE

Interference with the blood supply to the femoral head results in infarction that may involve the entire head; more frequently, it is limited to one segment. In the infarcted area, there is death of the marrow elements and of the osteocytes. Bone death is recognized histologically by the disappearance of osteocytes from their lacunae. Following infarction, there is an attempt at revascularization that extends inward from the adjacent viable bone. This revascularization process is very slow in the femoral head. The hyperemia of the surrounding bones causes osteoporosis of the living bone, while the infarcted bone retains its density and thus appears whiter or denser on the roentgenogram.

As vessels approach the necrotic area, osteoclastic resorption of the dead bone at the periphery of the infarct may so weaken the femoral head that a portion of it will collapse, resulting in an irregular articular surface that sets the stage for painful degenerative arthritis. The combination of osteoclastic resorption and new bone formation in the revascularized areas creates a roentgenographic appearance of mottled density. When collapse of a segment of necrotic bone occurs, the compression of more bone into a smaller area also produces increased roentgenographic density. Thus, there are several anatomic reasons for the increased density of necrotic bone as seen on the roentgenogram. Though avascular necrosis of the femoral head may occur at any age, there is some variation in the clinical and roentgenographic manifestations of this condition in different age groups. This change is probably due to differences in the pattern of epiphyseal circulation in various age groups as well as in individuals.

In the child, the treatment of avascular necrosis of the femoral head consists of protecting the hip from localized stress concentrations by maintaining complete coverage of the head by the acetabulum. By keeping the hip abducted and internally rotated, the weight is transmitted through the acetabulum over a wide area of the head, which prevents collapse of the bone. It takes from 2 to

3 years for complete reconstitution of the femoral head following avascular necrosis. In the adult, collapse and deformity of the femoral head usually result in severe degenerative arthritis and a painful hip that may require reconstructive surgery.

Avascular necrosis occurs in other bones, particularly the body of the talus, the scaphoid, the lunate, and the head of the second metatarsal. Occasionally, it develops in multiple areas in the same patient. This condition has been found to be a frequent complication of the prolonged steroid therapy used in patients with kidney transplants. Infarction can also occur in the shafts of the long bones, probably from emboli in the nutrient artery, as seen after caisson disease when nitrogen bubbles become entrapped in the marrow vessels. Such marrow infarcts do not result in a significant impairment of function, nor do they cause the damage and collapse seen with infarcts adjacent to joints. On rare occasions, a malignant bone tumor may develop in an area of an old marrow infarct.

CLINICAL CONDITIONS ASSOCIATED WITH INCREASED BLOOD FLOW TO BONE

The clinical conditions associated with increased blood flow to bone are less frequently encountered than those related to deprivation of blood supply. In the child, an increase in the blood flow to a long bone may stimulate longitudinal growth. Since fracture, infection, and arteriovenous fistulae are known to increase bone circulation, these conditions are often associated with overgrowth of the affected bone, sometimes amounting to several centimeters. In the adult, Paget's disease causes a significant increase in the blood flow of the involved bones. This increase may be so extensive, presumably in the form of small arteriovenous shunts, that cardiac output is significantly increased. Degenerative arthritis is associated with hypervascularity of the ends of bones. Whether this is a response to the disease or a factor in its etiology is not known.

As has been pointed out, the flow of blood in bone is significant. A knowledge not only of the general aspects of bone circulation but of the peculiar vascular anatomy in certain areas is important in understanding of the disease processes that affect bone. An awareness of and respect for the blood supply of bone is essential to the proper management of fractures.

SELECTED REFERENCES

Aegerter EE, Kirkpatrick JA Jr: Orthopaedic Diseases, 4th ed., Chap. 10. Philadelphia, W B Saunders, 1975

Trueta J: Studies of the Development and Decay of the Human Frame. Philadelphia, W B Saunders, 1968

Chapter 10

Metabolic Bone Diseases

Stephen A. Grubb and Roy V. Talmage

GOALS AND OBJECTIVES

Goals: To acquaint the reader with the pathologic changes that occur in bone as the result of malfunctions of the two basic bone physiologic processes, namely, (1) the control of calcium fluxes on the surface of bone by the osteocyte–osteoblast lining cell system and (2) the bone remodeling system

Objectives: On completion of this unit, and using the text as the standard reference, one should be able to evaluate, describe, list, or recognize the following:

1. The relationships of the osteocyte–osteoblast lining cell system and the bone remodeling system to bone pathologic processes
2. Pathologic processes occurring in bone as the result of abnormalities in the secretion, metabolism, or action of the calcium-regulating hormones (parathyroid hormone, $1,25(OH)_2D_3$, and calcitonin)
3. Pathologic processes occurring in bone that are a result of other endocrinopathies (hypercortisolism, hyperthyroidism, acromegaly)
4. Pathologic processes occurring in bone that are the result of abnormalities of bone formation (scurvy, osteogenesis imperfecta)
5. Pathologic processes occurring in bone that are the result of abnormal bone resorption (osteopetrosis)
6. Pathologic processes occurring in bone that result in decreased bone mass (postmenopausal osteoporosis)

OUTLINE

I. Generalized pathologic processes in bone

II. Endocrinopathies associated with the calcium-regulating hormones
  A. Hyperparathyroidism
  B. Hypoparathyroidism

- C. Abnormalities associated with $1,25(OH)_2D_3$
- D. Abnormalities associated with calcitonin

III. Other endocrinopathies
- A. Hyperthyroidism
- B. Hypercortisolism
- C. Acromegaly

IV. Malabsorption syndromes
V. Renal disease
VI. Multiple end-organ defects
VII. Abnormalities of bone formation
VIII. Abnormalities of bone resorption
IX. Abnormalities of bone remodeling
X. Postmenopausal osteoporosis

In order to understand the processes that cause generalized bone disease (metabolic bone disease), it is necessary to appreciate the complexity of the interrelationships between the skeletal, renal, gastrointestinal, and endocrine systems presented in the previous chapters as they relate to total calcium homeostasis. These systems are responsible for maintaining plasma calcium and phosphate homeostasis, and also for maintaining skeletal homeostasis. Since all mammals, including man, must maintain plasma calcium concentrations within a narrow range, abnormalities in either of these two homeostatic systems will be manifested in pathologic processes in bone before significant changes in plasma calcium levels occur. Defects in the osteo–renal–gastrointestinal–endocrine (ORGIE) balance will result in the development of generalized bone disease. Also, almost every systemic illness will eventually have an effect on bone. It is our primary goal to convey an understanding of the physiologic processes of bone and how abnormalities within any of these organ systems produce systemic bone disease.

GENERALIZED PATHOLOGIC PROCESSES IN BONE

The two primary physiologic processes of bone, namely, those associated with the osteocyte-lining cell system and with bone remodeling, are discussed in the previous chapter. These physiologic processes are involved with bone resorption and bone formation (modeling and remodeling), control of the internal milieu of the bone fluid compartment, and control of the relationship between bone and plasma ions, of which plasma calcium concentration is the most important. Plasma calcium concentration is very closely controlled, and errors in the controlling physiologic processes are corrected rapidly. The first compensation for these errors occurs within the osteocyte-lining cell system, but the skeletal homeostatic system may also be called on early to maintain plasma calcium levels. Errors in the plasma calcium homeostatic system are manifested clinically and pathologically by the development of metabolic bone disease. On the other hand, errors in the skeletal homeostatic system can lead to pathologic conditions in bone without affecting the maintenance of plasma calcium concentrations for years.

Pathologic processes in bone can result in osteopenia (a decrease in the quantity of bone), osteosclerosis (an increase in the quantity of bone), or abnormalities in the quality of bone (osteomalacia and certain genetic diseases). Metabolic bone disease can produce abnormalities either in the quantity or quality of bone, or both.

Generalized pathologic processes in bone can be best understood by understanding how these processes alter the normal sequence of bone remodeling as described in the previous chapter. Bone remodeling occurs in local groups of osteoblasts and osteoclasts called bone multicellular units (BMU). Each unit has a finite time for the completion of its remodeling cycle (sigma), beginning with the activation of a new unit and progressing through a bone resorptive phase followed by a bone formation phase. The end product is a new osteon replacing resorbed bone. This sequence is presented schematically in Figure 10-1. In normal bone, activation frequency, bone resorption rate, and bone formation rate are relatively constant. For this reason, a steady-state situation develops such that the total amount of bone "missing" due to bone remodeling at any one time is fairly constant. Any changes in the unit activation frequency, resorption rate, or formation rate will alter this steady-state situation. If a new constant rate for activation, resorption, and formation develops, then a new steady state will occur at the end of one sigma.

The time at which the maximal amount

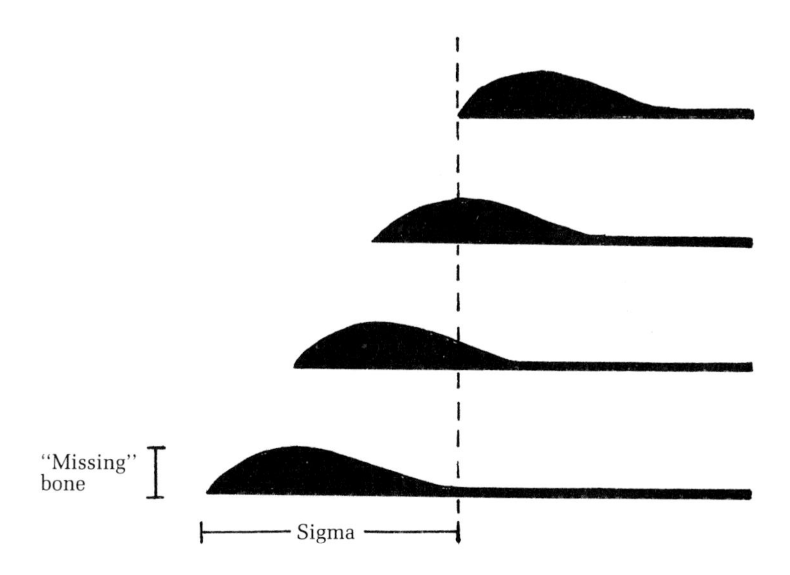

Fig. 10-1. Bone missing due to normal remodeling. The abscissa of each "whale" (BMU) represents the time from the activation of a new unit until a new osteon is formed (approximately 4 mo in a normal adult); the ordinate represents total bone missing at any one time during the sequence. The total amount of bone missing at the steady state is the sum of the bone missing from each of the remodeling units at the end of one sigma. (Irreversible bone loss is represented by the "tail" on each unit.)

of bone is missing in each BMU occurs approximately one third of the way through the cycle. In the adult, bone removed during each sigma is not 100% restored, and a small amount of bone is permanently lost. This gradual bone loss (failure to completely reform bone within each BMU) is a normal phenomenon in humans and accounts for the gradual loss of bone with age.

Pathologic conditions in bone may increase the amount of irreversible bone loss by either increasing the amount of irreversible bone loss in each BMU or by increasing the total number of BMUs. Increases in the irreversible bone loss per BMU can result from (1) overactivity of the osteoclasts so that more bone is resorbed than the "normal" osteoblasts can replace, or (2) a decreased capacity of the osteoblasts to reform the "missing" bone although resorption may be normal. This irreversible bone loss occurs both in cortical and trabecular bone. Except for the vascular spaces, all cortical bone resorbed could theoretically be replaced by the osteoblasts, and greater than 100% of the bone removed in trabecular bone could be replaced; however, in the normal adult, this degree of replacement does not occur. If greater bone formation than bone resorption could be induced, the treatment of osteopenic bone conditions would be greatly enhanced. Permanent increase in bone mass does not normally occur in the adult, except possibly in instances of periosteal bone formation owing to exercise.

A leading cause of metabolic bone disease is an increase in the activation frequency of new remodeling centers. There are many different types of stimuli that lead to this increase, the best studied being parathyroid hormone. Figure 10-2 illustrates the effect of an increase in activation frequency of the remodeling centers from the normal condition, with no change in either the rate of bone resorption or formation in any one of the remodeling centers. In the steady state, there is a net increase in the total amount of bone loss as noted by the vertical line at the end of one sigma in time. If the activation frequency were decreased to normal, the majority of the bone loss that occurred in this condition would be reversible. The only permanent (long-range) damage that would occur would be from the amount of irreversible bone loss. In mild hyperparathyroidism or hyperthyroidism, the net amount of irreversible bone loss is relatively small. In some situations, such as severe hyperparathyroidism, the increase in total bone resorption can be so great that bone formation cannot keep pace, and large quantities of bone can be lost.

Figure 10-3 illustrates the changes that occur when the activation frequency is decreased with no change in the rate of bone resorption or formation. Note that the total amount of bone missing at any one time from the remodeling process is decreased. In the adult, this loss would not lead to a significant change in the amount of bone, although the quality of bone might be affected. This situation could be serious in infancy or early

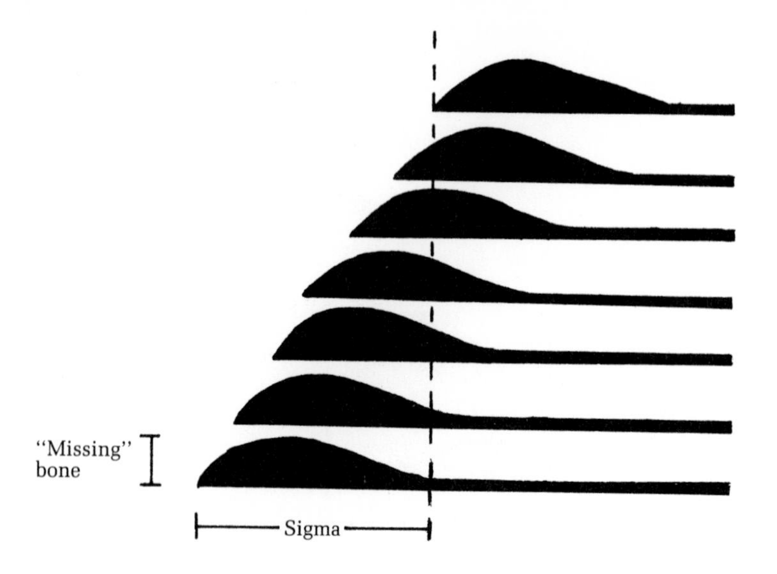

Fig. 10-2. Bone missing due to increased activation frequency. More BMUs are formed, so that more total bone is missing at the end of one sigma.

childhood where the frequency of remodeling centers in the metaphyseal area of long bones determines the efficiency of modeling and proper growth of this area.

Figure 10-4 illustrates the change that would occur if bone formation within each remodeling unit is decreased with little or no change in the bone resorption leading up to this formation. There is a significant lengthening of sigma (the length of the cycle). After the time period equal to one new sigma (*i.e.*, steady state), a cross section of bone through many remodeling units would show a marked decrease in total bone mass. This example of low turnover osteopenia is representative of the majority of patients with postmenopausal osteoporosis. By looking at these graphs, it becomes obvious that further inhibition of the remodeling cycle in low turnover osteoporosis would have a deleterious effect; however, inhibition of the remodeling cycle in high-turnover osteoporosis (as seen in Fig. 10-2) would have a positive effect.

There are hundreds of possible combinations of abnormalities in the bone-remodeling dynamics that could cause changes in total bone mass. In order to understand or

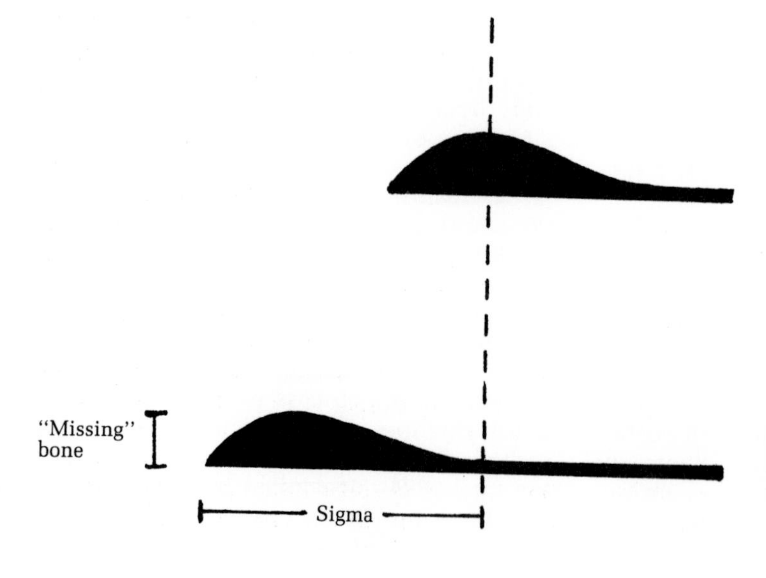

Fig. 10-3. Bone missing due to decreased activation frequecy. Fewer BMUs being formed result in less total bone missing at the end of one sigma.

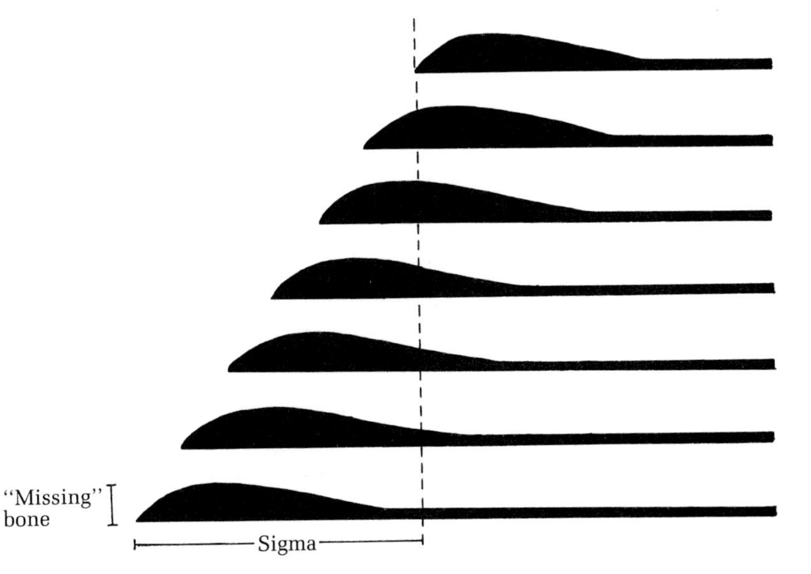

Fig. 10-4. Bone missing due to slowing of the bone formation rate. More total bone is missing due to a greater number of "unfinished" BMUs at the end of one sigma, which is lengthened.

treat metabolic bone diseases, it is important to determine which abnormalities in the BMU are present, which can best be done by histomorphometric analysis of bone biopsies. This technique permits quantification of rates of bone formation, resorption, and activation frequency after labeling of the bone with tetracycline, which serves as a dated fluorescent marker.

In the following sections, various abnormalities that lead to bone disorders are reviewed. These examples are given to demonstrate how abnormalities in the various components of the ORGIE system can cause metabolic bone disease by affecting the remodeling process.

ENDOCRINOPATHIES ASSOCIATED WITH THE CALCIUM-REGULATING HORMONES

Only a few of the endocrinopathies are discussed here, but with those discussed we hope to demonstrate how endocrinopathies can cause abnormal functioning of either the bone remodeling system, the osteocyte–osteoblast lining cell system, or both. We first describe abnormalities associated with the calcium-regulating hormones and then discuss three or four examples of other endocrinopathies.

Hyperparathyroidism. In order to understand the clinical manifestations of oversecretion of parathyroid hormone, one must have a thorough understanding of the function and actions of this hormone as discussed in the previous chapter. It should be reemphasized that all actions of parathyroid hormone are either directly or indirectly involved with maintaining the ionic calcium concentration in the blood. Hyperparathyroidism may result from (1) a primary defect of the parathyroid glands with hypersecretion of parathyroid hormone, as seen in adenomas of the parathyroid gland; (2) secondary causes, as any condition that produces abnormally low ionic plasma calcium levels and thereby stimulates the production of parathyroid hormone; or (3) tertiary conditions in which parathyroid hormone secretion has become autonomous after prolonged stimulation of the parathyroid glands owing to one of the secondary causes of hyperparathyroidism. The abnormalities seen are those that can be predicted from understanding the primary actions of parathyroid hormone. Those actions are (1) to increase the efflux of calcium from bone; (2) to indirectly increase the intestinal calcium absorption; (3) to increase the tubular reabsorption of calcium from the kidney; (4) to increase renal phosphate excretion by decreasing the renal tubular reabsorption of phosphate; and (5) to stimulate the bone remodeling system with an increase in the number of activation centers. The resultant biochemical changes are an increase in plasma calcium, a decrease in plasma phosphate, and an increase in the urinary phosphate excretion. In very mild cases of hyperparathyroidism, the urinary calcium excretion could be low, but in the majority of cases, the ability of the kidney to reabsorb the high calcium load is exceeded and there is a net increase in urinary calcium excretion. The stimulation of the bone remodeling system results primarily in an increase in the number of activation centers, with the rate of bone formation and resorption within any one remodeling center being affected only minimally. Due to the increase in the total number of remodeling centers, there is an increase in the total number of "bites" taken out of the bone at any one time, with an increase in the amount of bone that is missing at any one time. This type of bone loss is illustrated in Figure 10-2. Most of this bone loss is reversible, as previously discussed.

The biochemical and pathologic changes seen in secondary hyperparathyroidism are those that result from a combination of the effects of increased parathyroid hormone secretion and the primary disease.

Hypoparathyroidism. The most common cause of hypoparathyroidism is inadvertent damage or removal of the parathyroids during surgical removal of the thyroid. Congenital hypoparathyroidism and late-onset hypoparathyroidism from other causes in adulthood are rare conditions. In hypoparathyroidism, the clinical findings are (1) a decrease in the plasma calcium; (2) an increase in plasma phosphate; (3) an increase in renal tubular reabsorption of phosphate; and (4) a decrease in the activation frequency of the bone remodeling centers.

When hypoparathyroidism occurs in adulthood, there are very few abnormalities in bone, even though there are fewer "bites" taken out of bone by the remodeling centers. In addition, the majority of these patients are treated with relatively high-dose vitamin D to maintain their plasma calcium levels, which can, in itself, stimulate the bone remodeling system.

Abnormalities Associated With Vitamin D. It appears that the primary function of vitamin D ($1,25[OH]_2D_3$) is to maintain skeletal homeostasis. Secondarily, this vitamin is important for the maintenance of plasma calcium homeostasis. Vitamin D is important for maintaining adequate quantities of calcium and phosphorus for bone formation through its effects on the kidney and the gut. In addition, it may have a direct effect on bone formation. Proper functioning of the vitamin D system is necessary for parathyroid hormone to maintain plasma calcium effectively, although drops in the plasma calcium occur only with severe vitamin D depletion. It appears that only minute amounts of vitamin D are necessary for parathyroid hormone to carry out its actions on bone and kidney.

The primary effect of a lack of vitamin D is a decrease in the calcification of newly formed matrix. In addition, the rate of bone formation is decreaaed. The net result is less total bone and a marked change in the quality of bone. Two clinical diseases associated with inadequate amounts of vitamin D are osteomalacia and rickets, which may also be abetted by any condition resulting in a low plasma phosphate. The necessity of maintaining plasma calcium is so important to the organism, and the calcium conservation mechanisms are so great that only in severe calcium depletion is calcification of bone inhibited. The net result of calcium depletion is secondary hyperparathyroidism, although inadequate amounts of vitamin D and phosphate result in decreased calcification of newly formed matrix.

Osteomalacia is a disorder in which there is a relative increase in the amount of osteoid in bone owing to a decrease in primary mineralization. Rickets is a disease with impaired mineralization of cartilage in the growth plate, leading to arrest in the formation of the primary spongiosa during enchondral ossification. Therefore, rickets affects only the initial formation of enchondral bone. Rickets occurs prior to the closure of the epiphyseal plate, whereas osteomalacia can occur either before or after closure of the plate; therefore, rickets is confined to children, but osteomalacia can occur in either children or adults.

The primary reason for lack of enchondral bone formation in rickets is defective mineralization of the epiphyseal plate in the zone of calcification with continued cellular hypertrophy in this zone. Calcification is necessary to prevent development of additional hypertrophy of cells and to allow ingrowth of vessels into the plate area. The ingrowth of vessels brings osteoprogenitor cells to the area for formation of the first enchondral bone. In rickets, there is not only inhibition of growth but also progressive osseous deformity, probably more a result of abnormal growth at the epiphysel plates than of bending of the bones, although both may be involved. The clinical manifestations of osteomalacia are bone pain, tenderness, and fractures as the disease develops. In the severe forms of the disease, muscular weakness is often an early finding. Symptoms are usually minimal, and histologic examination is frequently necessary to provide the definitive diagnosis. Unique areas called Looser's zones can be identified roentgenographically in long bones related to areas of stress. These zones are caused by rapid resorption and slow mineralization; they are generally perpendicular to the bone cortex and may be surrounded by a collar of callus.

Abnormalities Associated With Calcitonin. The precise physiologic function of calcitonin is not yet known, and no specific metabolic bone disease has been attributed to either its overactivity or underactivity. Calcitonin is primarily involved with the "fine tuning" of the entire ORGIE system. As the integrator of this system, it is probably important in maintaining an appropriate balance between the skeletal homeostatic and the plasma calcium homeostatic systems. Calcitonin appears to be especially important in times of increased calcium demand, as indicated by the presence of higher calcitonin levels in neonates and children, and during pregnancy and lactation. In addition, levels are higher in men than in women, and lower in osteoporotic subjects than in nonosteoporotic subjects.

Recent experimental evidence suggests that the primary role of calcitonin is routing dietary calcium to certain portions of bone and conserving dietary calcium, particularly during periods of relatively low calcium intake. Abnormalities of the regulating system between the various components of the ORGIE system may be important in the production of osteopenic states. Calcitonin, as a primary coordinator of the various components of this system, may prove to play an important role in the pathogenesis of some osteopenic conditions.

OTHER ENDOCRINOPATHIES

Other endocrinopathies are presented briefly to demonstrate how systemic events can cause generalized bone disease and have different effects on the two basic physiologic bone systems: the osteocyte–osteoblast lining cell system and the bone remodeling system.

Hyperthyroidism. Hyperthyroidism produces a high-turnover-type osteopenia from increased activity of the remodeling system. High-turnover osteopenia occurs in both hyperthyroidism and hyperparathyroidism, although the abnormalities of calcium homeostasis seen in hyperparathyroidism do not occur in hyperthyroidism. Thyroid hormone probably also affects the osteocyte–osteoblast lining cell system, but this system is able to adjust adequately to these effects, and no net abnormality occurs.

Hypercortisolism. The bone changes following either long-term oversecretion of cortisol (Cushing's disease) or excessive corticosteroid administration are the same, namely, severe osteopenia. Steroids produce an increase in bone turnover and a high-turnover-type osteopenia, which is theorized to occur from steroid inhibition of the osteocyte–osteoblast lining cell system, with a resultant increase in parathyroid hormone secretion and bone turnover. Long-term administration of steroids or long-term oversecretion of cortisol results in a low-turnover-type osteopenia. The reasons for these differences in bone turnover states are not known.

Acromegaly. Acromegaly, which results from increased secretion of growth hormone in adulthood, produces a high-turnover osteopenia and, in addition, stimulates the periosteal envelope of bone, causing an increase in bone diameter. This is one of the very few conditions in which the periosteal bone envelope seems to be stimulated excessively in the adult. Other endocrinopathies do not have such a marked effect on this element of the bone modeling system.

MALABSORPTION SYNDROMES

Abnormalities of the gastrointestinal system can result in osteomalacia, rickets, or secondary hyperparathyroidism from lack of absorption of phosphate, vitamin D or calcium. In addition, subtle abnormalities of the integrators of gastrointestinal hormones and the calcium-regulating hormones may play a role in the development of certain osteopenic conditions; however, as yet no specific bone disease has been attributed to abnormalities in the integrators of the gastrointestinal hormones and the calcium-regulating hormones.

RENAL DISEASE

Abnormalities of renal function can produce profound bone disease. The bone disease seen in renal failure is called renal osteodystrophy. The clinical picture in the earlier stages of renal failure is primarily due to the action of parathyroid hormone on the osteocyte–osteoblast lining cell system, which is probably a result of decreased phosphate excretion by the kidney. With decreased phosphate excretion, there is elevation of plasma phosphate and complexing of calcium and phosphate in the bone fluid. As a result of this complexing, increasing amounts of parathyroid hormone are required to move the same amount of calcium from bone in order to maintain the plasma calcium at a constant level. The inhibition of the osteocyte–osteoblast lining cell system may also be caused by other inhibitors present in the uremic state. Owing to the elevated parathyroid hormone levels, there is an increase in the activation frequencies of the bone remodeling system and an increase in bone turnover.

Later in renal disease, the diminished ability of the kidney to hydroxylate vitamin D leads to a decrease in the circulating levels of $1,25(OH)_2D_3$. This deficiency of $1,25(OH)_2D_3$ produces a decrease in intestinal calcium absorption. Calcification of osteoid is inhibited owing to the deficiency of $1,25(OH)_2D_3$, and probably also owing to metabolic acidosis and other circulating inhibitors of mineralization that occur in the uremic state.

In late renal failure, when the glomerular filtration rate falls below 25% of normal, increased secretion of parathyroid hormone is no longer able to maintain normal phosphate levels, and the serum phosphate increases. Mineralization of previously osteomalacic bone then occurs, and osteosclerosis develops.

The net effect of renal disease on bone, then, is a combination of secondary hyperparathyroidism, osteomalacia, and osteosclerosis. Renal osteodystrophy is a complex disease with many pathologic features in bone that exemplify the dichotomy between the osteocyte–osteoblast lining cell system and the bone remodeling system.

MULTIPLE END-ORGAN DEFECTS

The lack of responsiveness of end-organs to a specific hormone can cause a clinical picture similar to the one seen in undersecretion of that hormone. Pseudohypoparathyroidism is a prime example of a metabolic bone disease resulting from multiple end-organ refractoriness at the biochemical level. Owing to the inability of bone and kidney to respond to parathyroid hormone, hypocalcemia and hyperphosphatemia occur in spite of elevated parathyroid levels. Patients with this disorder have a characteristic clinical appearance that includes short stature, round facies, and shortened fourth metacarpals.

ABNORMALITIES OF BONE FORMATION

Any systemic disease resulting in abnormal formation of the three basic elements of bone (collagen, ground substance, and hydroxyapatite) will result in abnormal bone formation. Examples of clinical diseases resulting from abnormal formation of the three basic bone elements are scurvy (absence of vitamin C), which results in inhibition of normal collagen formation; the mucopolysaccaridoses, which result in abnormal formation of ground substance; and osteomalacia or rickets, which result in abnormal formation of hydroxyapatite.

Osteogenesis imperfecta is an example of a disease resulting from the inability to form normal bone, owing primarily to a defect in osteoblastic function. With the formation of abnormal bone, there is a secondary, though not precisely understood, increase in the resorption of bone with a secondary increase in bone turnover. This process results in a marked loss of bone, with a significant lack of growth of bone in length, multiple fractures, and multiple deformities secondary to these fractures. Other abnormalities associated with abnormal collagen formation are evident, such as blue sclerae, abnormalities of tooth formation and skull shape, and occasional deafness.

ABNORMALITIES OF BONE RESORPTION

As discussed throughout this chapter, changes in the dynamics of bone resorption are seen in all metabolic bone diseases. However, one disease, osteopetrosis, results completely from the lack of osteoclastic resorption; abnormalities in the concentrations of the plasma calcium are not a factor. In this disease there is no bone remodeling owing to the absence of osteoclasts, which leads to thickened bones and exclusion of the marrow cavity. Associated with the inability to model and remodel bone is short stature. Owing to absence of marrow elements and the resultant immunoincompetency, patients with osteopetrosis are usually very susceptible to infectious diseases. This disease has recently been cured in mice and, in isolated instances, in humans with transfusions of the bone marrow elements necessary for the development of osteoclast progenitor cells.

ABNORMALITIES OF BONE REMODELING

Abnormalities of bone remodeling occur in all metabolic bone diseases; however, these abnormalities are secondary to other systemic factors. In Paget's disease, the primary defect is in the remodeling system itself. This disease, which recent evidence suggests may be caused by a virus, is frequently not a generalized bone disease but often involves only one or several bones. It is characterized by massive turnover of bone in localized areas with marked increase in both bone resorption and bone formation. Owing to the rapid turnover, the bone formed is immature bone. In patients with Paget's disease, the serum calcium and phosphorus are usually normal, but there is a marked increase in alkaline phosphatase, which reflects the increase in bone formation. In the bones affected, there may be either little change in the shape of the bone or very marked change in the bone contour resulting from both the lack of appropriate remodeling and the change in the quality of the bone.

POSTMENOPAUSAL OSTEOPOROSIS

By far the most common metabolic bone disease is postmenopausal osteoporosis, which costs our society billions of dollars every year and is responsible for tremendous morbidity and mortality. The exact etiology of this disease is not yet known. The fact that there is a rapid increase in bone loss after the menopause has led many clinicians to feel that this condition is caused primarily by loss of estrogens. However, all postmenopausal women have lost estrogens but not all develop postmenopausal osteoporosis. Dietary calcium deficiency has also been implicated, but again, there are women who have very low calcium intakes who do not develop postmenopausal osteoporosis. Perhaps as we better understand the normal physiologic processes in bone, we will be able to understand the pathophysiologic mechanisms that occur in the postmenopausal osteoporotic population.

SELECTED REFERENCES

DeGroot LJ, Cahill GF Jr, Odell WD et al: Endocrinology, Vol 2, pp. 551–906. New York, Grune & Stratton, 1979

Frost HM (ed): Bone Remodeling and Its Relationship to Metabolic Bone Diseases. Springfield, Charles C Thomas, 1973

Parfitt AM, Duncan H: Metabolic bone disease affecting the spine. In Rothman RH, Simeone FA (ed): The Spine, Vol 2, pp. 599–720. Philadelphia, WB Saunders, 1975

Chapter 11

Infections of Bones and Joints

H. Robert Brashear and Frank C. Wilson

GOALS AND OBJECTIVES

Goals: To familiarize the reader with infectious diseases of bones and joints, their pathogenesis, bacteriology, morbid anatomy, clinical course, and complications

Objectives: Upon completion of this unit, using the text as a standard reference, one should be able to describe, list or recognize the following:

1. Three methods by which osteomyelitis may be acquired
2. Microscopic structural features of bone that enhance infection
3. Three cellular responses of bone cells to infection
4. The site within bone of the primary focus of hematogenous osteomyelitis in childhood, and the vascular pathways by which organisms gain this site
5. The spread of bone infection from the original site
6. The pathogenesis of sequestra and involucra
7. Three possible clinical courses of acute osteomyelitis
8. Five complications of hematogenous osteomyelitis
9. Three causes of exogenous osteomyelitis
10. Five factors influencing the likelihood of osteomyelitis following an open fracture or penetrating wound
11. Two pathologic features common to exogenous osteomyelitis
12. Three methods by which joints may become infected
13. The most common organism causing infectious arthritis in children
14. The two organisms that most frequently cause infectious arthritis in adults
15. The microscopic changes of infectious arthritis in synovium and cartilage

16. The two most important laboratory studies in the diagnosis of infectious arthritis
17. Four clinical features of infectious arthritis
18. Three characteristics of joint fluid in infectious arthritis
19. Three complications of infectious arthritis

OUTLINE

I. Osteomyelitis
   A. Pathways of infection
   B. Pathologic features of bone infection
      1. The inflammatory response
      2. Host defense mechanisms
      3. Unique features of bone infection
   C. Hematogenous osteomyelitis
      1. Pathogenesis
      2. Bacteriology
      3. Pathology
      4. Roentgenographic manifestations
      5. Clinical course
      6. Complications
      7. Treatment
   D. Exogenous osteomyelitis
      1. Etiology
      2. Determining factors
      3. Pathology
      4. Clinical course
II. Infectious arthritis
   A. Etiology
   B. Bacteriology
   C. Pathogenesis
   D. Clinical features
   E. Diagnosis
   F. Treatment
   G. Complications

OSTEOMYELITIS

Osteomyelitis is infection of bone. The prefix *osteo* refers to bony tissue and *myelo* designates the marrow cavity, both of which are usually involved in this disease. Any pathogenic bacteria or fungi (and, rarely, even viruses) may cause osteomyelitis. Pathogenic agents reach bone in one of three ways: by way of the bloodstream from a focus of infection elsewhere in the body (hematogenous osteomyelitis); through their introduction directly into the bone from the external environment (exogenous osteomyelitis), as may occur following open fractures, penetrating wounds, or surgical procedures; or by direct extension from adjacent soft tissue.

The structure of bone (see Chap. 6) presents certain problems in the control of the spread of infection that are unique to this tissue. Because of the physical disability it produces and the expense and difficulty of successful treatment, bone infection is a major medical problem.

Pathologic Features of Bone Infection

Regardless of the source of the pathogen, many features of bone infection are similar to those of infection in other tissues. An inflammatory response, provoked by the invading organism and its products, leads to the production of chemotactic substances, which in turn attract leukocytes and stimulate phagocytosis. Toxins produced by the organisms cause the death of host cells, necrosis of tissue, hemolysis of red blood cells, localized thrombosis, and the breakdown of host proteins. In the case of a bacterial pathogen, antigens in the bacterial cell wall, as well as other foreign proteins produced or released by the organisms, stimulate the host's immune system. Lymphocytes respond by producing clones of plasma cells, which in turn manufacture specific antibodies to these bacterial products. The antibodies, in the form of immunoglobulins, combine with and neutralize the toxic products of the bacteria, attach to the bacterial cell walls, and stimulate the host complement system to aid in the destruction of the invader. The success of the host in limiting the infection is related to several factors that include the number and virulence of the offending organisms and the rapidity and adequacy of the host response (host resistance). An immediate and adequate response to a small inoculum of organisms of low virulence usually leads to rapid elimination of the infection. On the other hand, a delayed or inadequate response by the host to a large inoculum of virulent bacteria may lead to overwhelming infection and death.

These features are common to all infections. Bone, however, provides an environment that significantly alters the interaction between bacteria and host defenses in favor of the invader. Bone contains numerous microscopic channels, the walls of which are impermeable to such host defenses as the large molecules of immunoglobulins. Bacteria, once gaining a foothold in these minute channels, may be isolated from both the cellular and chemical elements of the host defenses and free to proliferate unimpeded. The microcirculation of bone within these channels is highly vulnerable to bacterial toxins, which may produce local thrombosis of these small vessels leading to the death of bone in the vicinity of the infection, which further impedes access by host defenses.

Bone cells have a limited capacity to respond to infection. Very early in the disease process, osteoclasts are activated and resorption of bone occurs. Resorption of the infected bone is helpful in that isolated channels are opened and host defenses may gain access to the otherwise protected bacteria. On the other hand, resorption is harmful in that the structural integrity of bone is weakened and pathologic fracture may result. Infection also stimulates bone formation in most instances, but this process lags behind bone destruction. The new bone formed as the result of infection is immature, woven, or fiber bone and is a hurried response to the loss of skeletal tissue resulting from osteoclastic resorption. Necrosis, or death of bone cells, occurs when infection destroys the precarious blood supply to these cells.

Bone resorption, bone formation, and necrosis are tissue responses seen in varying degrees in all bone infections. There are significant differences, however, in the degree and nature of the response in bone infections of hematogenous origin and in the exogenous form of osteomyelitis; therefore, these conditions are considered separately.

Hematogenous Osteomyelitis

Transient bacteremia is a common day-to-day occurrence. The source of the organisms may be any small focus such as a boil, a minor skin infection, or an upper respiratory infection. Bacteria released into the bloodstream are usually removed quickly by the macrophage systems in the liver, spleen, and lung. Occasionally, small clumps of blood-borne bacteria lodge in the vulnerable areas of bone, and osteomyelitis results.

Bacteriology. Any bacterium may spread by the bloodstream to bone. By far the most common organism responsible for hematogenous osteomyelitis is *Staphylococcus aureus. Streptococcus* and *Haemophilus influenzae* bone infections are seen in young children, and patients with sickle cell anemia are prone to bone infection by *Salmonella*. In older adults and in patients with compromised immune systems, bone infection by gram-negative organisms is common. Tubercle bacilli and fungi may also cause hematogenous osteomyelitis.

Pathology. In classical hematogenous osteomyelitis of childhood, organisms in the bloodstream gain access to bone by way of the nutrient artery and pass through branches of this vessel to the metaphysis (Fig. 11-1). Here, terminal vessels enter small, bone-lined channels on the metaphyseal side of the epiphyseal plate. These channels have a blind end, and each terminates in the last hypertrophic cartilage cell of the epiphyseal plate. On reaching the end of the tunnel, the capillary inside this channel must turn 180° and exit through the same passage by which it entered. It is in this area of sluggish circulation, in tunnels whose walls are essentially impermeable, that bacteria lodge and hematogenous osteomyelitis begins. Once the process starts, thrombosis of the small terminal vessel and exudate seal the entrance to the channel. In the depths of this bone tunnel the organisms begin to proliferate, unimpeded by the host defenses that are unable to reach them. Once the infection is established in one channel, it extends into the metaphysis and involves other channels. Where bacteria and their products contact host cells within the marrow spaces of the metaphysis, the inflammatory process described earlier expands. Hordes of polymorphonuclear cells are mobilized in the metaphysis, and cellular destruction occurs at a rapid rate (Fig. 11-2). Pus in the metaphyseal area expands under pressure and travels up the marrow cavity or passes out of the cortex through the many small metaphyseal openings (Fig. 11-3). The bones of children are encased in a tough periosteal sleeve; this sleeve is lifted away from the bone by dissecting pus. The periosteal sleeve is firmly attached to the bone in the region of the epiphyseal plate and forms a barrier to prevent spread of the infection to the adjacent

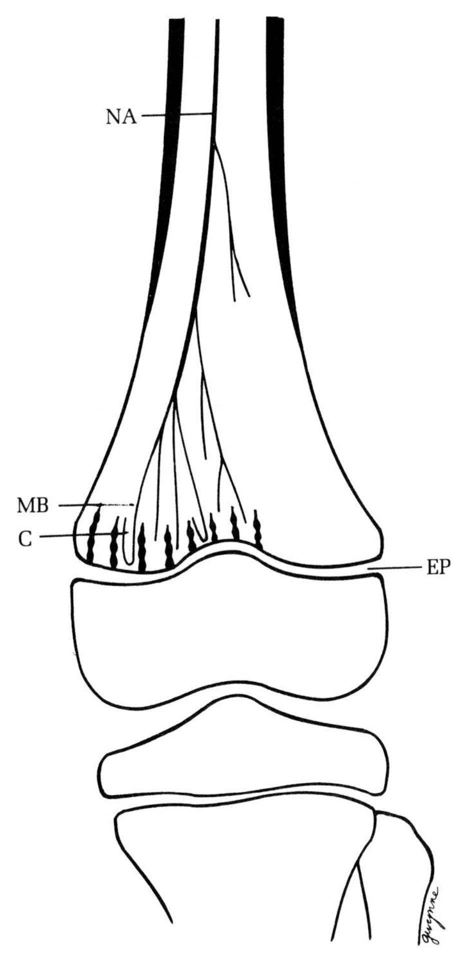

Fig. 11-1. Hematogenous osteomyelitis. Organisms traveling in the bloodstream enter the bone by way of the nutrient artery (NA), which divides into multiple metaphyseal branches (MB) that finally enter the small bone-lined channels (C) adjacent to the epiphyseal plate (EP). It is within these isolated channels that the original focus of hematogenous osteomyelitis develops.

joint. In certain areas such as the hip, where the epiphyseal plate is situated within the joint capsule, early joint involvement by infection is common (Fig. 11-4). In infants below the age of 1 year, some metaphyseal vessels may traverse the epiphyseal plate and permit spread of infection to the epiphysis and adjacent joint. At the knee, the joint is usually spared, and infections beginning in the distal femoral or proximal tibial metaphysis usually spread along the shaft of the bone moving away from the joint (Fig. 11-3).

As pus strips the periosteum from the shaft, it deprives the underlying bone of its periosteal blood supply (see Chap. 9). Pus within the bone may extend through the marrow cavity and destroy the endosteal circulation. If both endosteal and periosteal blood supplies are disrupted, the shaft becomes devoid of circulation and undergoes necrosis. Bone cells die, lyse, and disappear from their lacunae. Segments of dead bone surrounded by pus and granulation tissue are called *sequestra*. These range in size from microscopic to massive and may, in severe cases, include the entire shaft of the bone (Fig. 11-5). Haversian canals of these sequestra may harbour viable organisms for years in such protected areas.

The stripping of the periosteum from the shaft by pus stimulates an intense osteoblastic response. New immature bone is formed as a response to the periosteal stripping, and, in severe cases, the entire shaft may be encased in a sheath of new bone referred to as an *involucrum* (Fig. 11-5). Where a major portion of the shaft has been deprived of blood supply, the resulting sequestrum lies within this involucrum. Openings in the involucrum, called *cloacae*, may permit escape of pus from bone into surrounding soft tissue and ultimately through the skin by way of sinuses.

Roentgenographic Manifestations. Although swelling of soft tissues may be noted on early roentgenograms, the bone changes in osteomyelitis are usually not apparent for 8 to 12 days after the onset of clinical symptoms. The earliest bone changes are those of destruction or resorption, and are usually seen as mottled areas of decreased density in the metaphyseal area (Fig. 11-6). A short time later, a thin line of newly formed bone parallel to the shaft may be detected in the periosteal regions of the metaphysis. This new bone that results from infection progressing into the subperiosteal region gradually extends along the shaft; if the infection is not controlled, the new periosteal bone thickens over the succeeding few weeks to become an involucrum (Fig. 11-4). After several weeks have passed and the disease is in the chronic phase, sequestra may appear as opaque areas of bone, usually surrounded by a radiolucent zone consisting of exudate and granulation tissue.

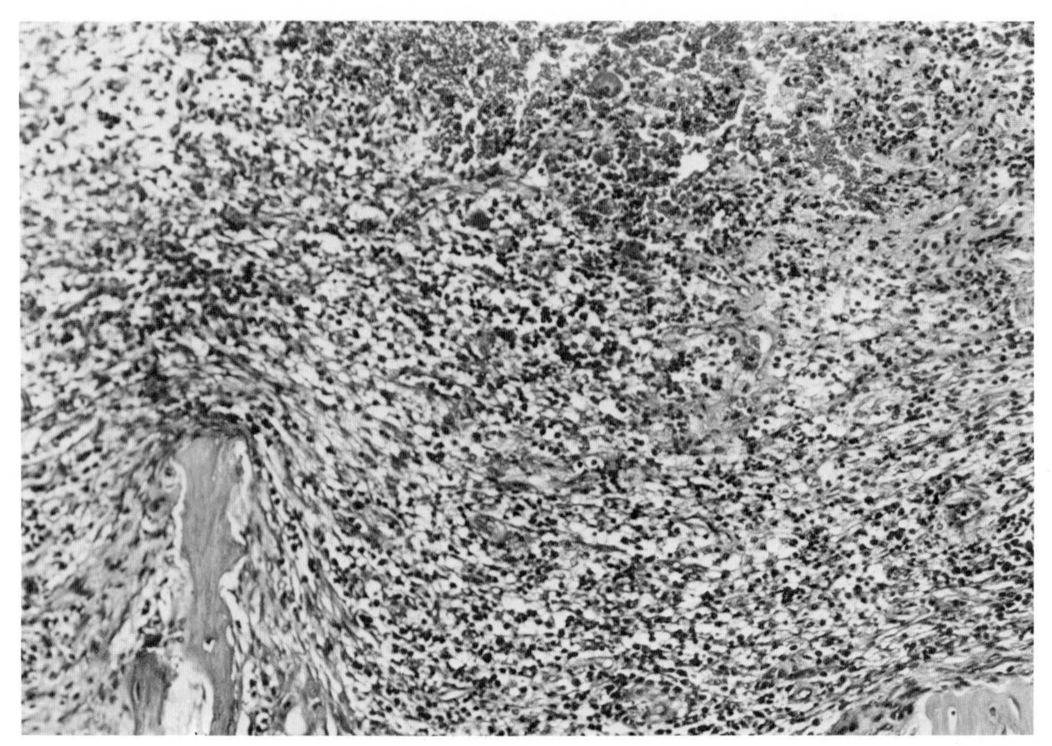

Fig. 11-2. Acute osteomyelitis results in extensive destruction of bone, which is replaced by an inflammatory infiltrate predominantly of segmented leukocytes. The marrow cavity becomes filled with pus.

Radioisotope scanning using technetium phosphate compounds can demonstrate acute osteomyelitis at an early stage before routine roentgenographic changes are apparent. Occasionally, presumably owing to the disruption of bone blood supply by the infection, bone uptake of the radioisotope may actually be impaired and result in a negative bone scan.

Clinical Course. The onset of acute hematogenous osteomyelitis is usually accompanied by pain and signs of systemic infection, including fever and elevation of the sedimentation rate and white blood count. The areas of bone most commonly affected are those adjacent to the most rapidly growing epiphyses, the distal femur, proximal tibia and proximal humerus. A careful history and examination will often reveal the primary source of infection in the skin, the upper respiratory tract, or another area. Frequently there is a history of minor trauma to the affected bone that antedates the infection. Pain and swelling in the area of infection increase rapidly and, in the case of the lower limb, the child usually refuses to walk. Localized tenderness can be detected in the metaphyseal area of the bone; later, when pus breaks out beneath the periosteum, the tenderness extends along the shaft. Blood cultures are frequently positive early in the disease.

Untreated, this disease may be fulminant, with overwhelming sepsis and death. The septicemia can cause bacterial seeding to other bones, leading to multiple sites of osteomyelitis. If the disease is treated early with appropriate antibiotics, septicemia is controlled, and there may be only limited bone damage. If, on the other hand, bone involvement is extensive, the disease may progress to a chronic phase. If large sequestra form, continued suppuration may result in the formation of sinus tracts that burrow through the soft tissues, exit through the skin, and result in the drainage of pus (Fig. 11-7). This chronic form of osteomyelitis is difficult to eradicate and can persist for many years. When chronic osteomyelitis is con-

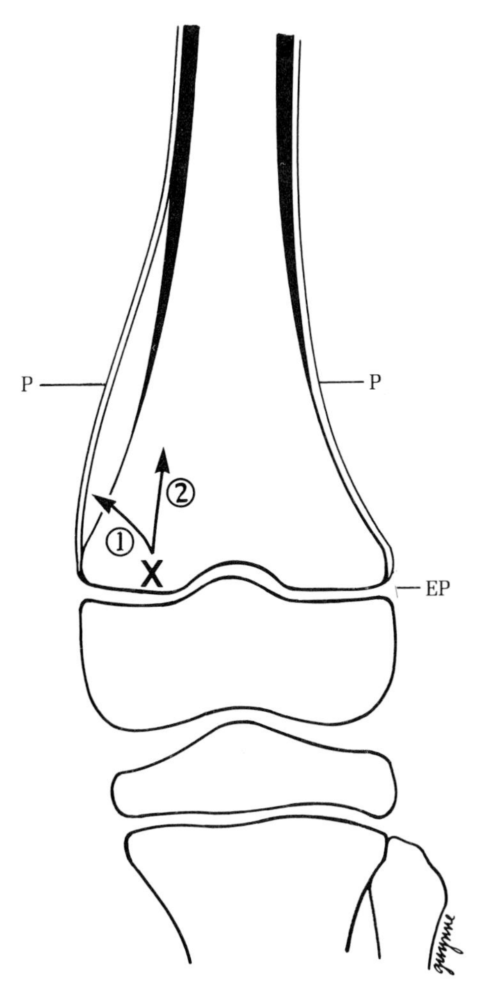

Fig. 11-3. The spread of acute hematogenous osteomyelitis from the original focus (X) is outward through metaphyseal vascular openings (1) beneath the periosteum (P), which is lifted from the shaft except where it is firmly attached to the periphery of the epiphyseal plate (EP). The infection also spreads up through the marrow cavity (2) away from the epiphyseal plate, which is a barrier to the infection.

trolled, the disease may become quiescent for long periods. Reactivation of quiescent osteomyelitis can occur many years after the original infection. The old adage, "Once an osteomyelitis always an osteomyelitis," unfortunately remains true in certain instances.

Occasionally, an acute metaphyseal osteomyelitis is contained locally by the host defenses. In such instances, the infection becomes surrounded by scar tissue and a rim of reactive bone. The resulting cavity or cyst is filled with pus, which may ultimately become sterile. The abscess resulting from this localized form of the disease is called a *Brodie's abscess.*

Complications. Complications of acute osteomyelitis include the seeding of other areas of the body with resulting infections of lung, kidneys or other bones, and septicemia that may be fatal. Extensive bone destruction resulting from osteoclastic resorption may provoke a *pathologic fracture.* Limbs affected by osteomyelitis must be protected by casts or splints, in order to prevent fracture, until adequate healing has occurred. *Infectious arthritis* may result from the spread of infection from the bone to an adjacent joint, most frequently in the hip and shoulder (Fig.

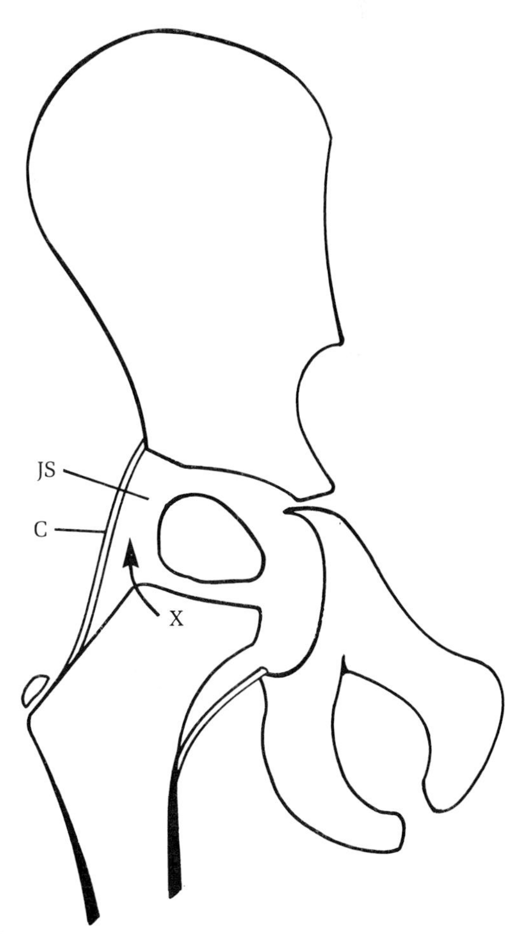

Fig. 11-4. In the case of the hip joint, the epiphyseal plate lies within the joint capsule (C) and pus spreads from the original metaphyseal focus (X) into the hip joint space (JS).

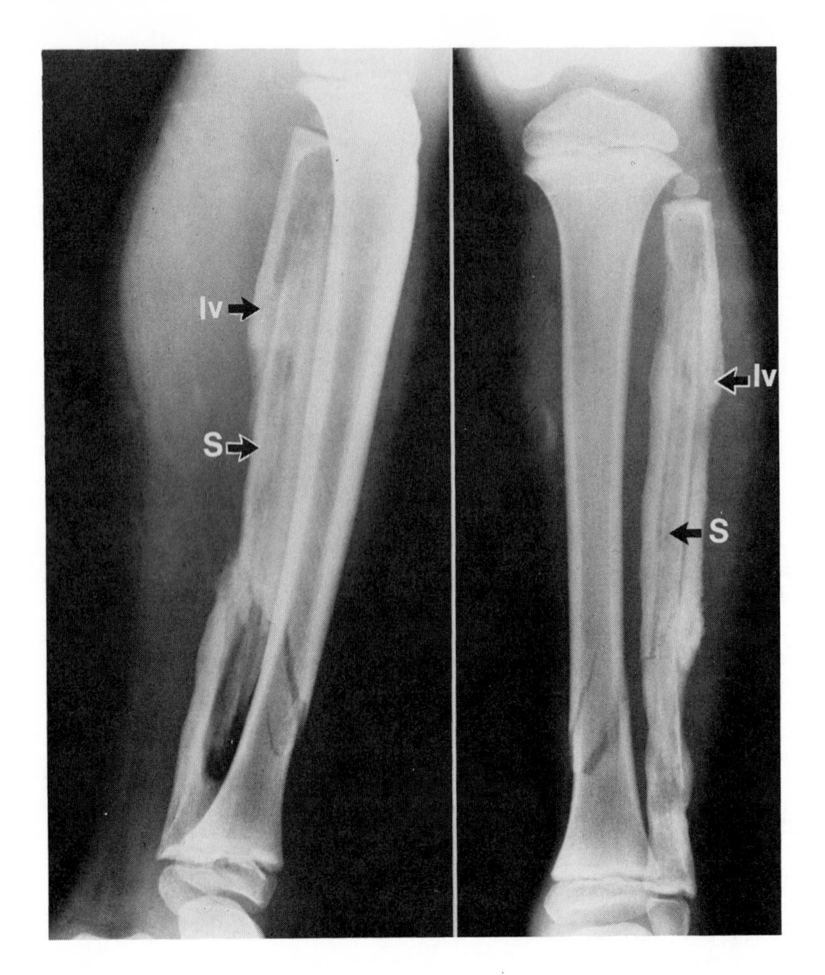

Fig. 11-5. Hematogenous osteomyelitis of the fibula of 3 mo duration. The entire shaft has been deprived of its blood supply and has become a sequestrum (S) surrounded by new immature bone, involucrum (IV). Pathologic fractures are present in the lower tibia and fibula.

11-4). The draining sinuses of chronic osteomyelitis may, after many years, become the site of *squamous cell carcinoma.*

Hematogenous osteomyelitis is seen less frequently in the adult than in the child. Since the adult does not have epiphyseal plates, the site of origin is different from that of childhood. The vertebral bodies are more frequently involved in adult hematogenous osteomyelitis. Such vertebral infections often follow genitourinary or gynecological surgery and result from the seeding of bacteria through the pelvic plexus of veins to the vertebra. Infections involving vertebral bodies frequently extend into and destroy adjacent intervertebral discs. Such involvement of the disc as noted on the roentgenogram is a helpful feature in distinguishing infections from tumors of vertebra. Osteomyelitis originating near the ends of long bones of adults can extend into the adjacent joint because there is no epiphyseal barrier to such extension, and the periosteum is a much thinner membrane in the adult.

Treatment. Successful therapy of bone infection involves the judicious use of antibiotics and surgery. In general, antibiotics should be specific and bactericidal. Early identification and sensitivity testing of the infectious organism is imperative. Antibiotics should be given early and in high doses until the indices of infection have returned to normal. Operative intervention is needed if the disease process cannot be controlled by antibiotics. It is usually necessary to drain abscesses and to remove sequestra if antibiotics are unsuccessful in preventing their development.

Exogenous Osteomyelitis

Exogenous osteomyelitis results from the contamination of bone from the external environment. The most common cause of this form of osteomyelitis is the open (compound) fracture. Other causes include penetrating wounds, such as splinters, nails or bullets, and infections occurring following operative procedures. Several factors are important in determining whether a given wound will become infected: the degree and type of contamination, the virulence of the infecting organism, the extent of tissue damage, host resistance, and the time lapse between introduction of the organism and institution of effective treatment.

Consider, for example, a person who twists his leg while taking a shower and sustains a spiral fracture of the tibia. A sharp fragment of bone punctures the skin creating a 2-mm hole. This is an open fracture occurring in clean surroundings and associated with minimal soft tissue damage. Infection is possible but unlikely. Compare that situation with a farmer whose leg is crushed under the wheel of a tractor in a barnyard sustaining an extensive soft tissue wound that exposes bone and muscle to massive contamination; this injury would very likely become infected.

The virulence of infecting organisms and host resistance are factors that are difficult to measure. There is no question that some strains of *Staphylococcus aureus*, for example, are much more virulent than others and may cause devastating infections. Host resistance cannot be easily quantitated, but chronically ill, diabetic, and alcoholic patients often exhibit lowered resistance to infections. Patients who are receiving large amounts of steroids or immunosuppressive drugs may have impaired ability to combat bacterial invasion. Specific defects in the immune systems can lead to infections with uncommon organisms, such as fungi.

Bone infection may follow surgical procedures, particularly those in which large foreign objects such as metallic plates or artificial joints are implanted. Such objects limit local tissue defense mechanisms, and infection about such implants is difficult to control. Since artificial joints are frequently used in patients with severe rheumatoid arthritis who may have compromised host resistance, the risk of bone infection is higher in this group.

Pathology. Osteomyelitis of exogenous origin differs from its hematogenous counterpart in that it usually remains localized to the site of original trauma, and it passes quickly from the acute to the chronic stage. Sequestra may develop, which, in the presence of foreign material, complicate and prolong the infection (Fig. 11-8). Draining sinuses frequently develop that lead from a skin opening directly to a sequestrum or foreign metallic implant. Bone destruction in localized areas is usual, and multiple small abscess cavities may develop within the affected bone. These areas are often surrounded by areas of sclerotic bone; these small isolated pockets of infected tissue make eradication of the osteomyelitis very difficult.

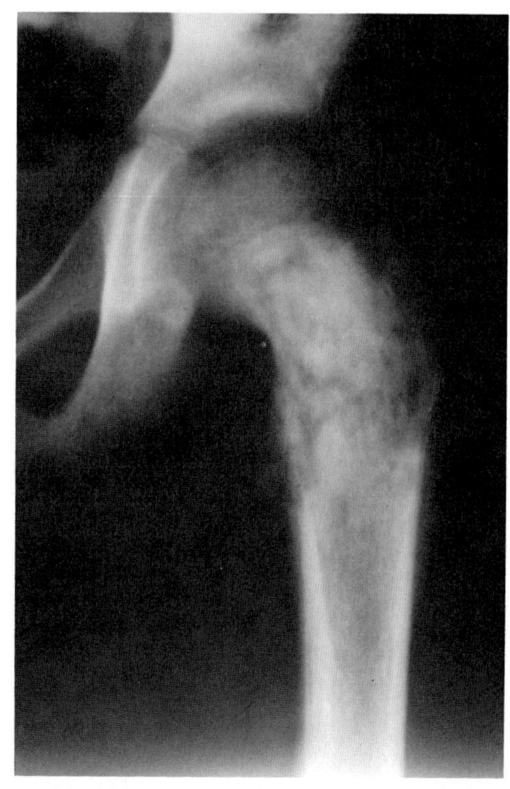

Fig. 11-6. Roentgenographic features of acute osteomyelitis 3 wk after onset of symptoms. Note the areas of lysis in the proximal femur and subperiosteal new bone formation adjacent to the cortex.

Clinical Course. Following an open fracture or surgical procedure, the early manifestations of infection are fever and increasing pain at the site of injury. Swelling and redness of the wound are followed by tissue breakdown and exudation. The systemic phase of the infection is usually quickly controlled by appropriate antibiotic treatment,

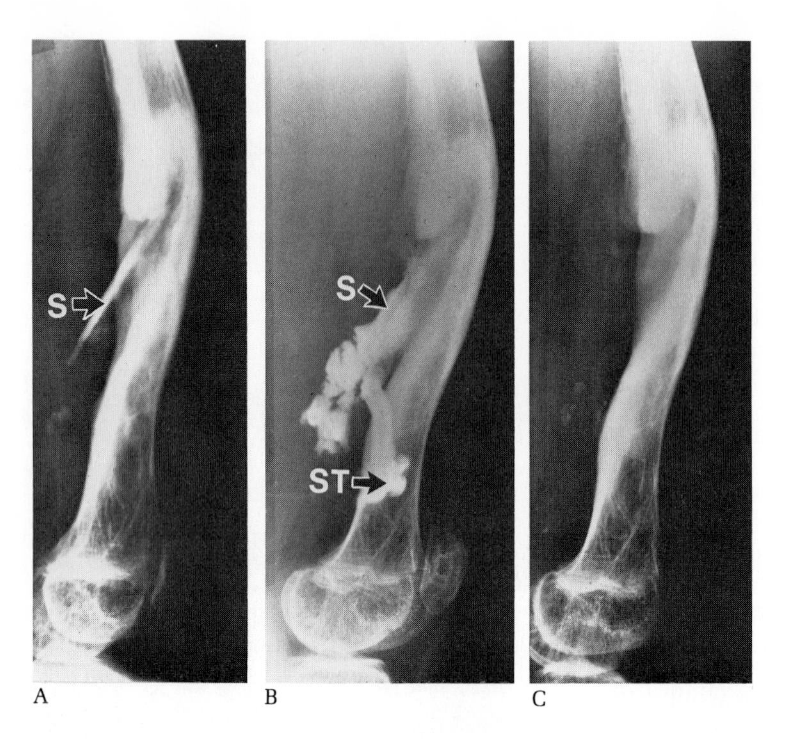

Fig. 11-7. Chronic osteomyelitis with sequestrum and sinus formation. The sequestrum (S), obvious in *A*, is outlined by the sinus tract ST in *B*, which is made visible by injecting radiopaque dye through the skin opening. *C* shows the femur after surgical removal of the sequestrum.

but, because of local tissue injury or the presence of foreign material, antibiotics frequently fail to control the local infection, which soon progresses to a chronic phase characterized by intermittent or chronic purulent drainage, periodic recurrence of pain, swelling, and local wound breakdown that may persist for years. In the case of fractures, infection inhibits healing and a nonunion of the fracture may result. Successful treatment of chronic bone infection may require several extensive surgical procedures combined with prolonged antibiotic therapy. Occasionally bone infections cannot be eradicated, and amputation or other radical surgical excision may be required.

INFECTIOUS ARTHRITIS

Infectious arthritis, also known as septic, suppurative, or pyogenic arthritis, is an acute inflammatory process involving synovium, synovial fluid, articular cartilage, and adjacent bone that results from the introduction of microorganisms (usually bacteria or fungi) into a joint.

The infecting organism may reach the joint in three ways: hematogenous seeding of the synovial membrane, extension from an adjacent focus of osteomyelitis, or direct implantation from a penetrating wound.

Bacteriology. Although almost any microorganism can cause infectious arthritis, most cases are produced by relatively few species of bacteria. In children, the most common agent is *Staphylococcus aureus;* however, *Hemophilus influenzae* is also frequent in children under 2 years of age. In adults, *Neisseria gonorrhoeae* accounts for many cases of septic arthritis, followed by *Staphylococcus aureus,* streptococci, and gram-negative bacilli, which account for most of the remainder. Mycobacteria and fungi are rare offenders but should be suspected when low-grade inflammation is associated with sterile cultures.

Pathogenesis. Staphylococci are found on the skin and in the nares of most persons throughout life. They are responsible for many common skin infections, and they are the most frequent colonizers of open wounds. Focal skin infections may lead to hematogenous seeding of other organs, including bones and joints. Although the organisms may be directly implanted into the synovial membrane, they may also reach the joint from a nearby osseous infection.

In response to an infectious inoculum, the synovial membrane becomes rapidly inflamed and thickened by an accumulation of polymorphonuclear leucocytes and edema. The supporting capsule and ligaments are distended by the production of increasingly purulent joint fluid. Necrosis of the synovium, which usually begins within 24 hours, is followed by necrosis of chondrocytes. Death of these cells leads to the failure of glycosaminoglycan production; as cartilage matrix becomes deficient, the collagen fibers become exposed and more susceptible to damage by joint friction. Nearby bone loss occurs as the result of hyperemia associated with the inflammatory response.

The formation of immune complexes potentiates the inflammatory response. Although this process is not fully understood, the events are probably similar to those occurring in the rheumatoid joint; an antigen (bacterial in this case) combines with IgG and IgM antibodies to form immune complexes that bind and activate the complement proteins. Additional immune-complex-like aggregates, formed by the coupling of protein A in the cell wall of *Staphylococci* with IgG, aids in the activation of complement. Complement activation produces chemotactic factors and other mediators of inflammation that enhance the inflammatory process through the mobilization and activation of polymorphonuclear and mononuclear cells. These cells phagocyticize the immune complexes, which leads to death of the cells. Cellular disintegration releases lysosomal enzymes (proteases and other hydrolytic enzymes) that injure chondrocytes and other structural components of the joint. Possibly, antigen–antibody immune complexes remain in the joint, even after eradication of the infectious agent, where they prolong the inflammatory response. In the healing phase of joint infections, extensive scar formation and fibrous adhesions within the joint lead to stiffness and impaired function.

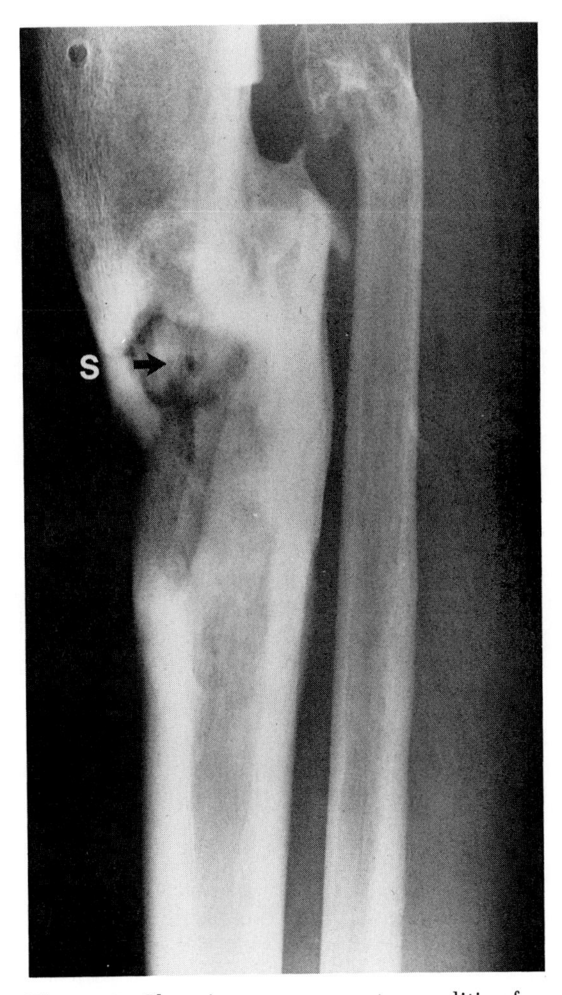

Fig. 11-8. Chronic exogenous osteomyelitis of the tibia resulting from an open fracture. The fracture has healed, but a sequestrum (S) is surrounded by pus and infected granulation tissue and causes chronic drainage.

Clinical Features. Infectious arthritis is typically monarticular; it favors the hip and knee in children because of the increased vascularity associated with rapid growth in these regions. Patients with impaired host defense mechanisms are susceptible. Diabetes mellitus, rheumatoid arthritis, and chronic granulomatous diseases are specific conditions associated with an increased incidence of septic arthritis.

The onset of pain in the affected joint is frequently sudden and often associated with chills and fever. The joint is swollen, warm, tender, and painful when moved. A careful search will often reveal a focus of infection elsewhere. Leukocytosis and elevation of the sedimentation rate are consistent laboratory findings.

Roentgenographically, capsular distention is followed by osteopenia, especially in the subchondral bone, narrowing of the cartilage space, and peripheral bone erosions (Fig. 11-9). Occasionally, bony ankylosis of

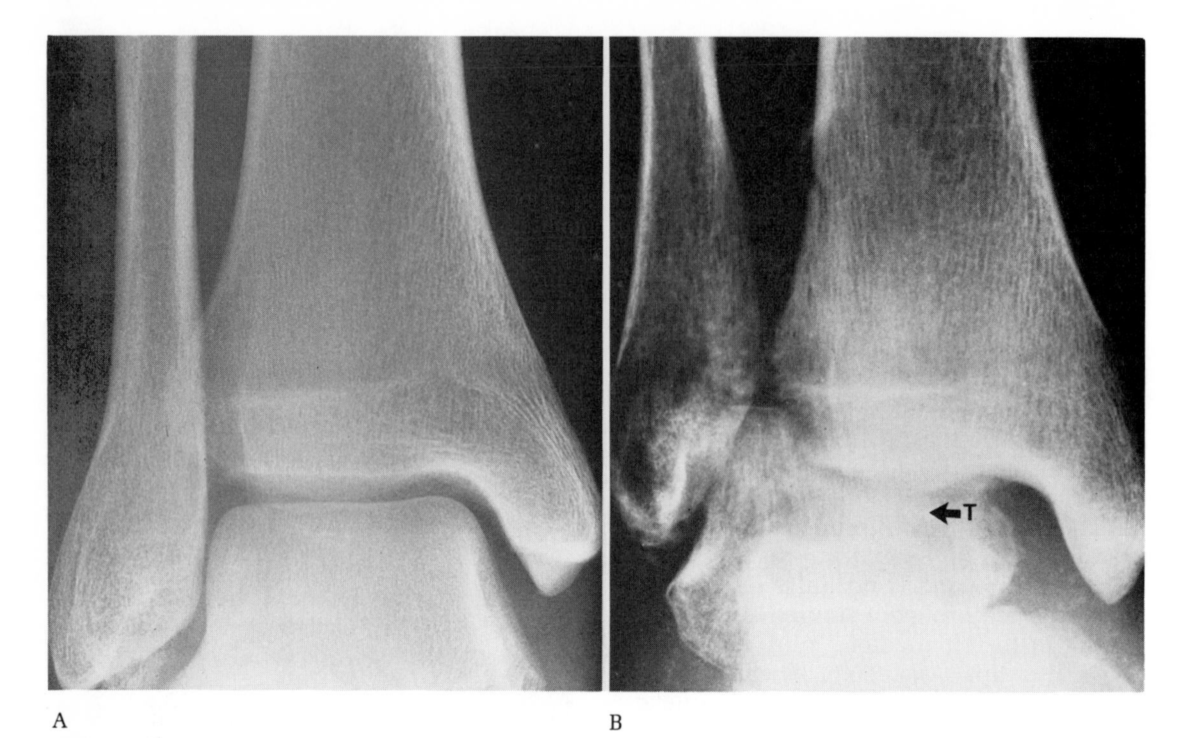

Fig. 11-9. Chronic infectious arthritis of the ankle resulting from an open fracture. A normal ankle is shown in *A*. In *B* there is loss of the cartilage space, and destruction and lateral subluxation of the talus resulting in permanent disability.

the joint follows infection; however, this is a later finding and is more common in spinal than in appendicular joints. Results of radioisotope scanning with technectium or gallium are positive early in the course of the infection, but other inflammatory joint conditions, such as rheumatoid arthritis or osteoarthritis, may produce a positive scan.

Diagnosis. Clinical suspicion of joint infection should be followed immediately by joint aspiration and microscopic examination and culture of the fluid obtained. Blood agar cultures are routinely obtained; chocolate agar should also be used when *Neisseria gonorrhoeae* and *Hemophilus influenzae* are suspected. Fungal media should be included when atypical low-grade findings are present.

In addition to bacteriologic data, the number of white blood cells and the glucose level in the joint should be determined. Although other conditions, including trauma, may lead to the presence of white cells in the joint fluid, levels above 75,000/mm^3 are usually the result of infectious arthritis. Fasting glucose levels are usually reduced to less than half of the simultaneously obtained blood levels. Gas chromatography is frequently used in the laboratory to identify specific infectious agents.

Treatment. Optimal treatment is based on early identification of the organism and its antibiotic sensitivities, followed by parenteral delivery of large concentrations of an appropriate bactericidal antibiotic to the joint until the organisms have been eradicated. Such treatment, if begun soon after the onset of symptoms, will usually cure the infection without serious sequelae, especially if the infection is caused by streptococci or gonococci. When the arthritis has been left untreated for a week or more, or when staphylococcal or gram-negative organisms are responsible, the prognosis is more guarded, and surgical drainage is more frequently necessary to control the infection. In superficial joints such as the knee, needle aspiration and irrigation on a daily basis may be a useful therapeutic adjunct. While the joint is acutely inflammed, it should be kept at rest, usually with a splint or cast.

Complications. Complications of joint infection, which usually reflect delayed diagnosis or inadequate treatment, include osteomyelitis, ankylosis, dislocation, or joint deformity. The development of a complication usually leads to a painful joint with limited function that may require surgical fusion or joint replacement.

SELECTED REFERENCES

Aegerter E, Kirkpatrick JA: Orthopedic Diseases, 4th ed. Philadelphia, WB Saunders, 1975

Edmonson AS, Crenshaw AH: Campbell's Operative Orthopaedics, 6th ed. St. Louis, CV Mosby, 1980

Jaffe HL: Metabolic, Degenerative, and Inflammatory Disease of Bone and Joints. Philadelphia, Lea & Febiger, 1972

Lovell WW, Winter RB: Pediatric Orthopaedics, Philadelphia, JB Lippincott, 1978

Trueta J: Studies of the Development and Decay of the Human Frame. Philadelphia, WB Saunders, 1968

Chapter 12

Tumors and Tumorlike Conditions of Bone

H. Robert Brashear

GOALS AND OBJECTIVES

Goals: To familiarize the reader with the more common benign and malignant tumors of bone and to give him an understanding of their classification, histology, roentgenography, and clinical behavior.

Objectives: On completion of this unit, and using the text as a standard reference, one should be able to evaluate, describe, or recognize the following:

1. Three features suggesting benignancy and three suggesting malignancy as seen in the roentgenogram of a bone tumor, and how the underlying pathologic process produces the roentgenographic findings.
2. A clinical, roentgenographic, and histologic finding pertinent to the diagnosis of the following bone tumors:
   a. Osteochondroma
   b. Osteoid osteoma
   c. Nonossifying fibroma
   d. Giant cell tumor
   e. Chondrosarcoma
   f. Osteogenic sarcoma
   g. Ewing's sarcoma
   h. Metastatic cancer
3. The principles of treatment of the following bone tumors as determined by the pathologic and clinical characteristics of the tumor:
   a. Osteoid osteoma
   b. Osteochondroma
   c. Bone cyst
   d. Osteogenic sarcoma
   e. Ewing's sarcoma
   f. Multiple myeloma

OUTLINE

I. General features of bone tumors
   A. Clinical features
      1. Pain

2. Mass
3. Pathologic fracture
4. Impairment of function

B. Roentgenographic features
1. Limitation of roentgenography
2. Osteolytic, osteoblastic, and mixed
3. Benign lesions
4. Malignant lesions

C. Microscopic features
1. Biopsy
2. Common cell ancestry: mesoderm
3. Histologic interpretation

D. Treatment
1. Observation and reassurance
2. Curettement and packing with bone
3. Excision
4. Radiation
5. Amputation
6. Chemotherapy

II. Classification of bone tumors
A. Significance and reason for classification
B. Table of bone tumors

III. Benign tumors
A. Osteochondroma
B. Enchondroma
C. Osteoid osteoma
D. Nonossifying fibroma
E. Aneurysmal bone cyst
F. Solitary bone cyst
G. Giant cell tumor

IV. Malignant tumors
A. Osteogenic sarcoma
B. Chondrosarcoma
C. Ewing's sarcoma
D. Multiple myeloma
E. Metastatic tumors

Tumors and tumorlike conditions of bone make up a fascinating group of lesions, the classification and understanding of which have been evolving slowly over the years. It has been appreciated only in the last 3 or 4 decades that painstaking correlation of the clinical, roentgenographic, and pathologic data, coupled with long-term follow-up studies, are the only means by which valid knowledge of this often confusing group of bone diseases can be obtained. There is a limited amount of information that can be derived from each of these three sources, but when it is assembled, a diagnosis can usually be established. There may come a time in the future when we will be able to quantitate the data obtained from clinical, roentgenographic, and pathologic studies, so that the diagnosis of bone tumors will be made by computer. Meanwhile, it is necessary to gather, put together, and carefully weigh all the information that can be obtained.

GENERAL FEATURES OF BONE TUMORS

The clinical features associated with bone tumors include pain, deformity, and impairment of function. Though there is little sex predilection in bone tumors, the *age* of the patient and the *location* of the lesion are highly important. An otherwise healthy 8-year-old with a pathologic fracture through the proximal humerus very likely has a simple bone cyst. It is most unlikely that he has a giant cell tumor, for these do not occur at this age and are uncommon in the humerus. A knowledge of what tumors occur where and at what age is very helpful in diagnosis.

Pain is a feature common to almost all malignant tumors of bone, but may or may not be present in benign lesions. For example, the simple bone cyst referred to above is usually asymptomatic until a pathologic fracture occurs. Whether or not a lesion is causing pain, and the type of pain experienced, are helpful in the diagnosis. Malignant bone tumors are usually associated with deep, aching pain, which, although not sharp and sometimes not severe, is quite distressing to the patient because of its constancy. Pain that persists at night and is not relieved by rest is suggestive of malignancy; however, certain benign tumors, notably osteoid osteoma, are characterized by nocturnal pain. Mild, dull, aching back pain that suddenly becomes excruciating with such insignificant trauma as sitting down a bit hard suggests a pathologic compression fracture in a vertebra involved by metastatic cancer.

Some bone tumors first make their presence known by the appearance of a *mass*. If the mass is not associated with pain, the chances are that the lesion is benign. A tumor that is commonly discovered by the patient because of a mass is the osteochondroma or exostosis. In this situation, the patient discovers a hard, nontender lump near a joint, which leads him to seek medical advice. On the other hand, if the mass is associated with pain, and especially if the patient is aware that the mass has been enlarging, malignancy, particularly osteosarcoma, is to be suspected. The discovery of a mass arising from bone is, of course, dictated in part by the location of the tumor. A small lump arising from the subcutaneous surface of the tibia would be easily discovered, whereas a tumor deep in the upper medial portion of the thigh might grow to a considerable size before it is detected. A tumor may cause a slow, diffuse enlargement of a part of a bone, and the patient only very gradually becomes aware of the difference in this bone and the one on the opposite side. Such is often the case with enchondromas, which are slow-growing cartilage tumors.

Many tumors gradually erode bone and weaken it to the extent that it cannot withstand the strain of ordinary use. In such situations, a very slight amount of trauma precipitates a *pathologic fracture.* Again, if there were no symptoms prior to the time of fracture, the chances are that the tumor is benign. The solitary bone cyst, fibrous dysplasia, nonossifying fibroma, and enchondromas are lesions that frequently are first noted because of fracture. On the other hand, if the fracture has been preceded by dull, aching pain, the possibility of a malignant primary bone tumor or a metastasis is likely.

Occasionally, the *impairment of function* is a presenting clinical symptom. A tumor near a joint may, either by mechanical pressure or through involvement of adjacent peripheral nerves, affect the function of the limb, and the patient seeks medical attention because of limp, weakness, or limitation of motion.

Some bone tumors cause no symptoms and are accidentally discovered when roentgenograms are made for some other reason, such as a sprain. These again are usually benign lesions, but a diagnosis must be established in such situations.

Roentgenograms are pictures of shadows, and there is a limit to the information that can be obtained from them. Some tumors, such as the typical osteochondroma, are so characteristic that the roentgenogram is sufficient to establish the diagnosis beyond any reasonable doubt. However, in the case of most bone tumors, and particularly those that destroy bone, the diagnosis cannot be established by roentgenographic means alone. The number of diagnostic possibilities can be limited, and certain lesions may be excluded, but the final diagnosis must await biopsy when the clinical, roentgenographic, and pathologic data can be assembled.

Roentgenographically, bone tumors are *osteolytic, osteoblastic,* or, as is most often the case, a combination of the two. *The position of a lesion in the bone* is highly important. Some tumors are found only in the epiphysis, whereas others are most frequently seen in the metaphysis; a smaller number are encountered in the diaphyseal region. Some lesions occur most frequently before epiphyseal closure, whereas others are seen only after the epiphyses have closed. There are roentgenographic features that suggest (but do not necessarily prove) that the changes present are benign in nature (Fig. 12-1). If the tumor is limited to the confines of the bone, if it has a well-demarcated border surrounded by a thin rim of sclerotic bone, and if it has not broken through the cortex, a benign process is suggested. Conversely, if the boundaries of the tumor are ill-defined, if there are no sharp borders, if the lesion has a mottled appearance, and if it has broken out of the confines of the bone and destroyed cortex, malignancy is to be suspected. Malignant tumor cells that extend through the cortex may elevate the periosteum and stimulate it to produce a small triangle of reactive bone (Codman's triangle) where the periosteum is lifted from the shaft. This feature is seen in osteogenic sarcoma and Ewing's sarcoma but can also be found in infections and hemorrhagic lesions.

The formation of new osseous tissue outside the involved bone is suggestive of malignancy but can also be found in cases of infection and in myositis ossificans. Small bony spicules radiating in a direction perpendicular to the shaft, the *sunray effect* (Fig. 12-1*B*), are frequently found in osteogenic sarcoma but may be caused by other malignant, and even by some benign, processes. Subperiosteal new bone formation, which has a laminated or *onionskin* appearance (Fig. 12-1*A*), is seen in Ewing's sarcoma, but it may also be found in other conditions that elevate the periosteum, such as infection. In addition to routine roentgenography, special techniques, such as laminography, arteriog-

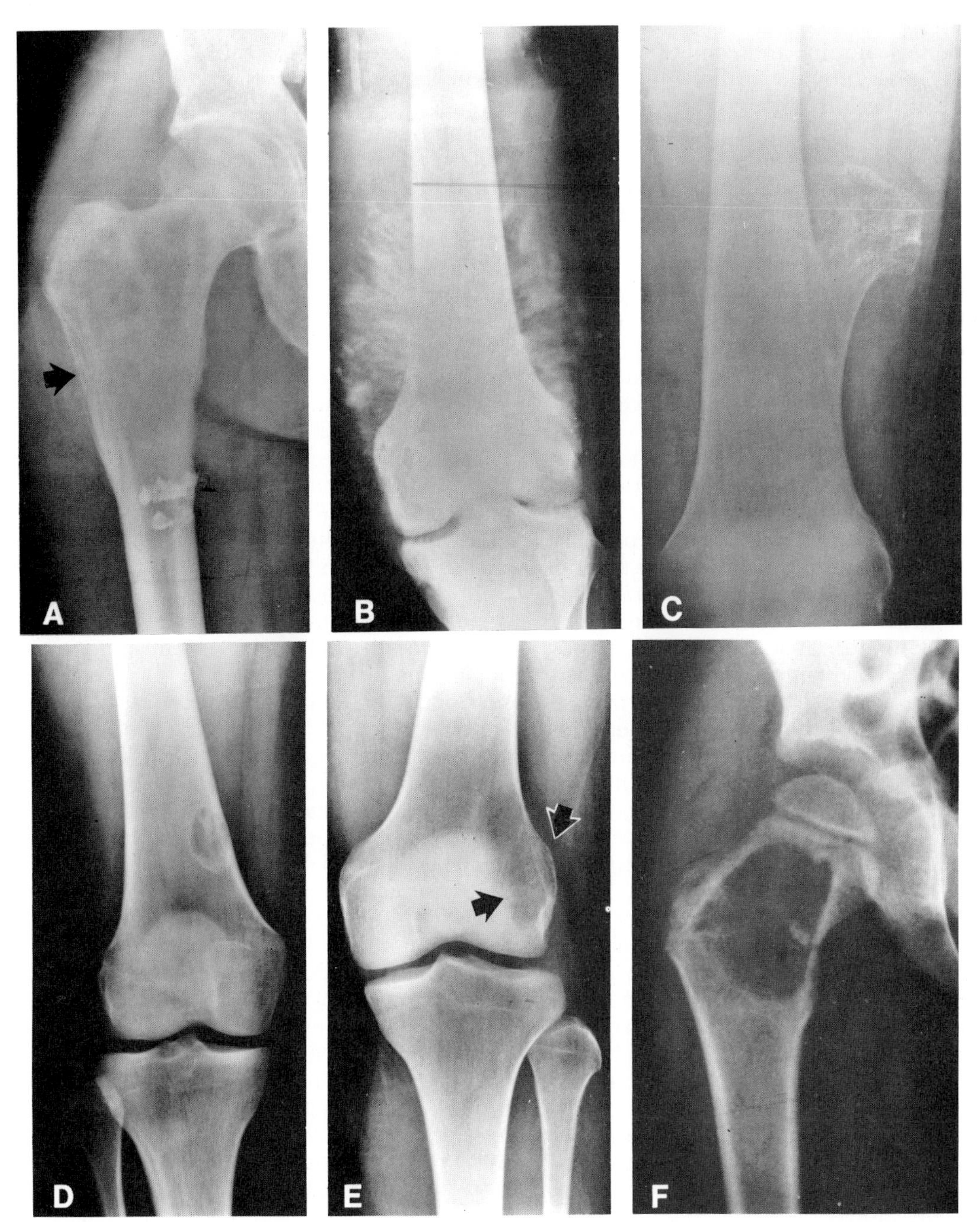

Fig. 12-1. Types of bone tumors. (*A*) Ewing's sarcoma of proximal femur. Note patchy bone destruction and periosteal elevation (*arrow*) parallel to shaft (onionskin effect). (*B*) Osteogenic sarcoma. The distal femur is the most frequent location. Note extensive bone formation outside of and in lines perpendicular to the shaft (sun ray effect). (*C*) Osteochondroma (exostosis) of the distal femoral metaphysis. The marrow cavity of the lesion is continuous with that of the femur. (*D*) Nonossifying fibroma. The lesion is in the metaphysis, eccentric in position, adjacent to the cortex. It is completely surrounded by a thin rim of bone, a sign of its benign nature. (*E*) Giant cell tumor. A lytic lesion involving both epiphysis and metaphysis after epiphyseal closure. (*F*) Simple bone cyst arising in the metaphysis adjacent to the growth plate. It is most frequently found in the proximal humerus. The proximal femoral location seen here is the second most common location.

raphy, bone scanning, and computerized tomography may provide further information about a bone lesion. Though the roentgenogram is of immense help in leading to the diagnosis, it is only for a few lesions of bone that a definitive diagnosis can be established by this means alone. In most instances, it is essential to obtain tissue for histologic evaluation.

Biopsy of bone tumors may be accomplished by means of a large needle or by open surgical methods. Each has its advantages. The *needle biopsy* involves less disturbance to the tissue and is usually a less extensive procedure. Where the bone lesion is accessible and near the surface, needle biopsy is often a simple matter. It is an especially helpful technique when the diagnosis can be made on the basis of a small number of cells, such as in metastatic cancer. Where several areas of a tumor must be evaluated, as is often the case with cartilage lesions, the larger sample obtained by open biopsy is to be preferred. Other disadvantages of needle biopsy are that the tissue obtained may be from a necrotic portion of the tumor and therefore not suitable for diagnosis, or the tissue may be reactive in nature and not representative of the actual tumor. An example of this is the Codman's triangle, which is reactive bone and may contain no tumor at all. In a few instances, immediate diagnosis on the basis of frozen sections can be made, but for most malignant lesions of bone it is advisable to await permanent paraffin sections.

Primary neoplasms of bone are derived from cells that have a common ancestry, the *mesoderm*. One group of bone tumors is produced by cells characterized by their ability to synthesize collagen; these are the osteogenic, the chondrogenic, and the fibrogenic tumors. Another group of lesions probably originates from the marrow reticulum and includes the various round cell tumors of bone such as Ewing's sarcoma and reticulum cell sarcoma. When this common ancestry of cells is appreciated, it is not surprising to find that several types of cells may be present in a single lesion. In a rapidly growing osteogenic sarcoma, some of the cells may appear to be malignant fibroblasts, and in other fields it is not unusual to find areas of malignant cartilage cells. Osteoclasts are found in most of the bone tumors, or at least there are multinucleated cells that look like osteoclasts. These cells are quite striking in appearance; in the past, there was a tendency to call almost any lesion that contained a substantial number of these multinucleated cells a giant cell tumor. This assumption proved to be quite wrong, for many of these tumors were so different in their incidence, appearance, and clinical behavior that it became obvious that they were different entities. Today the term *giant cell tumor* is restricted to a small and very specific group of lesions.

The *host bone* involved by a tumor reacts to it in a very limited manner. It may undergo resorption, which roentgenographically appears as a lytic or osteoporotic area. Such resorption is accomplished by osteoclasts that may be so abundant as to appear to be an integral part of the lesion rather than a reaction to it. Such is sometimes the case in the lining membrane of a solitary bone cyst. On the other hand, the host bone may respond to the presence of the tumor by forming more bone. This response is seen in the osteoblastic reaction to metastatic cancer of the prostate.

It is very important to determine whether the bone formed in a tumor is being produced by the actual tumor cells or by normal osteoblasts reacting to the tumor. Though there are several benign tumors which actually form bone, there is only one malignant bone-forming tumor, osteogenic sarcoma. In most situations, the host bone responds to a tumor by a combination of resorption and bone formation. Thus, in addition to the tumor cells and their supporting tissue, there may be an abundance of normal osteoclasts, osteoblasts, and newly formed bone in the lesion. If the reactive bone in a lesion is a hurried response to a rapidly growing tumor, this bone is of the primitive fiber type and may be confused with actual tumor bone. Reactive bone that forms the thin sclerotic lining of a slowly growing tumor may be mature lamellar bone.

The histologic interpretation of the tumor tissue may be quite difficult. Though the classic lesions offer little trouble, one frequently encounters tumors that are borderline, and the difference between the benign and the malignant is not clear. This difficulty is notoriously true of cartilage tumors, and even the most experienced bone pathologist may be hard pressed by this tissue. Another lesion that causes trouble is the giant cell tumor. Some of these are obviously malignant, and others are clearly benign, but there are some giant cell tumors in which the diagnosis of malignancy cannot be made with certainty. Even the osteogenic sarcoma can cause trouble, for bone which is being produced rapidly in response to injury, as seen in exuberant fracture callus or early myositis ossificans, can have the appearance of malignancy. In such situations, the clinical information and the roentgenographic findings can be of immense help to the pathologist, which serves to emphasize again the importance of having all three sources of information—clinical, roentgenographic, and pathological—available to make the proper diagnosis of osseous lesions. Although in some instances the diagnosis is clear on the basis of only one of these sources, the careful clinician, radiologist, or pathologist uses all of the material available. By so doing, the tragedy of a needless amputation or of failure to recognize malignancy may be avoided.

Once the diagnosis of a bone lesion has been established, treatment is based on a knowledge of the natural history of the particular tumor, on its location in the body, and on other factors such as the age and general health of the patient. Several alternatives may be available in some situations; in others, only one form of therapy may be acceptable. The simplest form of treatment is observation and reassurance. This approach can be used only when the exact nature of the lesion is unquestionable from the clinical and roentgenographic evaluation, as for example an obvious and asymptomatic osteochondroma or nonossifying fibroma.

Some lytic or cystic bone lesions respond to curettement and packing with autogenous bone chips. Solitary bone cysts and aneurysmal bone cysts frequently respond to this form of treatment, which has the advantage of not leaving a structural defect in the bone. Excision of such lesions as giant cell tumors and enchondromas of the major long bones is advisable where possible, but often these lesions occupy the entire width of the shaft, and excision leaves a serious structural defect. Such defects may sometimes be replaced by cadaver bone or by a metallic implant. Radiation is the treatment of choice for only a few bone tumors. Reticulum cell sarcoma, Ewing's sarcoma, and some benign lesions that are surgically inaccessible but potentially dangerous are treated by this method. Radiation should not be used for benign tumors where other forms of treatment are effective, since there is a small but recognized danger of postradiation sarcoma. Amputation is usually the treatment of choice in osteogenic sarcoma, but occasionally wide local resection may be feasible. Where possible, amputation should be done through the bone proximal to the one involved by the tumor, since it is impossible to be certain just how far the tumor has extended within the marrow cavity of the involved bone. Amputation should be followed by prolonged and intensive chemotherapy. Chemotherapy has been effective with bone tumors of the reticulum or myelogenic series such as Ewing's sarcoma and plasma cell myeloma. It is often used in combination with other forms of therapy.

CLASSIFICATION OF BONE TUMORS

Many classifications of bone tumors have been proposed but, as Jaffe has suggested, these are probably of little practical significance, since each tumor must be treated as an entity in itself with knowledge of its specific behavior, which may have little to do with the class in which it happens to be listed. However, a classification of bone tumors may be helpful as an introduction to help the student remember the different types of lesions. Before one can make a rational approach to diagnosis, one must be aware of the various possibilities. Table 12-1 is a simplified classification of the more important tumors and tumorlike conditions of bone. Those listed in capital letters are considered individually in the text.

In addition to the above, tumors of neurogenic, vascular, muscular, or fatty tissue origin may arise within bone. Many cancers may metastasize to bone, but the five most frequent sources of bone metastases are breast, prostate, lung, thyroid, and kidney.

Benign Tumors

Osteochondroma. The osteocartilaginous exostosis, the most common benign bone tumor (Fig. 12-1C), is a cartilage-capped projection of bone usually found in the metaph-

Table 12-1. Classification of Bone Tumors and Tumorlike Conditions

TISSUE	BENIGN	MALIGNANT
Cartilage	OSTEOCHONDROMA ENCHONDROMA Chondroblastoma Chondromyxoid fibroma Juxtacortical chondroma	CHONDROSARCOMA
Bone	OSTEOID OSTEOMA Osteoblastoma Osteoma	OSTEOGENIC SARCOMA (OSTEOSARCOMA) Parosteal osteosarcoma
Marrow elements		EWING'S SARCOMA Reticulum cell sarcoma MULTIPLE MYELOMA
Fibrous and connective tissue	NONOSSIFYING FIBROMA ANEURYSMAL BONE CYST SOLITARY BONE CYST GIANT CELL TUMORS Fibrous dysplasia Desmoplastic fibroma	Fibrosarcoma Malignant giant cell tumors Malignant fibrous histiocytoma

yses of long bones. The lesion grows by enchondral ossification of proliferating cartilage cells in its cap and usually stops growing at puberty. The diagnosis is easily made on clinical and roentgenographic findings of a firm, nontender, immovable mass arising near the end of the long bone. The lesions usually require no treatment unless they cause symptoms, in which case simple excision is usually curative. The incidence of malignant change in osteochondromas is probably less than 1%.

Enchondroma. As its name implies, the enchondroma is a benign cartilaginous tumor arising within the medullary cavity of bone. It is most frequently found in the small bones of the hands and feet; in these areas it rarely becomes malignant. The lesion is osteolytic in nature and appears cystic on the roentgenogram, although it may contain speckled densities of calcified cartilage. Not infrequently, it weakens the bone sufficiently to lead to fracture; in fact, the enchondroma is probably the most common cause of pathologic fracture of a finger. Enchondromas of the major long bones are more serious and carry a higher potential for malignant change.

Osteoid Osteoma. The osteoid osteoma tumor is a peculiar benign lesion of bone-forming cells. It may occur in almost any bone, is small in size (usually less than 2 cm in diameter), and is characterized by pain that is frequently worse at night and relieved by aspirin. The small radiolucent nidus is often surrounded by an extensive area of sclerotic bone. The nidus itself contains a vascular stroma with osteoid and numerous active osteoblasts and osteoclasts. In spite of its active appearance, the tumor remains stationary for many years and does not become malignant. Because of the pain, block excision of the lesion is the treatment of choice.

Nonossifying Fibroma. The nonossifying fibroma, a very common benign lesion of bone, has also been called a fibrous cortical defect. It usually causes no symptoms, and most are discovered incidentally when a roentgenogram of the knee or ankle is taken for an unrelated sprain. The majority of nonossifying fibromas occur in the metaphysis of the femur or tibia. The lesion is eccentrically placed against one cortex, elongated in the long axis of the bone, and usually surrounded by a thin sclerotic rim of bone (Fig. 12-1*D*). The cellular elements within the defect consist of whorled fibrous tissue, foam cells, and, occasionally, small elongated giant cells. Nonossifying fibromas are found in children and usually regress spontaneously by or after puberty. Occasionally, one may be of sufficient size to cause pathologic fracture. The roentgenographic findings of the nonossifying fibroma are usually typical enough not to require histologic confirmation, and smaller lesions are treated by reassurance to the parents and periodic observation until regression. Larger lesions that endanger the strength of bone are treated surgically. Malignant change in nonossifying fibroma is exceedingly rare.

Aneurysmal Bone Cyst. The aneurysmal bone cyst, an uncommon expansile osteolytic lesion of bone, contains large vascular channels separated by septa in which numerous giant cells are found. The lesion may grow rapidly, may attain considerable size, and can cause paraplegia when it involves the vertebrae. It is benign and usually responds to simple curettement, although resection is preferred where possible. In inaccessible areas, such as the vertebrae, roentgen therapy is effective. This tumor is one of the few benign bone lesions in which radiation may be used for treatment.

Solitary Bone Cyst. The solitary bone cyst, an osteolytic lesion of the metaphysis, is common in children and exceedingly rare in adults, so one may assume that it can regress spontaneously. Bone cysts are most often encountered in the proximal humerus and proximal end of the femur (Fig. 12-1*F*). They are usually asymptomatic until a pathologic fracture occurs. The cystic cavity is lined with a thin, fibrous tissue that frequently contains giant cells. The cavity itself contains a clear, yellow fluid unless there has been a recent fracture, in which case the fluid is amber or bloody. The treatment is usually curettement and packing of the cyst with bone chips. The injection of prednisolone into the cyst cavity has been effective on occasion. Recurrence is common in younger children, but by puberty most cysts are healed.

Giant Cell Tumor. Many bone lesions contain giant cells, but the true giant cell tumor is uncommon. Occurring in young adults after epiphyseal closure, it is an expansile lytic lesion that involves the epiphysis and metaphysis and frequently extends up to the subchondral bone (Fig. 12-1*E*). Scalloping and ridges in the wall of the tumor give it a "soap bubble" appearance on the roentgenogram. The lesion is found most frequently about the knee and the distal end of the radius. Microscopically, the tumor is characterized by slightly elongated stromal cells with oval nuclei and numerous multinucleated giant cells. The tumor is somewhat unpredictable. Those having a definitely malignant stroma behave in a malignant fashion, but occasionally lesions that are benign in appearance have metastasized. Because of this unpredictable nature, the treatment of choice in giant cell tumors is resection when feasible, although this treatment may cause serious mechanical dysfunction of the affected limb.

Malignant Tumors

Osteosarcoma. The osteosarcoma is the most common primary malignant bone tumor (excluding multiple myeloma). It occurs in the metaphyseal regions of the long bones, especially in the distal femur and proximal tibia. The presenting symptoms and signs are deep, aching pain and an enlarging, hard mass, usually just below or just above the knee joint. The diagnosis may be suspected from the roentgenogram and established by biopsy. The roentgenographic picture is that of a malignant tumor extending beyond the confines of bone, with both new bone formation and bone destruction. Elevation of the periosteum often produces a Codman's triangle, and spicules of new bone perpendicular to the periosteal surface (the sun ray effect) are frequently seen (Fig. 12-1*B*). The microscopic picture of malignant cells producing tumor osteoid or tumor bone is diagnostic.

The preferred treatment for osteosarcoma is amputation followed by an intense and prolonged course of chemotherapy. Osteosarcoma tends to metastasize by way of the bloodstream early in the course of the disease. Pulmonary metastases are usually detected within a year after the diagnosis has been made. Undetectable micrometastases are probably present in the lungs of most patients at the time they first seek medical attention. The survival rate for patients with osteosarcoma was formerly around 15%, but with current treatment it may be considerably higher.

A secondary form of osteosarcoma is seen

in a much older age group. The tumor may develop in bones affected by Paget's disease or other preexisting benign bone lesions. It may occur from 5 to 30 years following radiation therapy to benign bone tumors or to other lesions.

Chondrosarcoma. The chondrosarcoma, a malignant tumor of cartilage, grows more slowly and is less common and less aggressive than osteosarcoma. It is found in an older age group than is primary osteogenic sarcoma, the peak incidence occurring around 45 years of age. The majority of chondrosarcomas occur about the hip and pelvis. They are slow to metastasize and may grow to immense proportions. The tumor tends to destroy bone and to extend into the soft tissues beyond the confines of the bone of origin. Often, scattered calcification of the tumor cartilage is a prominent roentgenographic feature. The treatment for chondrosarcoma is either wide surgical resection or amputation. The tumor does not respond to radiation therapy or to currently available antineoplastic drugs. The long-term survival rate of patients with treated chondrosarcoma is about 50%.

Ewing's Sarcoma. Ewing's sarcoma is an uncommon bone tumor of uncertain origin; it probably arises from primitive reticulum cells of the marrow and, in this respect, may have some relationship to the lymphomas. It is a tumor of children and young adults, most cases occurring between the ages of 10 and 20 years. Ewing's sarcoma may mimic osteomyelitis clinically, the patients often having fever with an elevated white blood count and sedimentation rate. The roentgenogram may also suggest osteomyelitis (Fig. 12-1A). The tumor can occur in almost any bone but has a predilection for the femur, humerus, and ilium. The microscopic picture of Ewing's sarcoma is one of densely packed areas of small, round cells about twice the size of lymphocytes. It may be difficult to distinguish this tumor from reticulum cell sarcoma and from neuroblastoma. The current treatment for Ewing's sarcoma is radiation combined with chemotherapy; in some instances, amputation is advisable. Older statistics showed a 5-year survival rate of about 5%. However, the results of combined therapy may elevate this rate to above 40%.

Multiple Myeloma. Multiple myeloma, a common neoplasm also called plasma cell myeloma, accounts for over 40% of the primary malignant tumors of bone. It occasionally presents as a solitary lesion, but more often it is diffuse, involving multiple bones, most frequently the vertebrae, skull, pelvis, and femurs. It usually occurs in the sixth and seventh decades of life. The roentgenographic features are those of bone destruction associated with little or no reactive bone formation unless a pathologic fracture is present. The sharply delineated punched-out lesions of bone are seen best in the skull. Most patients with multiple myeloma have an elevated serum globulin with an abnormal serum electrophoretic pattern, usually showing a high monoclonal immunoglobulin peak. The serum calcium level is often high, and Bence Jones protein is frequently present in the urine. The microscopic picture consists of closely packed masses of cells that have many of the features of normal plasma cells. The prognosis in diffuse multiple myeloma is poor, but with adequate chemotherapy a survival time of 5 years or more is not uncommon.

Metastatic Tumors. Carcinoma metastatic to bone is the most common malignancy of osseous tissue. The tumors that frequently spread to the skeleton are breast, lung, prostate, kidney, and thyroid, although cancer from any organ may ultimately involve bone. Cancers may invade the skeleton by contiguous extension from the primary site, but widespread dissemination occurs through the bloodstream. The vertebral bodies are a very common site of metastases, but the skull, ribs, and pelvis are also frequently involved. The femur and humerus are the usual locations of metastases to the long bones, and involvement of bones distal to the knee or the elbow is unusual. Most skeletal metastases cause bone destruction and appear osteolytic on the roentgenogram. The bone destruction may be extensive enough to weaken the skeleton and cause a pathologic fracture. Occasionally, the tumor cells provoke an osteoblastic response, and the roentgenographic appearance of the lesion is then one of increased density; this picture is frequently seen in metastases from carcinoma of the prostate. The treatment of metastatic lesions to bone varies with the primary tumor. Roentgen therapy, chemotherapy, and hormonal treatment are often helpful but not curative. Pathologic fractures and impending fractures of the long bones are frequently most effectively treated by open reduction and internal fixation; this approach may prevent the cancer patient from becoming bedridden and enable him to maintain a functional state for a longer period.

SELECTED REFERENCES

Huvos AG: Bone tumors. Philadelphia, WB Saunders, 1979

Jaffe HL: Tumors and Tumorous Conditions of Bones and Joints. Philadelphia, Lea & Febiger, 1968

Lichtenstein L: Bone Tumors, 5th ed. St. Louis, CV Mosby, 1977

Spjut HJ et al: Tumors of Bone and Cartilage: Atlas of Tumor Pathology, 2nd series, Fascicle 5. Washington DC, American Registry of Pathology, Armed Forces Institute of Pathology, 1971

Part 5

BASIC PROCESSES IN MUSCLE

Chapter 13

Histology and Biochemistry of Muscle

Carole J. VanderWiel and Charles W. Hooker

GOALS AND OBJECTIVES

Goals: To review the gross anatomy and histology of muscle, with emphasis on skeletal muscle, and to acquaint the reader with the chemistry of skeletal muscle proteins and the biochemistry of skeletal muscle contraction

Objectives: Upon completion of this unit, and using the text as a standard reference, one should be able to evaluate, describe, list or recognize the

1. Three varieties of muscle as seen with a light microscope, and the significance of each
2. Vascular architecture and connective tissue sheaths of typical muscle, muscle–tendon and tendon–bone attachments
3. Innervation of a typical muscle
4. Major fine structural features of skeletal muscle
5. Primary proteins of muscle concerned with contraction
6. Role of the protein troponin in muscle contraction
7. Propagation of the nerve impulse through the muscle cell
8. Sources of energy for muscle contraction
9. Relationship of biochemical events to the morphological changes that occur in muscle contraction and relaxation
10. Role of calcium in the contractile event

OUTLINE

I. Types of muscle
   A. Smooth muscle
   B. Striated muscle

II. Gross anatomical features of skeletal muscle
  A. Connective tissue
  B. Tendons
  C. Blood supply
  D. Innervation
III. Histology of skeletal muscle
  A. The myofibril
  B. Morphological changes during contraction
IV. Chemistry of skeletal muscle
  A. Muscle proteins
    1. Myosin
    2. Actin
    3. Tropomyosin B
    4. Troponin
  B. Relationship of thick and thin filaments
V. Biochemistry of skeletal muscle contraction
  A. ATP and ATPase
  B. Stimulus for contraction
  C. Energy sources
  D. Metabolic sequence in muscle contraction and relaxation
  E. Physiologic and clinical relationships

Muscle has the histologic features and ultrastructural components that provide for contraction through a series of physiologic and biochemical events. Equally important, muscle has attributes that make it possible for its contraction to be translated into mechanical work. As seen with the naked eye, muscle is fibrous in nature, and the fibers (actually, bundles of fibers) are oriented parallel to the long axis of the muscle. It is attached at both ends to some other structure, such as bone, cartilage, fascia, or skin—that is, each muscle possesses the equivalent of an origin and insertion.

TYPES OF MUSCLE

Approximately half of the human body is made up of muscle, which occurs in two generalized forms, smooth muscle and striated muscle.

Smooth Muscle. Smooth muscle is found primarily in the walls of viscera, trachea, bronchi, and blood vessels. It exists as fusiform or spindle-shaped cells with an abundant cytoplasm and a single nucleus. The cytoplasm of each cell contains longitudinally coursing myofibrils, and the elongated nucleus contains many nucleoli. Smooth muscle gives a slow, sustained contraction and slow relaxation with its longitudinally aligned thick and thin filaments. Under the light microscope, these filaments are not as visible as those in skeletal muscle because there is no precise, orderly arrangement of the filaments.

Smooth muscle is nonstriated and involuntary. In certain sites, such as the intestine, smooth muscle possesses a degree of myogenic autorhythmicity with impulses conducted from cell to cell through specialized areas in closely approximated plasma membranes. In other locations, such as the walls of blood vessels, conduction between muscle cells has not been demonstrated, and contraction is provoked by neural stimulation. The motor innervation of smooth muscle is by the autonomic nervous system.

Striated Muscle. Striated muscle is made up of fibers containing many nuclei that resemble the nuclei of smooth muscle. The cytoplasm contains longitudinally oriented fibrils that, unlike those of smooth muscle, exhibit striations. This type of muscle occurs in two forms, cardiac and skeletal.

Cardiac muscle occurs in the walls of the heart and of the great veins in the thorax. It is striated but involuntary. Cardiac muscle is composed of single cells aligned end to end that characteristically branch and anastomose. Each cell has one or two centrally located nuclei and many mitochondria. Peculiar to cardiac muscle are the intercalated discs, which represent specialized cell junctions. Cardiac muscle contracts spontaneously and rhythmically, a property that can readily be observed in isolated cells and fibers from the embryonic or fetal heart. The rate and force of contraction are controlled by the autonomic nervous system.

Skeletal muscle is both striated and innervated by the voluntary nervous system. Contraction of the myofilaments requires neural stimulation. Because skeletal muscle is the main concern of the musculoskeletal system we discuss it in detail below.

GROSS ANATOMICAL FEATURES OF SKELETAL MUSCLE

Connective Tissue. Each muscle is enclosed in a sheath of fibrous connective tissue known as the epimysium or deep fascia. Projections of this connective tissue sheath into the substance of the muscle subdivide it into bundles of fibers or fascicles of various sizes. The sheath of each fascicle is the perimysium. Connective tissue fibers leave the perimysium to surround individual muscle fibers; this innermost sheath is known as the endomysium. The several sheaths are composed chiefly of collagenous fibers and fibrils, with the proportion of elastic fibers being greater in muscles that are in constant use, such as the diaphragm. The numbers and sizes of both collagenous and elastic fibers increase with age, a circumstance that accounts for the toughness of old beef. The perimysium and endomysium convey the blood vessels and nerves within a muscle. They also form tunnels in which bundles of fibers and individual fibers contract. Additionally, they provide attachments for many of the muscle fibers.

Tendons. The attachment of a muscle to its site of origin and insertion is usually provided by tendons. The arrangement of the fasciculi and their angle of attachment to a tendon vary according to the state of contraction. In its simplest arrangement, a muscle is fusiform in shape with a tendon at each end, the tendon of insertion typically being long when the points of attachment are widely separated, as in the flexor carpi ulnaris. In such a muscle, the fasciculi may extend the length of the muscle, and run parallel to each other and to the longitudinal axis of the muscle. This arrangement of fasciculi provides for great range of movement but limited power. The more powerful muscles with less range of movement have more fasciculi of decreased length that run parallel to each other but not to the long axis of the muscle–tendon complex. Muscle fasciculi situated on one side of a tendon that runs the entire length of the muscle form a unipennate muscle (e.g., vastus medialis, flexor pollicis longus). Fasciculi on two sides of a tendon that attach to it at an angle are referred to as bipennate muscles (e.g., rectus femoris). If the entire muscle is, in effect, largely a group of bipennate muscles converging to one or more tendons, it is a multipennate muscle (e.g., the deltoid).

The exact point of attachment of the muscle fibers to tendon fibers is difficult to locate. However, the reticular fibers of the sarcolemma aggregate into strands at the end of a muscle fiber, and these strands are continuous with collagenous fibers of the tendon. The reticular fibers also project into invaginations of the sarcolemma to attach the muscle firmly to the tendon.

A tendon is composed of heavy, parallel bundles of collagenous fibers packed to form an exceedingly dense tissue. Between bundles of fibers are fibroblasts, nerves, and blood vessels that supply the tendon. The bundles of tendon fibers are held together by connective tissue resembling perimysium. Surrounding the entire tendon is a dense but thin fibroelastic membrane, the epitendineum, a counterpart of the epimysium.

The large, parallel bundles of the tendon are composed of intertwining smaller bundles of fibers, particularly near their termination on bone. The intertwining bundles fan out to provide extensive attachment that spreads the contraction of even a portion of the muscle throughout the attachment. This method of attachment also provides a direct line of pull as the angle between tendon and bone changes with movement of the bone. Although tendons appear to blend with and terminate in the periosteum, it has been known, since Ranvier's observations with polarized light in 1880, that many tendon fibers continue into the matrix of the bone. Such fibers occurring in clumps constitute the well-known fibers of Sharpey. As the bone grows, it engulfs tendon fibers, which are then converted to bone.

The architecture of a bone at the point of insertion of a tendon seems to be determined by the orientation of the insertion. When the angle of insertion is acute and the pull of the muscle is parallel to the surface of the bone, the osseous lamellae in this region are also parallel to the surface of the bone. If the angle of insertion is less acute and the pull perpendicular to the surface of bone, the osseous lamellae are also roughly perpendicular to the surface of the bone. When the angle of insertion varies with the movement of the bone, the osseous lamellae radiate from the surface of the bone at varying angles. The sites of attachment of tendons to bone are characteristically elevated and rugose, whereas the sites of attachment of muscle directly to bone are smooth.

When a tendon is held in place by thickened fascia, or when its location could entail friction in rubbing against bone or other firm structures, the tendon may be enclosed in a sheath. The tendon sheath is a tube composed of two layers of connective tissue that are continuous with each other at the ends of the sheath. The outer, thicker layer is attached to surrounding structures, and the inner layer is applied to the tendon. The space between the two layers is comparable to a synovial cavity and contains fluid presumed to be a lubricant. Cartilage or a sesamoid bone may develop within the tendon at sites where friction is great.

Blood Supply. A rich circulation to muscle is provided by the arteries and veins that pierce the epimysium and course parallel to each other in the perimysium. The arteries in the perimysium form longitudinally anastomosing arrays when the artery or arteries supplying a muscle enter it toward one end, as in the gastrocnemius and soleus, and a radial pattern when the nutrient artery enters the muscle near its middle, as in the biceps brachii. Despite these anastomoses, necrosis of a portion of a muscle after interruption of a small artery suggests that collateral circulation is established quite slowly. Some muscles, notably the long flexors and extensors in the leg, are supplied by a series of arteries that form anastomosing arcades. When these arcades are derived from two parent arteries, the viability of the muscle is less threatened by injury than when a single parent artery furnishes the arcades.

The arteries give rise to plexuses of capillaries about individual muscle fibers. Typically, each muscle fiber is related to four or five capillaries, most of which parallel the muscle fiber and have cross connections resembling the rungs of a ladder. The blood flow capacity of these capillary beds and their ability to increase the number of patent capillaries by as much as 45% during exercise can significantly alter blood flow to other organs.

The veins in muscle are richly supplied with valves, a circumstance that may be of primary significance in promoting the great increase in blood flow during exercise. The lymphatic vessels appear to be present in the connective tissue sheaths and in tendons. They constitute a vast network in the perimysium and a finer network surrounding small fascicles. Lymph flow from the muscles is small when muscles are at rest and increases during exercise.

Innervation. The nerve or nerves supplying a muscle contain both efferent and afferent fibers. After piercing the epimysium, they course in the perimysium and branch into nerve fibers that course in the endomysium to reach their destinations. Each motor nerve fiber is distributed to a group of muscle fibers numbering from 1 to perhaps 200. A motor neuron and the group of muscle fibers it supplies is designated as a motor unit (Fig. 13-1). In muscles controlled with precision (e.g., ocular muscles), the motor unit is small; in muscles controlled with less precision, the motor unit is large.

It has suggested that perhaps as many as one half of the nerve fibers traced to a muscle are afferent fibers. Some of the afferent fibers have branched terminals with minute varicosities that surround muscle fibers; other nerve fibers have simpler free endings; still others end in pacinian corpuscles. These several endings are presumably receptors for tactile, pain, and pressure stimuli. The distinctive receptors in muscle are the muscle spindles.

Muscle spindles have been found in nearly all muscles and are more numerous in muscles of the limbs than in the muscles of the trunk. Each muscle spindle is of the order of 5 mm long and 200 μ in diameter (Fig. 13-2). It consists of a bundle of two to ten thin muscle fibers (intrafusal fibers) enclosed in an extensible sheath of loose connective tissue whose ends attach to endomysium surrounding regular (extrafusal) muscle fibers, to perimysium, or to tendon. The ends of the intrafusal fibers are striated and contractile. The midportion of the fiber, called the nuclear bag region, is a bit expanded and filled with nuclei; it lacks stria-

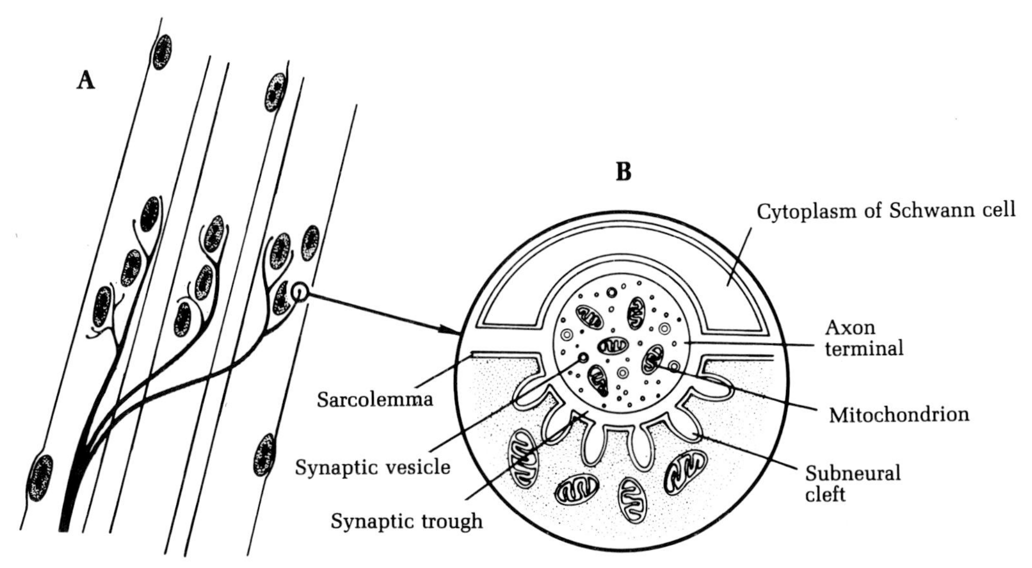

Fig. 13-1. (*A*) The myoneural junction as seen with a light microscope. (*B*) The myoneural junction at higher magnification.

tions and is probably noncontractile. For a short distance beyond the ends of the nuclear bag region, the nuclei are arranged in a centrally located chain; this portion of the intrafusal fiber is called the myotube region. A so-called lymph space surrounds the equatorial region of each intrafusal fiber from one myotube region to the other.

Intrafusal fibers are supplied by three types of nerve fibers. The first type are large afferent nerve fibers 8 to 20 μ in diameter that lose their myelin after penetrating the capsule of the spindle and end in helical terminals that encircle the nuclear bag region; these endings are known as annulospiral, primary, or nuclear bag endings. The second type are smaller afferent fibers 6 to 9 μ in diameter that end as rings, coils, or varicosities on one or both sides of the nuclear bag area; these endings are called myotube, secondary, or flower-spray endings. The third type are small efferent fibers 3 to 7 μ in diameter that terminate in end-plates on the striated poles of the intrafusal fiber; these fibers are known as gamma efferent fibers or fusimotor fibers, and they degenerate following section of the ventral (but not the dorsal) roots of appropriate spinal nerves.

Evidence has been presented that a muscle spindle may contain two varieties of intrafusal fibers. Nuclear bag fibers are relatively large (up to 25 μ in diameter) and stretch the full length of the spindle; nuclear chain fibers are smaller (12 μ in diameter) and much shorter. The latter exhibit a single chain of nuclei rather than a large collection of nuclei. Primary (annulospiral) endings are present in both varieties of intrafusal fiber, but secondary (flower-spray) endings are found primarily on nuclear chain fibers.

Most tendons are supplied with stretch receptors, the Golgi tendon organs. These receptors are located near the attachment of the tendon to its muscle, and each is composed of a number of tendon fasciculi enclosed in a cylindrical or fusiform fibrous capsule penetrated by one or two myelinated nerve fibers. Upon penetrating the capsule, the nerve fibers divide into progressively smaller branches, lose their myelin, and arborize in the tendon bundle. Tension on the tendon presumably distorts these endings and constitutes the stimulus for discharge of the receptor. These receptors apparently do not distinguish between tension produced by active contraction of muscle and that produced by passive pull on the muscle.

HISTOLOGY OF SKELETAL MUSCLE

Individual muscle fibers are cylindrical in shape and typically range from 10 to 50 μ in

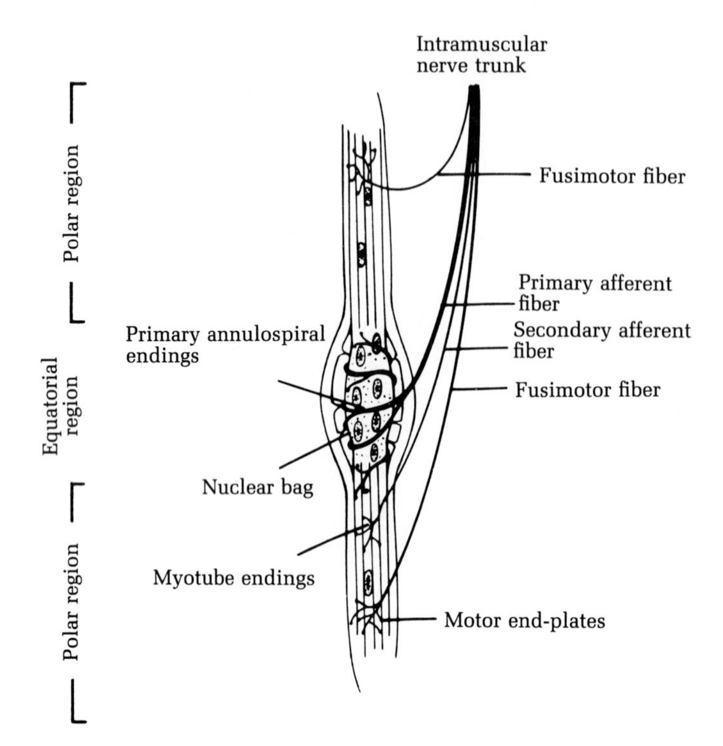

Fig. 13-2. An intrafusal fiber in a muscle spindle and its innervation.

diameter and 1 to 40 mm in length. Each fiber has a limiting plasma membrane, the sarcolemma. Within the sarcolemma, the fiber consists of a fluid material or sarcoplasm, great numbers of longitudinally oriented myofibrils, and many nuclei peripherally located near the sarcolemma. The sarcoplasm contains a Golgi apparatus, many mitochondria, ribosomes, sarcoplasmic reticulum, glycogen, and lipid droplets.

The sarcoplasmic reticulum is a network of cisternae or closed sacs of agranular endoplasmic reticulum that course between and around the myofibrils in a primarily longitudinal direction. Invaginations of the sarcolemma between each myofibril form the transverse tubules (Fig. 13-3). One transverse tubule and two terminal cisternae or lateral sacroplasmic reticular sacs constitute a triad (Fig. 13-4). Each sarcomere has two triads associated with it; in mammals, the triads are located at the level of each A-I junction in skeletal muscle and at the Z line in cardiac muscle.

The Myofibril. Each myofibril exhibits periodic cross striations so aligned with striations of other myofibrils that at a low magnification the entire fiber appears to be striated. These striations are alternating light and dark bands of isotropic and anisotropic materials, respectively. The isotropic band is conventionally designated the I band, and the anisotropic band, the A band. At somewhat higher magnification, each I band is bisected by a thin, dark line, the Z line (for the German word *zwischen,* meaning *between*); each A band is bisected by a light area, or H zone (for the German word *hell,* meaning *bright*). In favorable preparations, the H zone is seen to be crossed in its middle by a thin, dark line, the M line (for the German word *mittel,* meaning *middle*). One contractile unit is the sarcomere, which extends the length between two successive Z lines and is approximately 2.2 μ long in a resting muscle.

With use of the electron microscope, it has been observed that each myofibril contains arrays of longitudinally oriented, parallel, thick and thin myofilaments. The thin filaments are approximately 50 angstroms in diameter and 2 μ in length. They extend for 1 μ on either side of the Z line to the border of the H zone. The thick filaments are of the order of 100 angstroms in diameter and 1.5 μ in length; they span the midportion of the

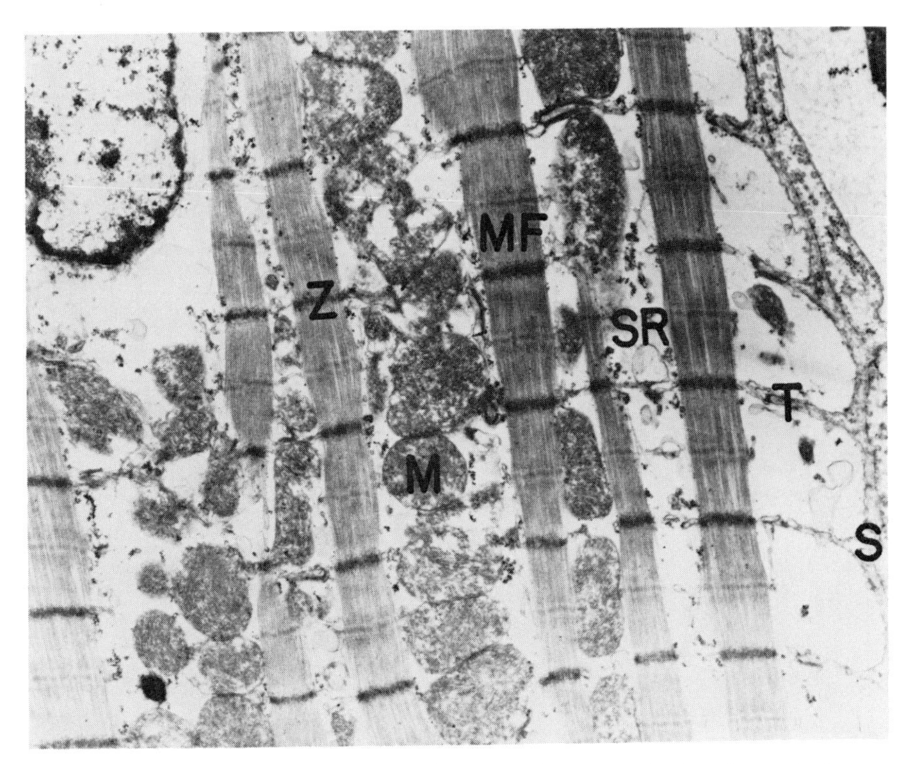

Fig. 13-3. Electron micrograph of cardiac muscle demonstrating the typical cross striation pattern of myofilaments (MF). The myofilaments are separated by many mitochondria (M) and the longitudinal tubules of the sarcoplasmic reticulum (SR). This relaxed muscle shows infoldings of the sarcolemma (S) to form the transverse tubules (T) that course toward the Z line (Z) of each sarcomere in cardiac muscle. In skeletal muscle, the transverse tubules are located at the level of the A-I junction. Original magnification × 8,000.

sarcomere in the A band. Thus, the I band contains only thin filaments, whereas the A band contains both thick and thin filaments, except in the H zone where only thick filaments are present.

Each sarcomere has a precise spacing of the myofilaments. In a cross section of an area where both thick and thin filaments overlap, each thin filament is surrounded by three thick filaments, and each thick filament is surrounded by six thin filaments in a hexagonal arrangement. (Fig. 13-5*D*). The distance between thick and thin filaments is on the order of 100 to 200 angstroms, and the space is bridged by regularly spaced, helically disposed projections of the thick filaments toward adjacent thin filaments.

Morphologic Changes During Contraction. When a muscle fiber contracts, each fiber and each sarcomere becomes shorter and broader. The thick and thin filaments are arranged so that they can slide without restriction past each other to change sarcomere length. Whether the sarcomere is contracted or relaxed, the thick and thin filaments always remain constant in their lengths; only the banding appearance changes (Fig. 13-5).

With maximal contraction, the sarcomere shortens 20% to 50% of its normal resting length. The I band becomes shorter and the H zone usually disappears. The A band does not change in length during contraction or relaxation. The sarcomere can extend to 120% of its length during passive stretching, and the I band becomes longer.

CHEMISTRY OF SKELETAL MUSCLE

Muscle Proteins. Smooth, cardiac, and skeletal muscle employ the same basic principle

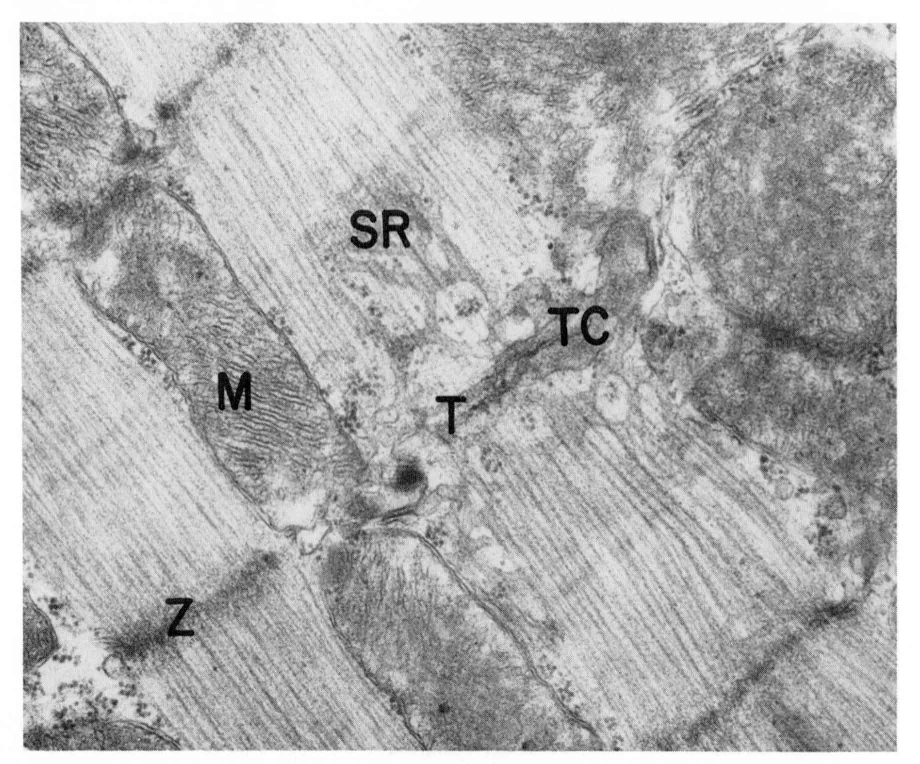

Fig. 13-4. Electron micrograph of striated muscle showing the longitudinal membranes of the sarcoplasmic reticulum (SR) that course over the sarcomere. The transverse tubules (T) cross over each Z line (Z) to meet with the sarcoplasmic reticular sacs or terminal cisternae (TC) to form a triad. Many mitochondria (M) fill the spaces between the myofilaments. Original magnification × 30,000.

of contraction, and all have four water-insoluble proteins that comprise their myofibrils. These proteins make up the contractile units of the cell and include approximately 80% of all muscle protein mass. While once known collectively as the actinomysins, they can be subdivided into discrete proteins with specific functions.

Myosin. Myosin is the largest of the myofibrillar proteins, and it makes up over 50% of the muscle mass. It constitutes the thick filament of the contractile unit. Each subunit consists of two individual single-chain proteins, each with a molecular weight of 225,000. These two proteins are coiled together in a double helical structure, each containing 1800 amino-acid residues. The myosin molecule resembles a thin rod with two small, globular heads. The heads of the chains, or SF_1 filaments, are not coiled, and they protrude from the thick filament (Fig. 13-6). The molecules of this filament are so arranged that these heads protrude at regular intervals along the length of the filament. There are several important characteristics of this head. It has marked ATPase activity in the presence of ionic calcium, and it is this portion of the molecule that serves as a cross-bridge binding myosin with actin.

Actin. The I band, or thin filament, is made up of three proteins. The major component of the thin filament is actin, which consists of two polymers. G-actin, or globular actin, is the usual purified form, a single-chain amino acid with a molecular weight of about 46,000. On binding with ATP, it polymerizes to the F form, or fibrous actin. F-actin binds calcium tightly. These polymers of actin are small, spherical particles arrayed in the thin filament, giving the appearance of a twisted double strand of beads.

Tropomyosin B. Tropomyosin B, also existing as two chains in alpha-helical configuration, is a component of the thin filament

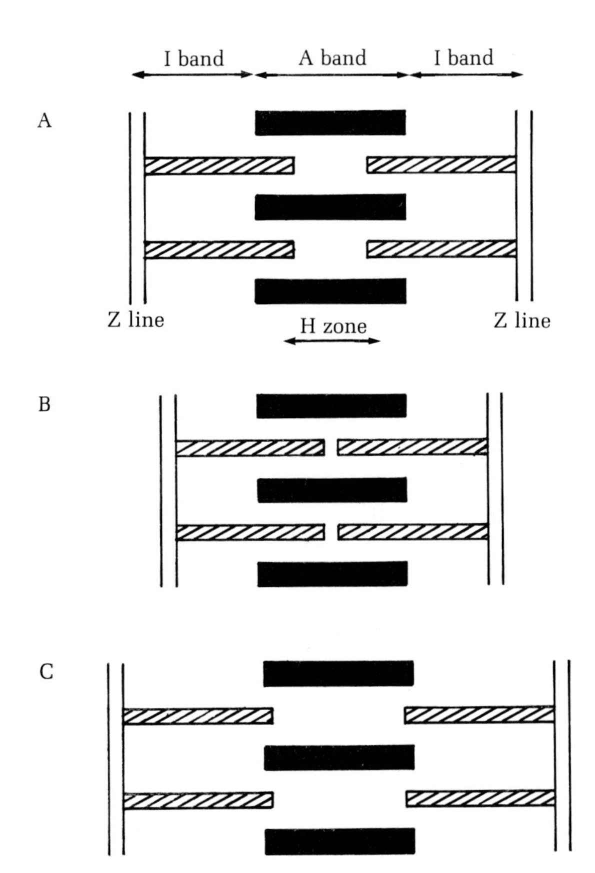

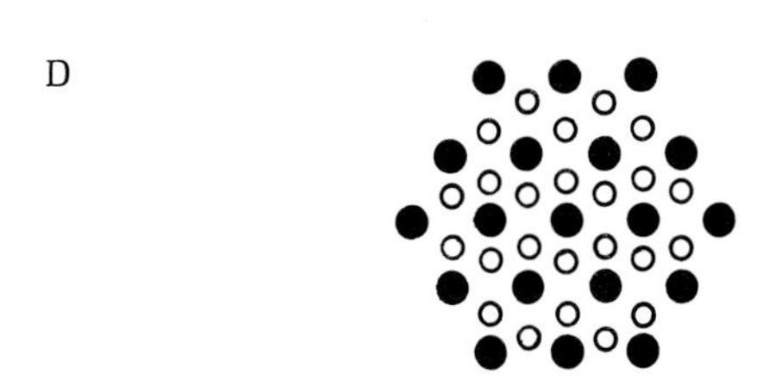

Fig. 13-5. Diagram showing the myofilaments within a fibril. (*A*) relaxed muscle; (*B*) contracted muscle; (*C*) stretched muscle; (*D*) arrangement of myofilaments as seen in cross section at the A-I overlap.

and is complexed with molecules of F-actin. Each molecule has a molecular weight of 70,000. This protein exists primarily in the I zone of the thin filament. Tropomyosin A is not found in mammalian muscle.

Troponin. The fourth muscle protein and the smallest component of the thin filament is troponin. This protein, with a molecular weight of 86,000, was considered until recently a minor component of the thin filament, comprising less than 10% of the filament by weight. However, it has a high affinity for calcium with which it complexes and from which it dissociates rapidly. This protein is now considered to be the key to the contractility of the unit.

Thus, the thin filament contains 300 to 400 actin, 40 to 60 tropomyosin, and 40 to 60 troponin molecules. One tropomyosin molecule extends over seven actin polymers with one troponin astride each tropomyosin B strand.

Relationship of Thick and Thin Filaments. The A band consists of the entire thick filament, the myosin proteins, which are considered to be stationary. It also contains one end of the thin filament. Under appropriate conditions, discussed later, heads of the myosin molecules form a strong bond with units of actin in the thin filament.

The I band consists of the remainder of the thin filament. At the Z line, it is attached to branches of the transverse tubules and is closely associated with the terminal cisternae of the sarcoplasmic reticulum.

BIOCHEMISTRY OF SKELETAL MUSCLE CONTRACTION

ATP and ATPase. There are two important points concerning the ATP of skeletal muscle. First, the actual ATP content in muscle changes little during the process of contraction. Since ATP is used rapidly during contraction, it must also be rapidly replaced. The high-energy compound responsible for this is phosphocreatine, which is present at four to five times the concentration of ATP in muscle. As ADP is formed, it is rephosphorylated by a transfer of phosphate from phosphocreatine. In the reaction (phosphocreatine + ADP $\leftrightarrows$ creatine + ATP), ATP formation is favored at the expense of phosphocreatine at the normal *p*H of the sarcoplasm.

The second point is that ATP readily attaches to the heads of the myosin molecules and produces a connection, or cross-bridge, with actin whenever reactive sites on that molecule are in proper alignment. However, in the presence of active ATPase, also located on the head or SF_1 portions of the myosin molecule, the ATP is reduced and

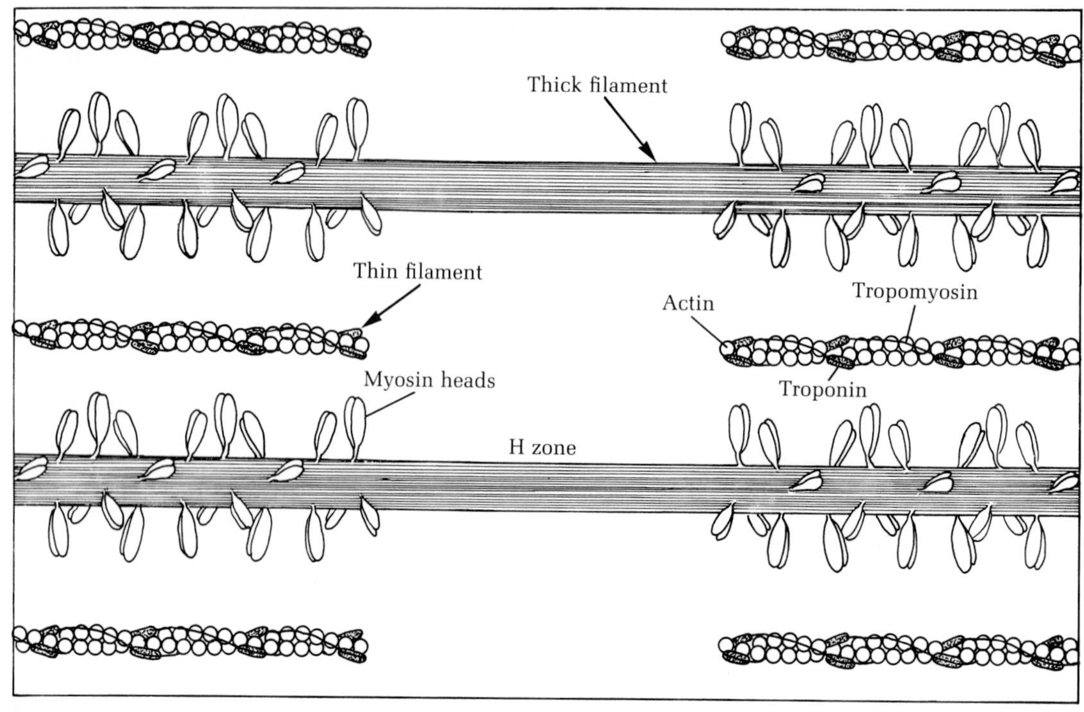

Fig. 13-6. Diagram showing interdigitation of thick and thin filaments and relationship of muscle proteins to each other. (Modified from Murray J, Weber A: The cooperative action of muscle proteins. Sci Am 230:58, 1974)

energy is released, shifting the angle of the cross-bridge between the two filaments. This ATPase is activated by an intracellular calcium ion concentration in the range of 10^{-6} M, but the enzyme is inactive at the resting muscle-cell calcium-ion concentration of 10^{-7} M. The ADP formed by the reaction with ATPase is immediately rephosphorylated to ATP, breaking the cross-bridge between actin and myosin and forming a new one at a different site on the actin molecule. Cross-bridge sites in the same plane on the thick filament are located at intervals of approximately 430 angstroms. At any moment, a majority of these sites remain in contact with the actin molecule in the thin filament. It is generally assumed, largely from the work of Huxley, that the making and breaking of these bonds is the driving force for the contraction of the sarcomere, that is, the sliding of the thin filament along the thick filament. The mechanical sliding of the filaments, or isotonic contraction, involves conformational changes in the head of the myosin molecule, changing the angle of the bridge attachment between the two filaments.

A second ATPase is located in the membranes of the sarcoplasmic reticulum. This system reverses the calcium flow and returns calcium into storage. This ATPase is also calcium sensitive and is activated at the same molar concentration as is the ATPase attached to myosin.

The Stimulus for Contraction. The contractile impulse causes a depolarization of the cell membrane, including the transverse tubules. This process is thought to be similar to the passage of an impulse down an axon. The actual movement of potassium and sodium ions within the tubules is discussed in Chapter 14. The permeability of the cell membrane to cations increases, and ionized calcium can then enter the cell.

Skeletal muscle cannot depend upon this method alone for the calcium needed to initiate contraction. Therefore, the relationship of the triad, that is, the location of transverse tubules near the calcium stores in the terminal cisternae, is of great importance. This calcium can be visualized by special techniques at the electron microscopic level. The impulse for depolarization must be passed on to these calcium storage sites.

The stimulus for muscle contraction is an electrical impulse from a motor nerve at the motor end-plate or neuromuscular junction. When the sarcolemma is excited by an incoming impulse, sodium, potassium, and chloride ions move about within the transverse tubules to spread the impulse and depolarize membranes. This depolarization rapidly spreads to the terminal cisternae, which release calcium ions into the sarcoplasm. The electrical impulse depolarizes the entire transverse tubular system instantaneously so that all filaments in a muscle fiber contract together. It is noteworthy that, during depolarization, the cell membrane may also become more permeable to other substances, such as glucose and amino acids.

Energy Sources. The immediate energy reserve is provided by phosphocreatine stores, because the level of ATP in muscle would only allow for a muscle contraction lasting about 0.5 sec. Phosphocreatine stores, however, provide energy for only a few seconds of contraction. The ultimate source of energy for rephosphorylation of ADP is from normal metabolic pathways, glycolysis and respiration. The more active the muscle, the more it must depend on respiration and the higher its content of myoglobin and cytochromes, which give it a red color. In red muscle, the myofibrils are less numerous, the cross-striations are less regular, and nuclei appear scattered through the fiber instead of being largely subsarcolemmal in location. Red fibers contract and relax more slowly than white muscle fibers and predominate in muscles that sustain prolonged contraction. Respiration serves as their chief source of energy for rephosphorylation of ADP by means of oxidative phosphorylation in mitochondria. The more inactive, or white, muscle uses glycolysis as its main energy source.

The rates of respiration and glycolysis are regulated by a metabolic series of feedback controls, particularly by the activities of the enzymes phosphofructokinase (glycolysis) and isocitrate dehydrogenase (respiration; Fig. 13-7). With maximum activity, the oxygen consumption may increase by as much as twentyfold, with an accompanying increase in the utilization of glucose or glycogen. These two activities result in the formation of excessive lactic acid, which diffuses from muscle and is eventually oxidized by means of the tricarboxylic acid (TCA) cycle in the liver. During recovery, additional oxygen is taken into the body by continued rapid breathing to provide an amount equivalent to that necessary to oxidize excessive lactic acid (the oxygen debt).

The energy sources required for both the duration and extent of muscular activity have been thoroughly studied. Obviously, the first source is phosphocreatine, which provides the initial ATP supply. The second source is through an increase in the oxidative processes, glycolysis, and the activity of the tricarboxylic acid cycle. If these sources are insufficient, the anaerobic glycolytic pathways provide additional energy sources but lead to increased lactic acid production, which increases the oxygen debt.

There are several methods by which increased energy for sustained muscle activity may be derived. One is by increasing the stores of phosphocreatine, which makes only a minor contribution. The primary method occurs in highly conditioned athletes through their ability to obtain an unusual share of their energy needs from increased oxygen consumption, so that lactic acid production begins at a higher level of exertion. This effect could be due to improved cardiovascular output, improved microcirculation in muscle, and increased cytochrome supplies for more rapid oxygen utilization and ATP formation in muscle itself.

Metabolic Sequence in Muscle Contraction and Relaxation. Muscle contraction starts with the release of ionic calcium, primarily from the terminal cisternae into the sarcoplasm. Although the amount of calcium released is sufficient, if it remains ionized, to raise the calcium ion level from its resting concentration of 10^{-7} M to 10^{-4} M, most of the calcium is immediately complexed by intracellular proteins. Complexing of calcium by troponin shifts the protein conformations in the thin filament and brings the reactive sites on actin in spatial relationship

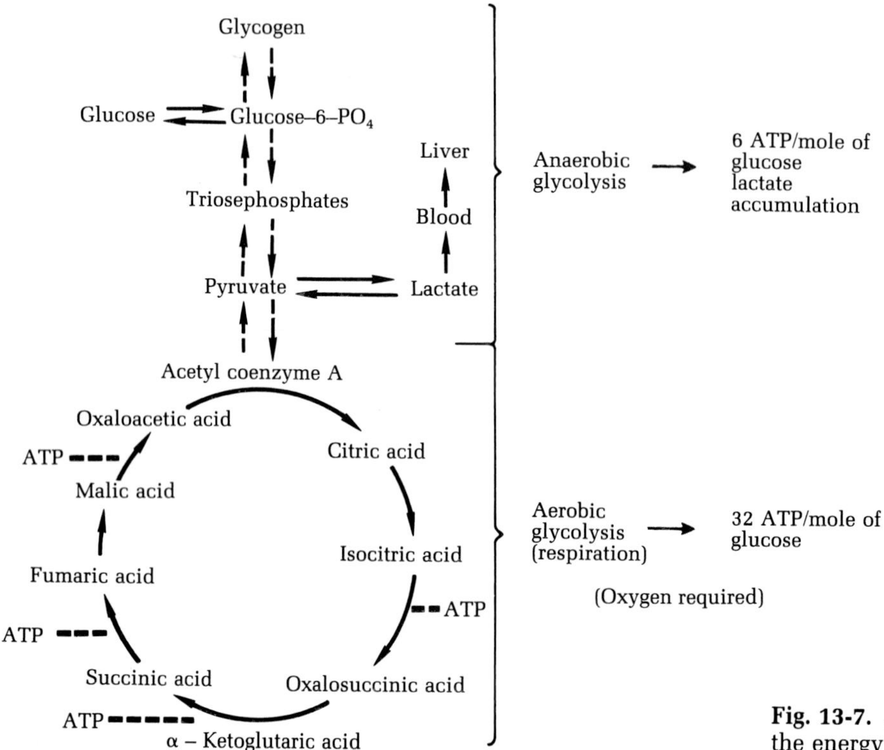

Fig. 13-7. A simplification of the energy sources in muscle.

to the receptive SF_1 units of myosin, forming cross-bridges between the two filaments. At the same time, the high ionic calcium activates the ATPase located in these units, reducing the ATP and supplying energy for the conformational change in the cross-bridge, which moves the actin molecule up the long axis of the myosin filament. Since additional ATP is immediately supplied, the cross-bridge is rapidly broken and reestablished at a different site along the actin molecule.

The driving force for the sliding of thick and thin filaments comes from cross-bridges on the thick filament that attach to the thin filament at a certain angle, then swivel to a new angle, thus pulling the thin filaments past the thick filaments. The cross-bridges on opposite sides of the H zone swivel in opposite directions, and each cross-bridge must attach, swivel, detach, and then reattach at a new point further along the thin filament. Contraction of the muscle is like a rowing action of many oars, attaching and reattaching to pull the filaments into a greater overlap, thus decreasing the distance between Z lines and shortening the muscle. One single cycle of attachment, swiveling, and detaching causes a relative movement of the two filaments of about 100 angstroms, so the muscle will shorten about 1% of its total length.

Making and breaking cross-bridges permits sliding of the thin filament along the thick filament while providing the force for isometric contraction. As long as the calcium concentration in the cell is maintained in the range of 10^{-6} M, both the conformation of troponin and the ATPase activity of myosin permit the fibril to stay in its contracted form, rapidly depleting ATP stores.

The ionic calcium concurrently activates the second ATPase system concentrated on the sarcoplasmic reticulum and the plasma membrane. An ATP-dependent calcium pump located within the membranes of the sarcoplasmic reticulum returns intracellular calcium back into storage areas in the terminal cisternae and in mitochondria. This is a rather ineffectual system as long as the nerve impulse maintains the high permeability of these membranes to calcium (the concentration of calcium in extracellular fluids is 1.5×10^{-3} M). However, when the energizing impulse terminates, calcium is rapidly

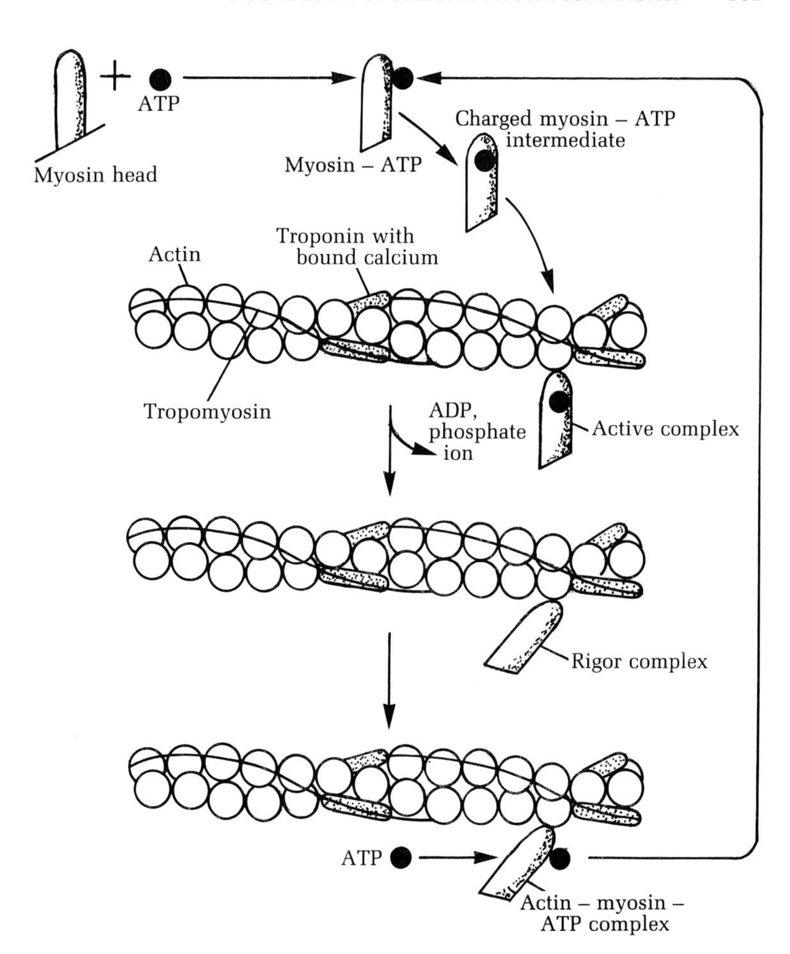

Fig. 13-8. Diagram of the chemical events of the muscle contraction cycle. (Modified from Murray J, Weber A: Chemical events of muscle-contraction cycle. Sci Am 230:58, 1974)

pumped out of the sarcoplasm. As the ionic concentration drops, calcium is withdrawn from troponin, and when sufficiently low, the ATPase on myosin is inactivated. When completely at rest, the ionic calcium concentration in the cell returns to its base level of 10^{-7} M, calcium stores are replaced in the sarcoplasmic reticulum, and the troponin–actin–tropomyosin B complex is such that bridges between actin and myosin are no longer possible.

The actual chemical events that occur in muscle contraction are illustrated in Fig. 13-8. ATP readily attaches to the head of a myosin molecule to make a charged myosin–ATP intermediate form. In healthy muscle, every myosin head will bind an ATP molecule. The intermediate form has a strong tendency to bind to actin to form an active complex with a high-energy state; this complex is short-lived. ATPase also located on the myosin head will split ATP into ADP and inorganic phosphate with a release of energy. The complex left is a low-energy complex, referréd to as a rigor complex, which remains intact until a new ATP molecule binds to the myosin head. In this manner, the myosin–ATP is recycled and recharged, and once again undergoes hydrolysis.

Muscle contraction is regulated by calcium ions, which will change the thin filament into an activated state by binding to troponin. Calcium must turn on actin in order for the charged myosin–ATP intermediate to bind with actin; then hydrolysis of ATP proceeds. Formation of the rigor complex is not sensitive to calcium control. Whether the thin filament is turned on or off, a myosin head can always combine with actin to form the rigor complex. In the absence of calcium, troponin and tropomyosin block the formation of active complexes. In the absence of ATP, myosin and actin form rigor complexes whether or not calcium is present. After death, there is a gradual decrease in ATP concentration, so less ATP is available to disassociate the myosin head in a rigor complex from the actin molecule. The extreme rigidity in muscles, or rigor mortis, results from the formation of more and more rigor complexes with not enough ATP present to dissociate them.

The importance of the proper calcium concentration throughout the process of muscle contraction should be emphasized. First, calcium is needed to bind to troponin so that the tropomyosin molecule can transmit a message to its seven actin molecules to activate them. Next, calcium is required to activate ATPase on the myosin head, which reduces ATP and supplies the energy needed for the conformational changes in the crossbridges to slide filaments along each other. Last, ionic calcium activates the ATPase in sarcoplasmic reticulum and on plasma membranes to generate the calcium pumps that pulls calcium back into the storage area.

Physiologic and Clinical Relationships. Despite the recent clarification of many of the biochemical steps in muscle contraction, there are many physiologic responses of muscle that are not clearly understood. For example, Starling's law states that a stretched muscle fiber has greater strength of contraction than the same fiber in a less stretched condition. The usual explanation given is that in the stretched condition, the impulse for depolarization is more rapidly and uniformly spread, permitting more myofibrils and their filaments to move the calcium needed for contraction. This phenomenon, also occurring in skeletal muscle, has an obvious practical application exemplified by the strength of the heartbeat during exercise, which is due to the more complete filling and stretching of the heart during diastole.

One of the more interesting phenomena is that an excessively low plasma calcium concentration leads to tetanic muscle contraction. This apparent paradox is due to the fact that skeletal muscle cells do not depend upon extracellular fluid calcium for their immediate needs and contraction, but the cell membranes of the neuromuscular complex and the muscle cells themselves are sensitive to loss of extracellular fluid calcium. With the decrease in membrane calcium, spontaneous firing may occur, which leads to a continuous and more complete depolarization of muscle cell membranes, causing tetanic contraction. Continuous, long-lasting dietary calcium deficiency will eventually lead to diminution of calcium in muscle, but these cells do not readily give up their calcium.

Cardiac muscle contraction is, however, immediately affected by changes in extracellular fluid calcium concentrations. This is because cardiac muscle uses calcium from the extracellular fluid as an immediate supply for contraction owing to its lack of calcium storage sites and dilated terminal cisternae. Although the use of calcium in emergency treatment of cardiac arrest is explained by this need for calcium in and on cardiac cell membranes, excessively high plasma calcium concentrations (as in acute hyperparathyroidism) can also cause cardiac arrest. This effect is probably produced by excessive calcium accumulation on cardiac muscle cell membranes, which reduces their permeability to sodium. The result is a failure of the membrane to depolarize properly on receipt of a stimulus. Excessive calcium prevents what the cell requires for contraction: an intracellular movement of calcium produced by the depolarization of its membrane.

The difficulties in accurately explaining the above phenomenon are due to the complexity of the effect of calcium accumulation on, or loss from, specific cell membranes, and to the importance of proper calcium movement within the cell for muscular contraction.

From a clinical standpoint, one of the most important attributes of muscle is its ability to develop tension, which is related to the length of the muscle at the time of contraction. The active contractile force of a muscle increases with the length of the muscle until the resting length of the muscle is achieved. Thereafter, the contractility of the muscle is supplemented by the elasticity of the fibrous tissue and sarcolemma of the muscle fibers until the muscle is torn. Clinical application of this information is found in the field of tendon surgery. In tendon grafting operations, it is important to determine the resting length of the musculotendinous unit, so that a tendon graft may be placed under the proper tension (usually the

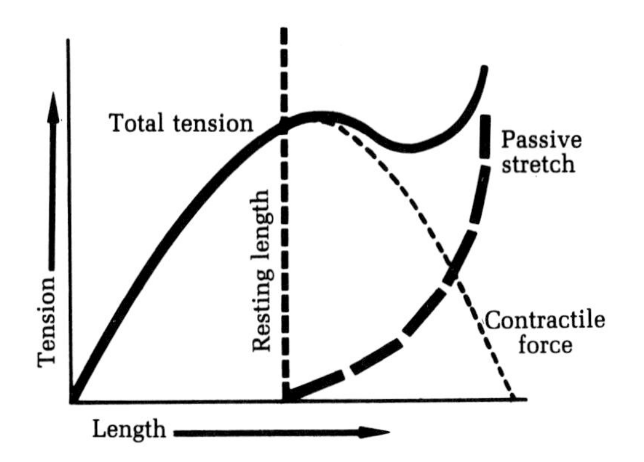

Fig. 13-9. The Blix curve. After the resting length of the muscle is reached, its contractile force decreases, but the total muscle tension increases with continued lengthening of the muscle as a result of the elasticity in its fibrous elements.

resting length of the muscle) to develop its strongest and most efficient contractile force. These relationships have been plotted in a curve by Blix (Fig. 13-9).

SELECTED REFERENCES

Bourne GH: The structure and function of muscle, Vol I and II. New York, Academic Press, 1960

Franzini-Armstrong C: Sarcolemmal invaginations and the T-system in skeletal muscle fibers. J Cell Biol 19:24A, 1963

Goss CM: The attachment of skeletal muscle fibers. Am J Anat 74:259, 1944

Huxley HE: The mechanism of muscle contraction. Science 104:1356, 1969

Lehninger AL: Biochemistry, pp 583–602. New York, Worth Publishers, Inc., 1970

Murray JM, Weber A: The cooperative action of muscle proteins. Sci Am 230:58, 1974

Physiology Symposium: Excitation-contraction coupling in skeletal muscle. Fed Proc 24:1112, 1965

Sandow A: Skeletal muscle. Annu Rev Physiol 32:87, 1970

Winegrad S: Intracellular calcium movements of frog skeletal muscle during recovery from tetanies. J Gen Physiol 51:1, 1968

Chapter 14

Physiology of Muscle

Colin D. Hall
and Timothy N. Taft

GOALS AND OBJECTIVES

Goals: To introduce the reader to the basic physiology of muscle contraction, to the physiologic variability found within fibers of skeletal muscle, and to the factors involved in increasing muscle bulk and in muscle atrophy

Objectives: On completion of this unit, and using the text as a standard reference, one should be able to describe, list, draw or recognize the

1. Propagation of an action potential from the anterior horn cell of the spinal cord along the nerve axon to the muscle fiber
2. Physiologic events in muscle contraction
3. Different forms of axoplasmic flow to and from the muscles
4. Different types of muscle fibers and their properties
5. Patterns of recruitment and fatigue of muscle fibers during exercise
6. Features of muscle hypertrophy and atrophy

OUTLINE

I. The physiologic process of muscle contraction
   A. Propagation of the nerve action potential
   B. Neuromuscular transmission
   C. Propagation of the muscle membrane potential
   D. Muscle contraction
II. Axoplasmic flow
   A. Centrifugal flow
      1. Fast axoplasmic flow
      2. Slow axoplasmic flow
   B. Centripetal flow

III. Muscle fiber types
IV. Recruitment of motor units
V. Fatigue
VI. Muscle hypertrophy
VII. Muscle atrophy

This chapter deals almost exclusively with physiologic changes in skeletal muscle. Several different types of fibers are present in each human skeletal muscle, but the basic physiologic process causing contraction of the myofibril is essentially the same in all, and these events are discussed first. The sequence is schematically represented in Figure 14-1.

THE PHYSIOLOGIC PROCESS OF MUSCLE CONTRACTION

Muscle contraction results from a voluntary impulse transmitted from cortical neurons, or from a reflex impulse arising in lower or upper motor neurons. In either case, muscle action is initiated by firing of the motor neurons, cell bodies which lie in the gray matter of the anterior horn of the spinal cord. Each motor neuron has several dendrites that pick up afferent input to the cell, and one axon that transmits the efferent impulse through the anterior root to the neuromuscular junction. In small muscles, for example, the extraocular muscles, each axon may supply only three or four individual muscle fibers; in large skeletal muscles, an axon may supply up to two thousand individual muscle fibers. Each axon has an all-or-nothing effect on the muscle it supplies, although the number of axons fired at any one time is under voluntary control, thus allowing graded responses by the muscle during voluntary action. Initiation of the least possible contraction of a muscle causes one single axon to commence firing and the fibers associated with it to contract. With gradual increase in effort, that axon increases its firing rate. As effort is further increased, more axons start firing, thus increasing muscle response by both an increase in the number of contractions of each fiber and an increase in the number of fibers contracting.

Propagation of the Nerve Action Potential

The mammalian nerve cell has a resting electrical potential across the membrane, the exterior having a potential of −85 millivolts (mv) as compared with the interior. When the nerve cell fires, the electrical potential is carried along the axon in a characteristic manner: the permeability of the external membrane to sodium increases, permitting sodium to flow into the cell and depolarize the membrane, followed by an efflux of potassium to restore the negative membrane potential. At rest, the membrane pump actively extrudes sodium, allowing potassium to reenter the cell and restore the balance in preparation for the next impulse. The pump uses adenosinetriphosphate as an energy source. As depolarization occurs across a portion of the membrane, the immediately adjacent membrane surface is also stimulated and depolarizes. In this way, the action potential is conducted along the axon to reach the muscle. However, motor axons constitute some of the longest cells of the body, running the entire length of the peripheral nerve, and to activate them throughout their length in this way would be both time and energy consuming. These cells have developed a method of reducing energy demands and decreasing conduction velocity while transmitting their impulses; this method is called *saltatory conduction*. Schwann cells develop a multilayered lipid coating, the *myelin sheath*, that tightly encases each axon throughout its length. At approximately every thousand micrometers along the axon, there is a break in the myelin sheath called the *node of Ranvier*, where the axon becomes exposed. Current can flow between the axon and the myelin sheath without the necessity of depolarizing each molecular level of the underlying axon, and the axon is only depolarized at the exposed nodes of Ranvier. Thus, on depolarization of the anterior horn cell, the impulse is rapidly and efficiently conducted to the neuromuscular junction.

Neuromuscular Transmission

As the motor axon enters the muscle, it ramifies into many individual processes, each of which makes contact with, and is responsible for, the initiation of firing in an individual muscle fiber. The architecture of the neuromuscular junction is discussed in the previous chapter. The nerve splays out over

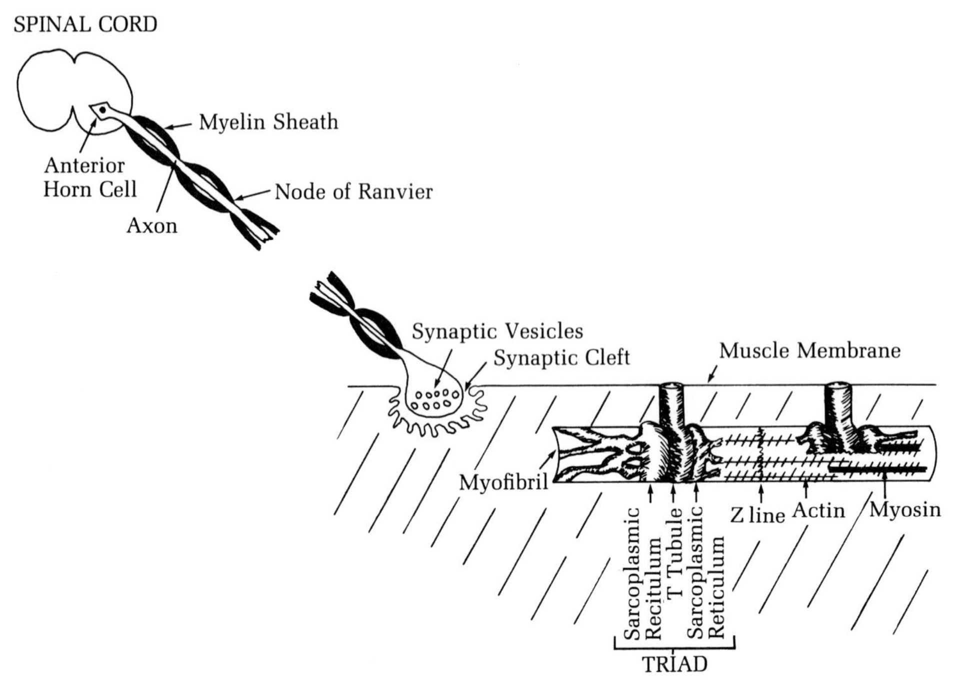

Fig. 14-1. Schematic representation of propagation of action potential from spinal anterior horn cell to muscle fiber resulting in muscle contraction. See text for explanation.

an area on the surface of the muscle like the sucker of a tentacle, but there is a small space between the terminal axon and the muscle fiber called the synaptic cleft. Chemical rather than electrical transmission occurs across this cleft. The chemical mediator is acetylcholine. It has long been believed that acetylcholine is stored in small packets, called vesicles, in the axon terminal, and that these packets are liberated with the propagation of a nerve impulse, resulting in release of acetylcholine into the synaptic cleft. This process occurs, but it has also become obvious that there are even larger amounts of free acetylcholine in the axon terminal that are also extruded into the cleft with the arrival of the nerve action potential. The roles of these two mechanisms are not fully understood.

Whatever their importance, the two sources allow acetylcholine to float across the synaptic cleft and to land on receptor sites that are clustered in this area of the muscle membrane. This chemical response causes depolarization of the muscle fiber membrane. The enzyme acetylcholinesterase then breaks the acetylcholine molecule down to choline and acetate, terminating the impulse on the receptor site and allowing the constituents to be recycled to form more presynaptic acetylcholine, which prepares the mechanism for the next impulse.

Propagation of the Muscle Membrane Potential

As with nerve, muscle has a resting membrane potential on its exterior of −85 mv. The arrival of acetylcholine on the postsynaptic receptor sites allows a sodium influx and a potassium efflux that reverses this potential. As with other mammalian cells, this electrical response is transmitted along the membrane into adjacent areas. A unique feature of the muscle cell is the way it enables this current to be transmitted to the interior of the cell, eventually causing stimulation and contraction of the myofibrils. Electron microscopic studies have shown holes in the external membrane that lead to hollow shafts plunging into the depths of the muscle fiber, called the T tubular system (Fig. 14-1). The external membrane continues into these shafts. Each T tubule runs down and encircles an underlying myofibril. As it runs around the myofibril, it is in close connection with dilated sacs of the sarcoplasmic reticulum. Thus, the sarcoplasmic reticulum at these points, known as *triads*, is in contact with the continuation of the external surface membrane of the muscle. The sarcoplasmic reticulum, as discussed in Chapter 13, forms a network of longitudinal channels surrounding the myofibrils and connecting them with their neighbors. The triads circle the myofibril over the junctions of the A and I bands.

Muscle Contraction

The microanatomy of the muscle fiber is discussed in the previous chapter. Actin and myosin filaments overlap each other. When contraction takes place, the head of the myosin fiber temporarily attaches itself to a receptor in the actin filament, then flexes, sliding the actin filament towards it. It detaches, attaches to the next receptor site on the filament, and repeats the process, thus sliding the two fibers along each other and shortening the muscle. Each "flexion" of the myosin or actin requires one molecule of adenosinetriphosphate as an energy source.

The actin filament has long, thin fibers on its surface, called tropomyosin fibers. Each tropomyosin strand has a globular molecule of the protein troponin near its end. It appears that the tropomyosin strands may physically impede the cross-bridges between actin and myosin, thus inhibiting contraction of the muscle. The troponin molecule in some way locks the tropomyosin in place. Calcium is required to negate this action. Calcium ions combine with troponin molecules, neutralizing their effect and "unlocking" the tropomyosin, which moves to a neutral position, allows coupling of the actin and myosin, and muscle contraction results.

The sarcoplasmic reticulum stores calcium in its interior. Depolarization of the muscle membrane along the T tubular system causes a release of calcium in the closely adjacent sarcoplasmic reticulum; these calcium ions are then available to uncouple the tropomyosin. After muscle contraction occurs, there is reuptake of calcium into the sarcoplasmic reticulum and reactivation of the blocking effect of the tropomyosin. Reuptake by the sarcoplasmic reticulum may be inhibited if there is insufficient energy available, which may lead to muscle contraction without electrical stimulation, as is seen in some glycogen storage diseases and malignant hyperthermia.

AXOPLASMIC FLOW

Electrical impulses generated by alterations in membrane potential are not the only things conducted along the axon that affect the muscle. Various chemical compounds also migrate along the nerve fiber, both toward the muscle and toward the anterior horn cell. These substances seem to have a profound effect on the functioning of the lower motor neuron. This migration of chemical messengers is known as axoplasmic flow.

Centrifugal Flow

The flow of axoplasm toward the muscle may be fast or slow.

Fast Axoplasmic Flow. Fast axoplasmic flow can be observed by injecting radioactive leucine into the ventral gray column of the spinal cord or by cooling a segment of the nerve and watching the rapid accumulation of substances above the cooled area. Proteins, lipids, and polysaccharides may be conducted down the axon at a rate of up to 40 cm per day. Most of these substances are transported in the form of mitochondria.

Slow Axoplasmic Flow. A very mild degree of compression on the nerve results, over a period of weeks, in the accumulation of conducted substances proximal to the constriction; removal of the compression then allows these materials to be passed along the nerve. Again, radio-labelled leucine injected into the ventral column of the spinal cord will be taken up by proteins and conducted along the nerve in a way that can be followed. This movement occurs at the rate of approximately 1 mm per day.

Centripetal Flow

Substances are also transmitted from muscle to the anterior horn cell; interruption of flow in this direction leads to a trophic effect on the motor neuron. This effect can be demonstrated by the injection of Evans blue dye into muscle and the appearance of that substance some hours later in the anterior horn cell of the spinal cord. Centripetal flow is carried out at an intermediate velocity, between the fast and slow centrifugal conduction speeds.

MUSCLE FIBER TYPES

The above physiologic processes are common to all motor units and muscle fibers. However, the study of muscle with a variety of histochemical stains has shown that there are significant biologic and physiologic variations in different muscle fibers. Exactly how many different types of muscle fibers there are is subject to controversy, and there is no universally accepted nomenclature for these different types. However, in the study of human physiology and disease, it is most useful to divide muscle into two major fiber types, type I and type II fibers. Type II fibers are subdivided into at least two types, type IIa and type IIb. In lower mammals and other animals, muscles are generally composed entirely of either type I or type II fibers. However, each human muscle is made up of a mixture of type I and type II fibers, in varying percentages, which gives a mosaic or checkerboard appearance when colored with appropriate differentiating histologic stains (Fig. 14-2).

There are significant differences in the fiber types. Type I muscle fibers are rich in the enzymes necessary for oxidative metabolism and are darker in appearance. When stimulated, they have a slow contraction or "twitch" time. Type IIa fibers are pale in appearance. They are rich in the enzymes necessary to promote glycolytic metabolism and show a rapid twitch time. Type IIb fibers have an admixture of glycolytic and oxidative enzymes and show an intermediate twitch time. Type I fibers thus appear particularly well suited for activities related to physical effort requiring strength and endurance that depend for energy metabolism on oxidative processes. Type II fibers, on the other hand, obtain their energy through the much faster glycolytic process; but as glycogen stores may be more rapidly depleted than oxygen supplies, they are less suited to continuous types of activity and more to rapid alternating ef-

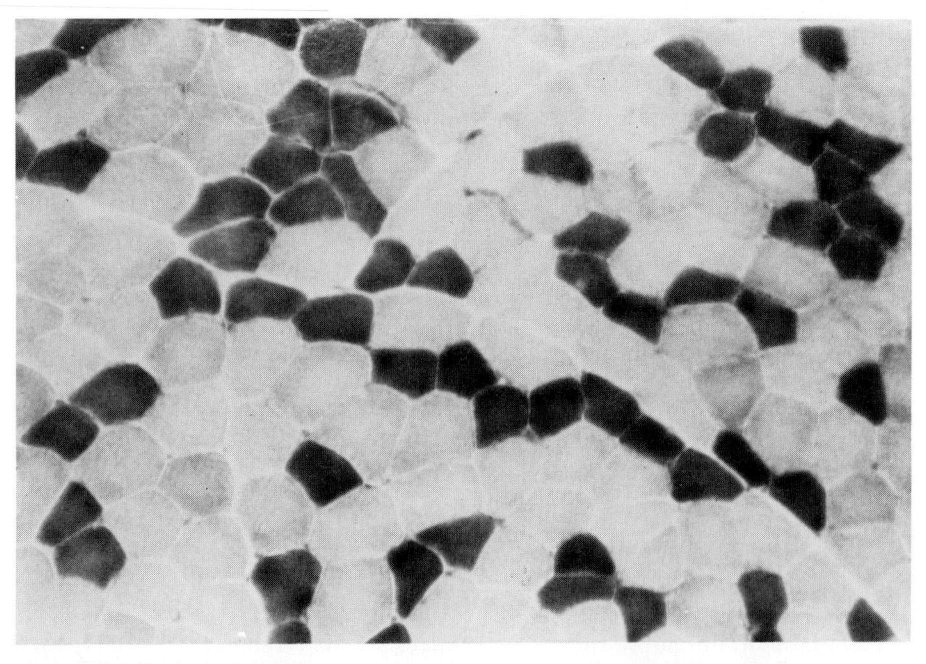

Fig. 14-2. Checkerboard appearance resulting from differential histochemical staining of muscle fibers. Type I fibers are dark, type II fibers light. (Adenosine triphosphate stain, pH 9.5)

fort. Indeed, gravity-related muscles in many animals, such as the thigh muscles of the chicken, are composed entirely of type I fibers, whereas muscles requiring repetitive rapid action, such as the wing muscles, are composed entirely of type II fibers. Even in humans, those muscles most accustomed to slow, continuous work have a higher percentage of type I muscle fibers.

There is some evidence that type II fibers are more prone to anatomic changes following altered energy demands than are type I. Type II fibers tend to be smaller than type I in children and in adults who do not carry out strenuous physical exercise, although they increase in size with repeated physical demands on the muscle. They also degenerate rapidly when the muscle is not used, as is discussed in the next chapter.

Fiber Type Determination. The muscle fiber type depends not on any intrinsic feature of the fiber itself but on the motor neuron supplying that particular fiber. Thus, all muscle fibers supplied by one particular axon will be of either type I or type II. This fact can be demonstrated by the simple experiment of cross-transplanting the nerve to a muscle composed entirely of type I fibers with the nerve to a muscle composed entirely of type II fibers. As the nerves reinnervate their new muscles, the fiber types completely reverse until the nerve that supplied type I muscle does so again, and *vice versa*. The importance of this factor in neuropathic disease is discussed in the next chapter.

RECRUITMENT OF MOTOR UNITS

As physical effort increases, more motor neurons and their muscle fibers are brought into play. The earliest fiber recruited generally fires at 5 to 10 Hz (cycles per second). As effort is increased, the unit speeds up to a maximum firing rate of around 100 Hz. Long before this time, usually when its firing rate passes 10 Hz, other units are recruited that also increase their firing rate with increased effort. Eventually, all units supplying the muscle fire, resulting in maximal voluntary effort. Some very large units appear to fire only in short bursts during the time of highest demand. The increase in force engendered by the muscle depends much more on the increased firing rate than it does on the recruitment of additional units, particularly at high levels of effort. With isometric exercise, the muscle develops increased tension without movement of its points of attachment, and the energy produced is dissipated as heat. With isotonic exercise, there is movement of the points of muscle attachment, and the work done can be measured by multiplying the load moved by the distance through which it is moved. The physiologic process is the same in both cases. The units recruited first are type I fibers with slow twitch that depend on oxidative energy sources. They are almost entirely responsible for the first 20% of contractile strength. Then there is an increasing demand on type II fibers with more rapid and phasic bursts of activity. At really high levels of effort, the type II fibers play the major role and are the first to fatigue.

FATIGUE

Even in the most fully trained athlete, continuous or repeated effort leads to fatigue of the neuromuscular system. Several factors appear to be responsible. Motor neurons are unable to maintain their high firing rate for a protracted period. Although the firing rate is approximately 100 Hz at the beginning of maximal effort, it rapidly diminishes to about 20 Hz after approximately 30 sec of activity. In addition, there is physiologic fatigue of the contractile mechanism of the muscle itself, resulting in less efficient functioning after protracted effort. Another factor, particularly during isometric exercise, is an increase in the pressure in the muscle above arterial blood pressure, which reduces the nutrient blood flow, and thereby the energy source, available to the muscle.

MUSCLE HYPERTROPHY

It is common knowledge that muscle increases in bulk and strength throughout childhood and puberty to reach a peak in young adulthood. It is also obvious that increased demand on the muscle leads to rapid increase in its bulk and work capacity, as witnessed by the results of physical fitness programs. There is evidence that the number of fibers in human muscle does not increase after birth. The increase in size appears to be due almost entirely to an increase in the number of myofibrils within each muscle fiber. During childhood, this increase appears to be at least partially under the control of growth hormone, and a further spurt at puberty appears to be due to testosterone. The potential of muscle to grow under the influence of testosterone-like anabolic steroids is maintained into adulthood and has been frequently used, and misused, in athletic circles.

The physiologic process causing myofibrillar increase following physical exercise is not fully understood. There is greater and more rapid increase in muscle bulk with isometric exercises than with isotonic exercises. With isometric exercise, there is muscle contraction with shortening of some myofibrils, or parts of myofibrils, as a result of the sliding filaments of actin and myosin. However, when myofibrils shorten, there must be a compensatory stretching of others since the two end points of the muscle do not move. This stretching process also takes place at the onset of isotonic exercise, before movement occurs, and, in general, the heavier the weight moved, the longer the initial isometric phase after contraction starts and before movement occurs. This stretching seems to be very important in producing the increase in myofibrils. It is postulated that, because the myofibrils are unable to cope readily with continuing demands, they go through a process of forking or splitting, where they divide centrally, and two or more new myofibrils form from the original. Evidence that stretching is an important feature has been gained from experiments where limbs are splinted in a position that causes continuous stretch of a muscle without associated work demand. When limbs are casted in this fashion, fiber splitting will again develop. In muscle damaged by various pathologic processes, residual undamaged myofibrils may split, presumably in an effort to compensate for their malfunctioning companions (see Chap. 15, Fig. 15-5).

MUSCLE ATROPHY

Muscle fibers atrophy during starvation, presumably owing to a lack of necessary nutrients. There is also diminution in muscle strength and bulk following protracted disuse, which is a significant clinical problem when limbs are immobilized, as occurs during the treatment of fractures or following tendon operations. Type II fibers are particularly prone to atrophy in these circumstances (see above).

The most dramatic atrophy of muscle, however, follows interruption of the neuronal supply to that particular muscle, which may be due to death of the anterior horn cell (see Chap. 15) or, more commonly, to severing of the peripheral nerve. The degeneration could result from the loss of electrical activity to the muscle or loss of axoplasmic flow. Whichever mechanism is primarily responsible, both electrical and nutritional transmission along the nerve to the muscle are important in maintaining muscle bulk.

SELECTED REFERENCES

Junge D: Nerve and Muscle Excitation. Sunderland, Massachusetts, Sinauer Associates, 1976

Katz B: Nerve Muscle and Synapse. New York, McGraw-Hill, 1966

McComas J: Neuromuscular Function and Disorders. Boston, Butterworth & Co, 1977

Part Six

PATHOLOGIC PROCESSES IN MUSCLE

Chapter 15

Disorders of Muscle

Colin D. Hall
and Walter B. Greene

GOALS AND OBJECTIVES

Goals: To describe the major disease processes that affect skeletal muscles so that the reader may be able to identify the major clinical and laboratory abnormalities found in patients suffering from diseases of the anterior horn cell, peripheral nerve, and muscle

Objectives: On completion of this unit, and using the text as a standard reference, one should be able to describe, list, draw, or recognize the following:

1. The clinical and pathologic features of spinal muscular atrophy, amyotrophic lateral sclerosis, and poliomyelitis
2. The pathologic findings in muscle biopsies of patients with diseases of the peripheral nerves
3. Diseases involving the neuromuscular junction
4. The clinical and pathologic features of the major forms of muscular dystrophy and other inherited myopathies
5. The clinical and pathologic features of the major acquired diseases of muscle
6. The two major forms of rhabdomyosarcoma

OUTLINE

I. Patient evaluation
  A. History
  B. Physical examination
  C. Laboratory studies
II. Diseases involving the anterior horn cell
  A. Spinal muscular atrophy
  B. Amyotrophic lateral sclerosis
  C. Poliomyelitis
III. Peripheral neuropathies
IV. Disorders of the neuromuscular junction
  A. Myasthenia gravis

- B. The myasthenic syndrome
- C. Botulism
- D. Tick paralysis

V. Myopathic disorders
- A. Muscular dystrophies
- B. The congenital myopathies
- C. Inflammatory myopathies
- D. Toxic myopathies
- E. Metabolic myopathies

VI. Neoplasia
- A. Rhabdomyoma
- B. Rhabdomyosarcoma

Pathologic processes involving either the upper or the lower motor neuron may result in dysfunction of the muscles. Generally it is easy to differentiate upper motor neuron lesions by their characteristic distribution as hemiplegias or paraplegias associated with increased deep tendon reflexes, spasticity, and extensor plantar responses. These disorders are not further considered in this chapter.

The neuromuscular system can be regarded as a unit including the anterior horn cell of the spinal cord, the peripheral nerve with its roots into and out of the spinal cord, the neuromuscular junction, and the muscle itself. When a neuromuscular disorder is present, it is important to differentiate which of these areas is involved. As is true in most facets of clinical medicine, this can best be determined by a thorough history and a physical examination, with reinforcement from appropriate laboratory studies.

PATIENT EVALUATION

History

The most common presenting feature of neuromuscular disease is a history of weakness that is usually gradual in onset and progression. The weakness of peripheral nerve diseases often starts in the distal musculature of the hands and feet and progresses proximally. Diseases of muscle generally begin in the proximal musculature of the hip and shoulder girdle and progress distally. Anterior horn cell disease results in weakness of muscles supplied by the segments involved and may be proximal, distal, or both. The most characteristic feature of weakness resulting from defects at the neuromuscular junction is its fluctuating nature, often changing dramatically over minutes or hours, and usually closely related to exercise.

Although muscle weakness is usually the presenting feature, most patients with neuromuscular disease complain of diminished ability to perform daily activities rather than decreased muscle strength. It is often difficult for the patient to be certain when the weakness started. In addition, he may not notice weakness in muscles that are not commonly used. Generally, when proximal muscle weakness involves the lower limbs, it leads to progressive difficulty in climbing stairs, running, getting up from seats, and, eventually, walking; in the upper limbs it produces increasing difficulty in putting objects on shelves above the head, combing the hair, and shaving. Distal muscle weakness makes the patient liable to trip over rugs and uneven ground, causes difficulty opening jars, turning door handles, and carrying out fine movements with the hands, such as buttoning clothes or writing.

Pain is a common complaint in diseases involving the peripheral nerves and nerve roots. It may be tingling, burning, or aching and is often worse at rest or when the skin is stimulated by sensory input. Pain in diseases of muscle is more commonly associated with exercise and is seen most frequently with inflammatory myopathies and with enzyme deficiencies that compromise the muscle's energy sources.

The history must include a careful search for possible exposure to toxic or infectious agents. Any associated medical diseases must also be thoroughly investigated, as they may be the precipitating cause of the neuromuscular symptoms.

Genetically determined neuromuscular disease is very common, and a complete and thorough family history, usually linked with examination of other members of the family, is mandatory.

Physical Examination

When examining the patient, sequentially evaluate the different parts of the body. Inspection may reveal abnormal muscle bulk, fasciculations, or postural adaptation to muscle weakness, often with resulting skeletal deformities. Palpation often demonstrates abnormalities of muscle consistency and tone, and may reveal areas of tenderness. Evaluate muscle strength by formal testing of the particular muscle. You may gain additional information by watching the patient perform certain functional tasks such as walking, running, stepping onto a stool or chair, arising from the floor, and lifting the hands above the head. The patient with neuromuscular weakness performs these tasks in a characteristically abnormal fashion.

Laboratory Studies

Laboratory data can only be adequately interpreted when combined with the clinical features. There are very few laboratory studies that are specific for any individual neuromuscular disease, and it is imperative that the clinician, electrodiagnostician, pathologist, and biochemist collaborate on the interpretation of their results. Serum levels of creatine phosphokinase (CPK), lactic dehydrogenase (LDH), aldolase, and glutamic-oxaloacetic transaminase (SGOT) may be markedly elevated with necrosis of striated muscle. The ischemic lactate test is performed by rendering the arm ischemic by inflating a blood pressure cuff on the upper arm to above systolic pressure. The forearm muscles are then exercised for one minute. In normal subjects, there is a significant rise in serum lactate levels; in certain enzyme deficiencies, this rise does not occur. In other enzyme deficiencies, prolonged fasting may cause abnormal fluctuations in serum lipids. Electromyography and nerve conduction studies are helpful in determining whether disease comes from the anterior horn cell, the peripheral nerve, the neuromuscular junction, or the muscle cell. A muscle biopsy, if properly selected and prepared, will usually differentiate disorders involving the anterior horn cell or the peripheral nerve from diseases that primarily involve muscle. It may also help to further differentiate muscle disease into primary dystrophies or secondary diseases caused by toxic, inflammatory, or metabolic agents.

DISEASES INVOLVING THE ANTERIOR HORN CELL

The most common forms of anterior horn cell disease are spinal muscular atrophy and amyotrophic lateral sclerosis, or motor neuron disease. Poliomyelitis, once the most common and devastating disease to involve the anterior horn cells, is now rare in western society.

Spinal Muscular Atrophy. Spinal muscular atrophy (SMA) is a disease of infancy and childhood that is generally transmitted as an autosomal recessive trait. The disease is variable in its severity and progression. Its most severe form, Werdnig-Hoffman disease, may be noted at birth or in early infancy and usually leads to death within months. The most striking finding is muscle weakness; the child generally shows only the feeblest of leg movements and tends to lie on his back in a "frog leg" position. Weakness progresses rapidly to the upper limbs and eventually to the muscles of respiration; death is due to respiratory compromise. Fasciculations of the tongue are common.

Some children present with a similar but less severe clinical picture. In this intermediate form, progression of the muscle weakness either stops or is very slow. Although these patients may sit, muscle weakness leads to joint contractures, bony abnormalities, and scoliosis. Appropriate physical therapy, bracing, and surgery may prevent severe deformities and allow the patient to function as a wheelchair ambulator.

An even less severe form of SMA is known as Kugelberg-Welander disease. This disorder usually manifests itself late in the first decade of life; it is clinically similar to muscular dystrophy with slowly progressive weakness and wasting of the proximal limb muscles. This form may be associated with a slight rise in the level of serum "muscle" enzymes.

Amyotrophic Lateral Sclerosis. Amyotrophic lateral sclerosis (ALS) is an acquired disease of unknown etiology that destroys anterior horn cells and descending corticospinal fibers, leading to progressive muscle wasting, weakness, and fasciculations. It may affect persons of any age but is most common in middle and later life. Muscles are affected in a random fashion, but eventually the muscles supplied by the bulbar cranial nerves degenerate; death is usually due to respiratory failure.

Poliomyelitis. Poliomyelitis is caused by destruction of the anterior horn cells of the spinal cord or brain stem by an acute viral infection. Usually the disease is transmitted by a type I, II, or III poliomyelitis virus. Initial infection with poliomyelitis spreads from the respiratory and gastrointestinal tracts by way of the bloodstream to the anterior horn cells, where acute destruction takes place. There is fever, stiffness of the neck, and a pleocytosis in the cerebrospinal fluid. Profound, usually asymmetrical muscle weakness develops. The initial acute phase may be followed by some recovery of muscle strength, but permanent weakness results from necrosis of the anterior horn cells.

Muscle biopsy is particularly useful in the diagnosis of spinal muscular atrophy or amyotrophic lateral sclerosis. Diseases of the anterior horn cells or peripheral nerves cause degeneration in the muscle fibers they supply. As single motor neurons die, degeneration in the small clusters of fibers results in a picture called small group atrophy (Fig. 15-1). As the process continues, larger numbers of axons are affected, causing more fibers to degenerate. However, those fibers supplied by axons not yet involved remain normal. This process leads to large group atrophy, with many fibers, or even whole fascicles, of muscle degenerating, whereas the surrounding fibers look normal (Fig. 15-2). In neuropathic disease, the individual muscle cells affected become thin and angulated (Fig. 15-1).

PERIPHERAL NEUROPATHIES

There are many acute and chronic conditions that affect peripheral nerves. Those that primarily affect the myelin sheath surrounding the nerve, the segmental demyelinating neuropathies, lead to slowing of nerve conduction velocity; those that primarily affect the axon cause a reduction in size of the electrical potential from the muscle when the nerve is stimulated, without marked reduction in the conduction velocity. Histologic changes in the muscles are similar with the different neuropathies. Individual fiber atrophy progresses to small and, in the more chronic forms, large group atrophy. A feature that may represent attempted regeneration in neuropathies is the "target fiber," which has a degenerated center that may appear as a bull's eye with various histochemical stains.

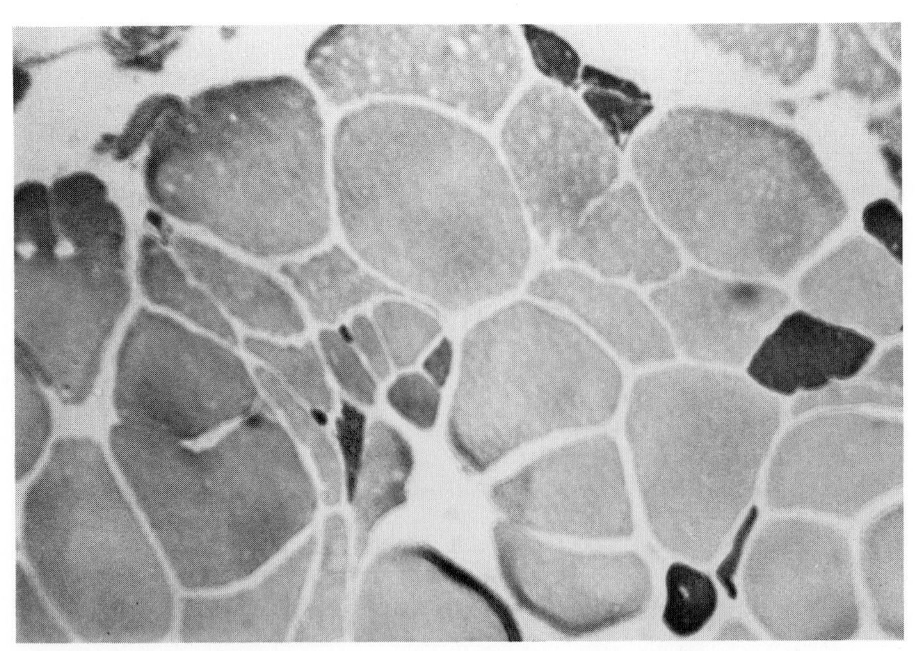

Fig. 15-1. Peripheral neuropathy. A small group of thin, angulated, atrophied muscle fibers is seen in the center of the field, surrounded by relatively normal fibers. (H. and E. stain)

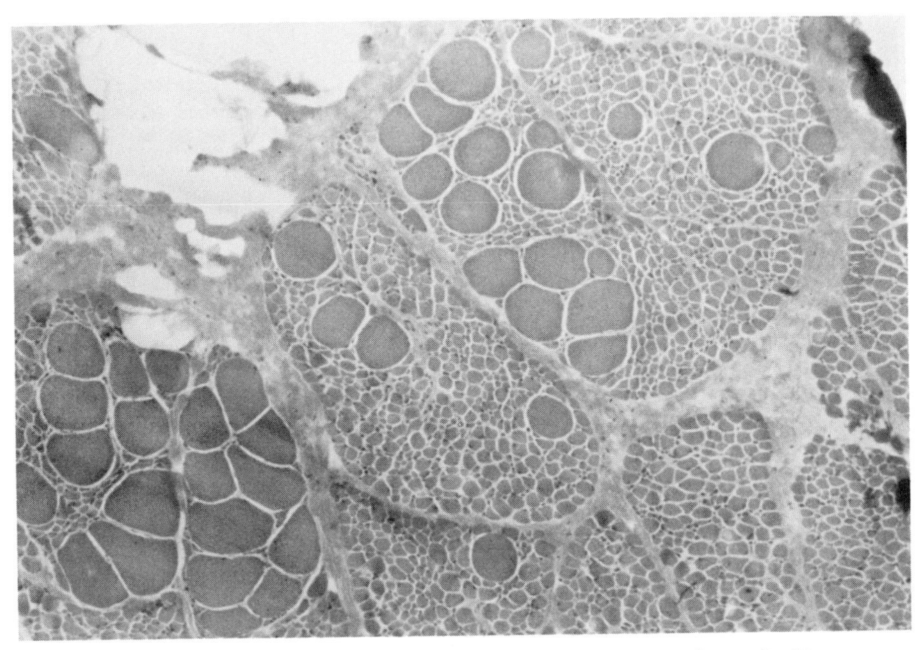

Fig. 15-2. Spinal muscular atrophy. Two distinct groups of muscle fibers are present, some of normal configuration and many large groups of tiny atrophied fibers, some occupying whole fascicles of the muscle. (H. and E. stain)

Recovery from peripheral neuropathy may lead to fiber type grouping, wherein all the type I or type II fibers (see previous chapter) in a particular biopsy site have degenerated and been replaced during recovery with fibers of the other type. This evolution leads to large, normal-looking groups comprised of one individual fiber type (Fig. 15-3).

A misleading feature occasionally found in biopsies from patients with chronic neuropathic disease is areas of muscle that appear to have myopathic changes. This finding is believed to be due to the greater stress put on these particular fibers to compensate for their atrophied neighbors.

DISORDERS OF THE NEUROMUSCULAR JUNCTION

Defects of the neuromuscular junction may be defined by electrodiagnostic techniques. Frequently there is an abnormal increment or decrement in the size of the compound action potential obtained from the muscle with repetitive stimulation of the nerve. Often muscle enzymes are normal, and muscle biopsy is normal or shows only nonspecific abnormalities.

Myasthenia Gravis. Myasthenia gravis is the most common neuromuscular junction defect. It results from damage to the postsynaptic acetylcholine receptor sites found on the muscle membrane. It is manifested as a fluctuating weakness of muscle, markedly exacerbated by exercise, which usually first involves the extraocular muscles and muscles of the eyelids. It progresses to involve any muscle group in the body. It affects any age group but is more common in young women and older adults of both sexes. Muscle bulk and reflexes are generally spared until late in the disease. The greatest danger to the patient is the advent of a "myasthenic crisis" with severe involvement of the bulbar and respiratory muscles. This event may be precipitated by intercurrent infection, other illness, or the injudicious use of medication.

Patients with myasthenia gravis may be greatly helped by various therapies, including anticholinergic medications, the use of corticosteroids and immunosuppressant drugs, plasmapheresis with the removal of harmful circulating antibodies, and thymectomy, which may remove the source of these antibodies.

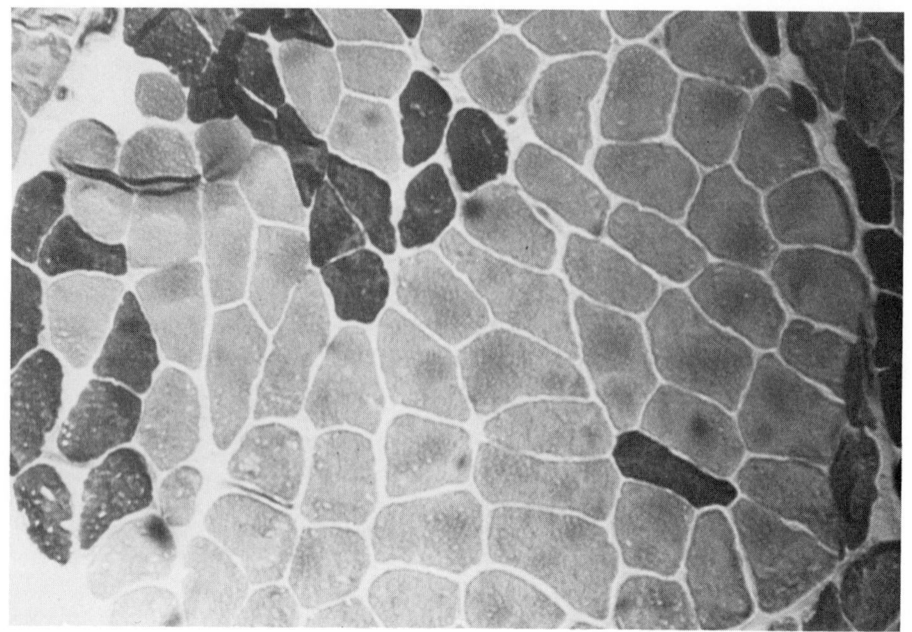

Fig. 15-3. Recovered neuropathy. Instead of the normal mosaic pattern of type I or type II fibers, a large group of type I and two small groups of type II fibers are seen. The biopsy otherwise shows normal features. (ATPase stain at *p*H 9.4)

The Myasthenic Syndrome (Eaton-Lambert Syndrome). The myasthenic syndrome, or Eaton-Lambert syndrome, is a rare disease usually found in association with occult neoplasms of the lung or other organs. The basic defect appears to be in the release of acetylcholine from the prejunctional axon terminals. The result is a fluctuating weakness that usually involves the proximal limb girdle. In contradistinction to myasthenia gravis, the weakness is often worse on initiating exercise and improves as the muscle is used more. The various therapeutic regimens have not greatly helped this disease; fortunately, the muscle weakness tends to be relatively slight, and the main danger to the patients is the manifestation of the underlying neoplasm.

Botulism. The botulinus toxin acts to prevent adequate liberation of acetylcholine at the neuromuscular junction. Acute botulism, usually acquired by the ingestion of contaminated food, leads to rapid and progressive muscle weakness that starts in the muscles supplied by the cranial nerves and progresses to the respiratory and limb muscles. The prompt administration of botulinus antitoxin may be of value. Supportive care of respiratory function until the immediate crisis is past is the preferred mode of therapy.

Tick Paralysis. An embedded tick may liberate a toxin that appears to disrupt the neuromuscular junction, which, in young children, may cause a progressive paralysis of muscle that is reversed by removal of the tick.

MYOPATHIC DISORDERS

The classification of a muscle disease depends on the clinical presentation. Laboratory studies are used to confirm that the pathologic process is in the muscle itself, and only rarely will they be specific enough in themselves to establish or confirm a definitive diagnosis. Muscle enzymes are frequently elevated, and the degree of their rise usually represents the degree of damage to muscle membranes. Nerve conduction velocities are normal. Needle electromyographic examination of the muscle shows characteristic alterations in the configuration of the electrical responses produced from firing of the muscle unit and in the overall pattern of firing of motor units in the muscle. Microscopic examination of the muscle helps confirm the presence of a myopathy and, at times, assists further differentiation into subgroups. With muscle disease, individual fibers are affected in random fashion throughout the body of the muscle without any particular grouping of atrophic fibers. Individual muscle fibers become rounded, and, although some fibers shrink in size, some become larger, possibly in an attempt to compensate for the weakness of their neighbors (Fig. 15-4). The nuclei frequently migrate centrally (Fig. 15-4, 15-5). The extra demand on the muscle fibers leads to division of single fibers into two or more fibers, which is called fiber splitting (Fig. 15-5). Mitochondrial stains show marked degeneration of the internal structure of individual fibers, giving a moth-eaten or whorled appearance (Fig. 15-6). Degeneration of fibers in either myopathic or neuropathic disease is associated with phagocytosis of individual cells (Fig. 15-7). Active regeneration of fibers is frequent in myopathic disease and rare in neuropathic disease. It is recognized by increased basophilic staining of fibers and swelling of the nucleus, which is therefore said to be "vesicular" (Fig. 15-8).

The changes in histochemical fiber types (see previous chapter) vary in different diseases. Type II fibers are more susceptible to atrophy than are type I. A variety of disorders, usually associated with lack of exercise of the muscle, leads to type II fiber atrophy (Fig. 15-9). These conditions include disuse, upper motor neuron disease involving the muscle, and even neoplasms in other organs of the body. Type II fibers are also more frequently involved in the muscular dystrophies. Type I fibers show more atrophy in congenital myopathies and in myotonic dystrophy.

Muscular Dystrophies

The recognition of muscular dystrophy is relatively easy when other family members are or have been involved. However, the diagnosis may be very difficult in sporadic cases of progressive muscle weakness and wasting. Again, accurate diagnosis depends

(Text continues on p. 202)

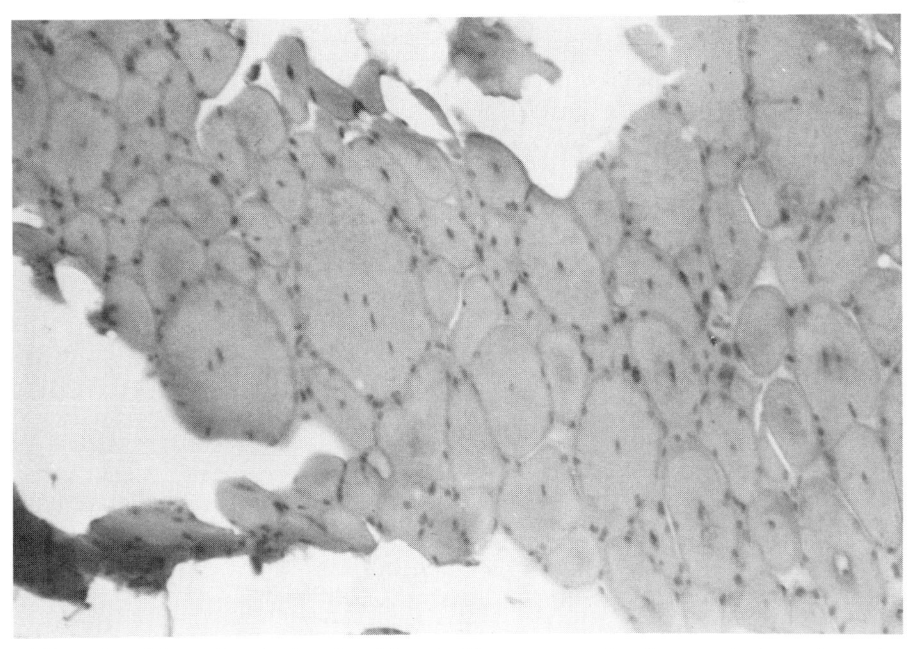

Fig. 15-4. Muscular dystrophy. Muscle fibers are randomly rounded or of varying size with central nuclei. (H. and E. stain)

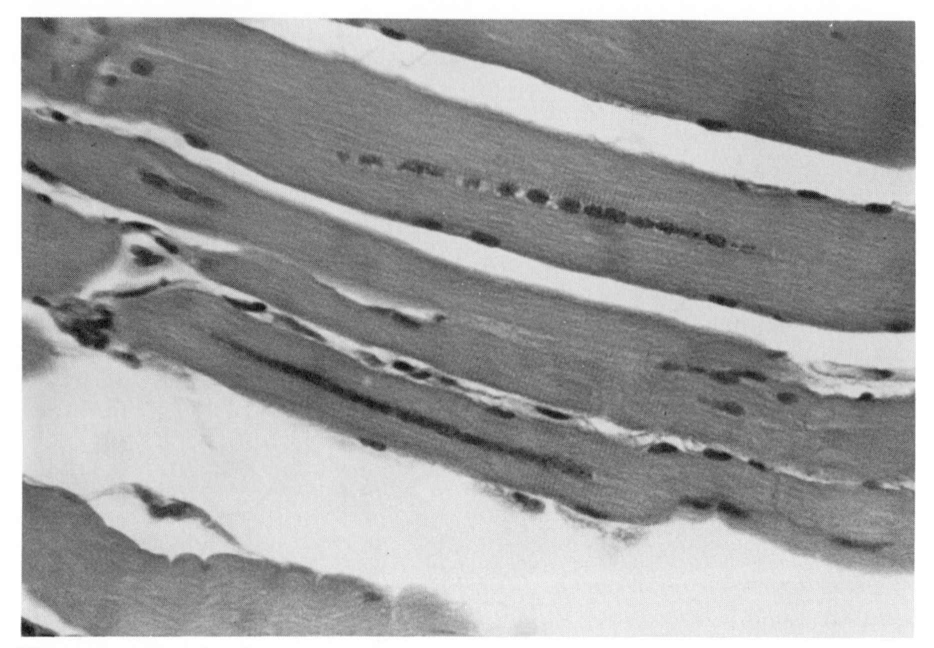

Fig. 15-5. Muscular dystrophy. Longitudinal section showing splitting of the fiber in the center of the field and two chains of central nuclei. (H. and E. stain)

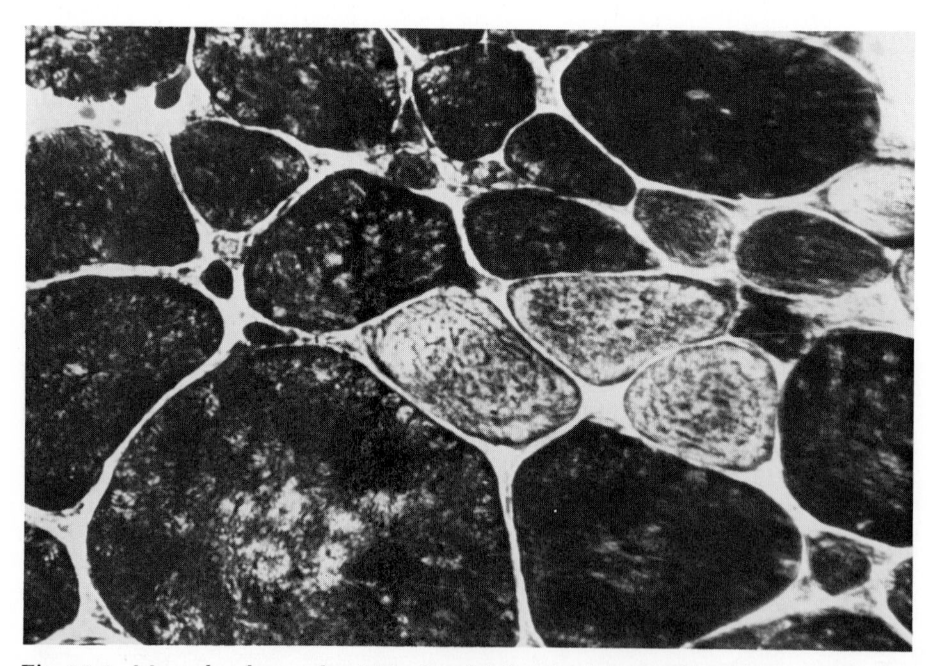

Fig. 15-6. Muscular dystrophy. Mitochondrial stain showing disruption of internal structure of fibers. These patterns are described as "moth-eaten" and "whorled." (NADH stain)

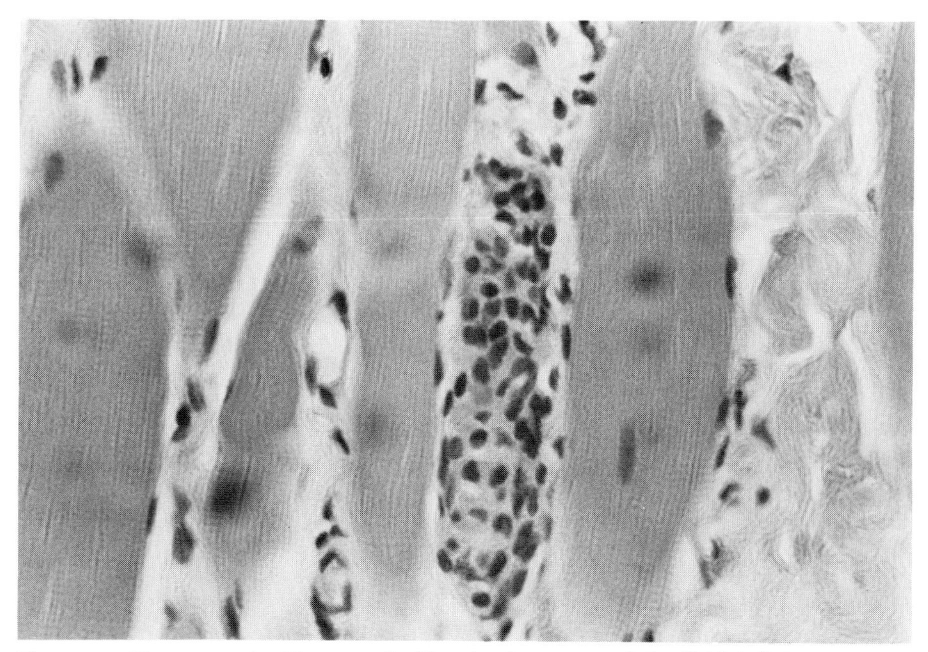

Fig. 15-7. Phagocytosis. The muscle fiber in the center of the field is being engulfed by mononuclear cells. (H. and E. stain)

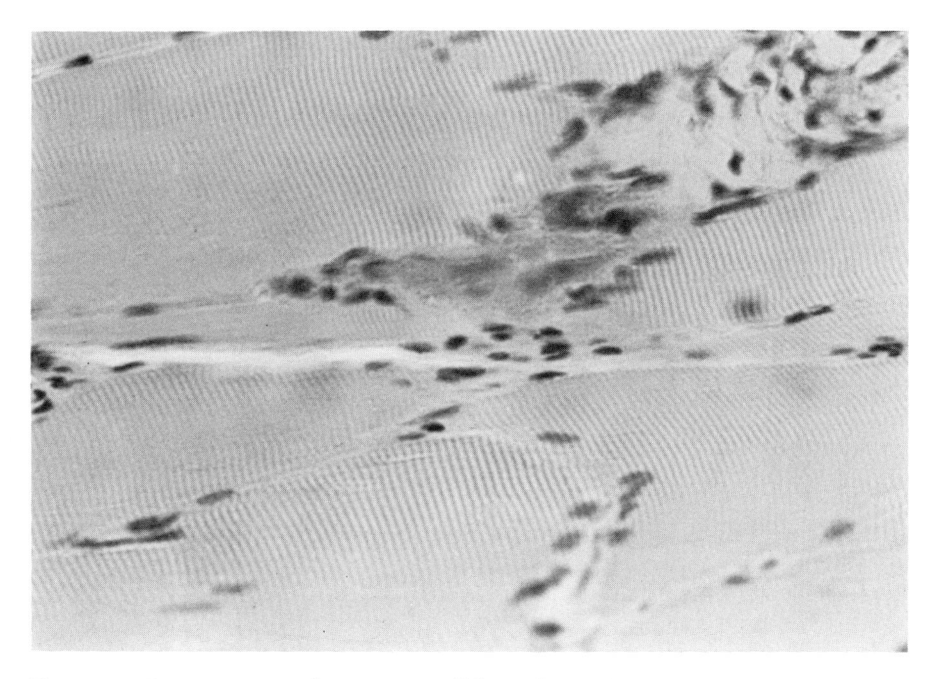

Fig. 15-8. Regeneration. There is a small basophilic fiber with large "fluffy" nuclei in the upper center of the field. (H. and E. stain)

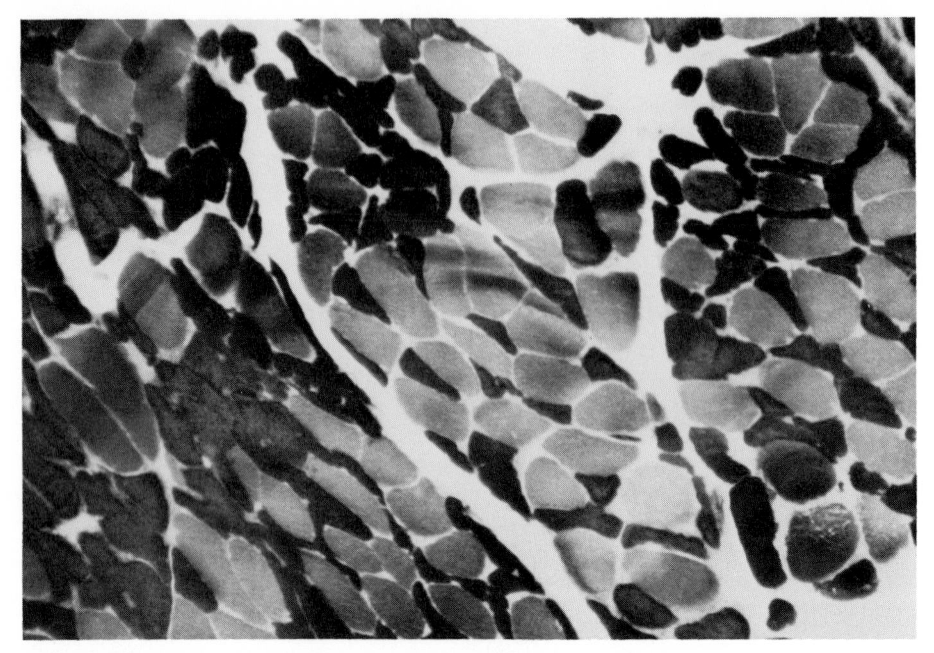

Fig. 15-9. Disuse atrophy. This muscle was stained with ATPase at a *p*H of 9.4, differentiating lightly staining type I from darkly staining type II fibers. The type II fibers are almost universally atrophied. (ATPase stain)

upon the clinical rather than the laboratory features.

Duchenne Muscular Dystrophy. Duchenne muscular dystrophy is the most severe and, unfortunately, the most common of the dystrophies. It is transmitted as an X-linked recessive disease. Females are carriers and show no, or only very mild, clinical effects, but males are severely incapacitated. The disease is present at birth and is associated with very high serum levels of enzymes found in muscle. These early levels gradually fall but commonly remain elevated throughout life. Clinical manifestations are usually obvious by 3 years of age, with the child experiencing particular difficulty in running and climbing. The proximal muscles are more severely affected than the distal. Some muscles, particularly the gastrocnemii, may be large and bulky, although weak, a condition termed pseudohypertrophy. Proximal muscle weakness progresses; the child is often restricted to a wheelchair before 10 years of age and succumbs to respiratory or cardiac complications by the age of 20. There is no effective therapy for the primary defect, but, as with other neuromuscular diseases, supportive treatment is very important.

Muscle biopsy shows the myopathic features described above. A finding that is prominent, but not unique, in this disease is the presence of large, rounded, flocculated "hyalin fibers" throughout the biopsy.

Becker Muscular Dystrophy. Becker muscular dystrophy is an X-linked recessive dystrophy that shares many of the features of Duchenne muscular dystrophy, including pseudohypertrophy of the muscles. The main clinical difference is that the course is more protracted; patients are usually able to walk as late as early adulthood and often live into their 30s and 40s.

Facioscapulohumeral Muscular Dystrophy. Facioscapulohumeral muscular dystrophy is transmitted as an autosomal dominant condition. Most patients show relatively slow progression of weakness involving primarily the muscles of facial expression and the proximal upper limbs. Whistling and sucking through a straw may be impossible, and the patients cannot fully bury their eyelashes when they close their eyes. Although their arms become gradually weaker from adolescence on, patients can usually work into later life. There is a subgroup with the disease in whom more severe muscle weakness is present from the first decade, which leads to significant restriction of mobility by early adulthood.

Myotonic Muscular Dystrophy. Myotonic muscular dystrophy is an autosomal dominant disease. There is widespread involvement of organ systems, which includes weakness and wasting of the muscles, cataracts of the posterior lens, endocrine abnormalities including hypogonadism and abnormalities of glucose metabolism, cardiac conduction defects, premature frontal balding in males, and, frequently, a nonprogressive intellectual dysfunction. The muscle wasting and weakness are unlike those found in most dystrophies in that they start in the distal parts of the limbs and progress proximally. There is also bulbar involvement with difficulties in speech and swallowing. The feature that gives the disease its name is myotonia, the inability of a muscle to relax following contraction. Myotonia is seen when the patient is asked to squeeze his fist hard and then open it quickly. The fingers will straighten only gradually. It may also be elicited by percussing a muscle with a tendon hammer, which elicits a muscle contraction visible as a slow dimpling beneath the skin. These features are exacerbated by cold and sometimes abolished by heat or repetitive exercise. Myotonia may be associated with discomfort. Myotonic dystrophy varies in severity among different family members and has a variable, but generally progressive, course. Patients are usually able to continue walking for many years, although heavy physical exercise becomes impossible. Sudden cardiac dysrhythmias may cause death but are preventable by the use of a cardiac pacemaker. Myotonia may be relieved by various medications.

The muscle biopsy in myotonic dystrophy shows more specific changes than other dystrophies. Early signs are atrophy of type I fibers with hypertrophy of type II fibers and a significant increase in the number of central nuclei. As with the other dystrophies, progression leads to marked myopathic changes. A feature that occurs frequently but is not unique to this disease is the ring fiber, a fiber in which the axis of the outer myofibrils is rotated at 90° to the main body, thus giving the appearance of an external ring around the fiber.

Limb-Girdle Muscular Dystrophy. Limb-girdle muscular dystrophy covers an extremely varied group of clinical diseases that are usually transmitted in an autosomal recessive mode. Patients show various degrees of proximal muscle weakness, often asymmetric and slowly progressive. As our knowledge increases, these disorders will almost certainly prove to be due to a wide variety of different defects.

Ocular Muscular Dystrophy. Ocular muscular dystrophy is also a term that embraces several different conditions. All show progressive ptosis and weakness of the extraocular muscles, but they may, in addition, have cardiac defects, skeletal muscle dysfunction, and central nervous system difficulties. They show variable genetic patterns. A frequent finding on muscle biopsy is the "ragged red" fiber, a name descriptive of their irregular appearance and reddish color on a Gomori trichrome stain. The defect is in the mitochondria of the cells.

The Congenital Myopathies

The congenital myopathies are a group of different conditions, with variable genetic patterns of inheritance, that lead to muscle weakness in infancy and early childhood. They include central core disease, nemaline myopathy, myotubular myopathy, congenital fiber type disproportion, and centronuclear myopathy. Children with congenital myopathies present as "floppy" babies in whom weakness leads to failure to achieve normal motor milestones. Generally they improve with age, but the children are never very athletically adept, and they may deteriorate and die of respiratory failure. Some show associated skeletal deformities. These conditions are frequently named after pathologic features found through light or electron microscopy. With many it is not clear how specific the different abnormalities are.

Inflammatory Myopathies

There are many different diseases that may result in similar morphologic changes in the muscle, including myopathic degeneration and regeneration with infiltration of mononuclear cells and lymphocytes, particularly around intramuscular blood vessels. These diseases include rheumatoid arthritis, systemic lupus erythematosus, polyarteritis and the other collagen vascular diseases, postviral myositides, and granulomatous disease. Biopsy is of great diagnostic importance in these conditions because specific medical treatment is of great help in controlling many of them.

Dermatomyositis and Polymyositis. Dermatomyositis and polymyositis are the commonest of the collagen vascular diseases to affect muscle significantly. Any age group may be affected, and there is sometimes a history of viral infection. In adults there is a significantly increased incidence of occult cancer. The patient is systemically ill with muscle tenderness and progressive weakness, often starting in the proximal limb muscles, that frequently progresses to involve respiratory muscles and the bulbar musculature. Serum muscle enzymes and the erythrocyte sedimentation rate are frequently elevated. In dermatomyositis, there is skin involvement with a characteristic heliotrope rash around the eyelids and erythematous and telangiectatic changes, particularly over nail beds, knuckles, other joints, and areas exposed to sunlight. The course is typically downhill, more rapidly in the first few weeks to months and more slowly thereafter, unless medical therapy is instituted. Steroid and immunosuppressive medications may improve the clinical picture greatly.

The most striking feature of the muscle biopsy is perivascular infiltrates of mononuclear cells that may eventually involve the entire muscle (Fig. 15-10). In addition, there is widespread patchy muscle degeneration, with regenerating fibers also frequently present. One problem in diagnosis is that these abnormalities may coexist with normal areas in the same or in other muscles; therefore, biopsy of more than one area is occasionally necessary to establish the diagnosis.

Sarcoid Myopathy. Sarcoidosis may show myopathic features as one of its clinical presentations. In addition, patients with sarcoidosis frequently have granulomatous changes in muscle without clinical manifestations of

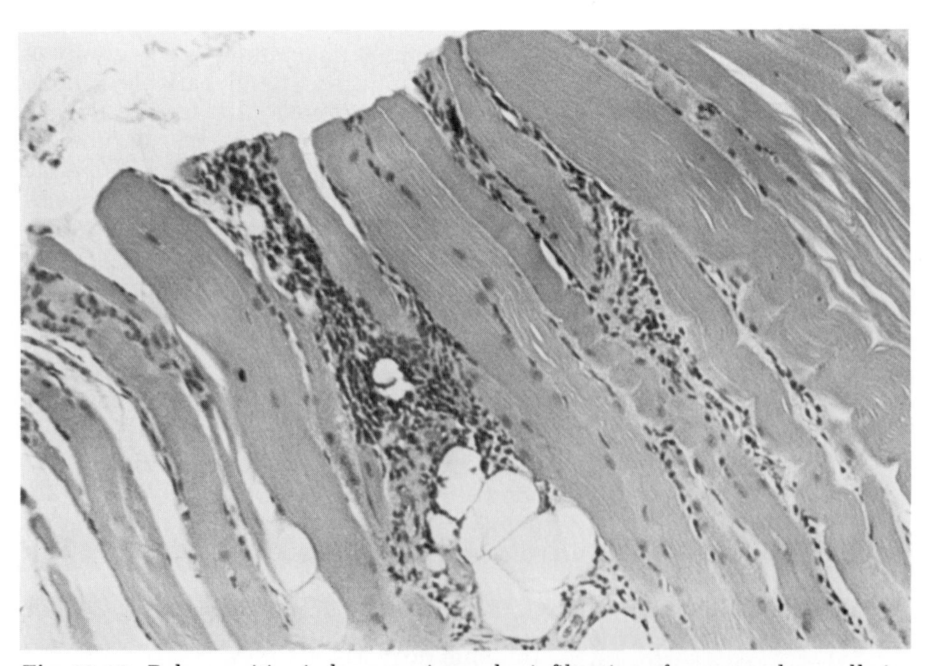

Fig. 15-10. Polymyositis. A dense perivascular infiltration of mononuclear cells is present in the left center of the field. There are scattered infiltrating mononuclear cells and degenerating muscle cells throughout the section. (H. and E. stain)

muscle disease; the biopsy is, therefore, an important diagnostic aid.

Trichinosis. Trichinosis is acquired by the ingestion of the nematode *Trichinella spiralis,* which is usually found in inadequately cooked pork. Larvae migrate from the duodenum and lodge in body organs, including skeletal muscle, causing muscle pain and necrosis, often in association with a systemic illness and marked eosinophilia. In addition to the changes of an inflammatory myopathy, the organisms may be identified in muscle tissue.

Toxic Myopathies

A variety of different agents, including narcotics and other drugs, alcohol, and toxic industrial agents, cause acute destructive changes in muscle. Again, there are somewhat nonspecific myopathic features, with phagocytosis and regeneration of muscle cells, mononuclear infiltration, and occasionally large areas of cell necrosis.

Steroid Myopathy. The administration of high doses of steroids, particularly the fluorinated steroids, over protracted periods may lead to proximal muscle weakness. Biopsy findings are usually limited to atrophy of type II fibers, which cannot be distinguished from the pathologic findings seen in disuse of muscle.

Metabolic Myopathies

Endocrine Myopathies. Myopathic features may result from any of the endocrine diseases, with variable, but usually mild, muscle abnormalities. Biopsy changes are usually nonspecific and minor.

The Periodic Paralyses. The periodic paralyses present as acute muscle weakness with or without aching, often precipitated during rest following physical exercise or by heavy carbohydrate loads. They may be associated with fluctuations in the serum potassium level. There is a genetic predisposition toward these diseases. Vacuolar changes may be seen on muscle biopsy, particularly after repeated episodes of weakness.

Enzymatic Defects. Several enzyme deficiencies can cause abnormalities of muscle energy metabolism. These conditions include three defects in the glycogen metabolism chain: a deficiency of acid maltase, resulting in Pompe's disease; a deficiency of phosphofructokinase, resulting in Tauri's disease; and a deficiency of myophosphorylase, resulting in McArdle's disease. There is also a defect in fat metabolism resulting from deficiency of the enzyme carnitine palmityl transferase. Another recently described enzyme deficiency is that of myoadenylate deaminase. The clinical features of these diseases vary, but pain frequently occurs after protracted muscle exercise, with subsequent necrosis of muscle owing to its inability to obtain an adequate energy supply. This necrosis leads to a rise in serum muscle enzymes and the liberation of myoglobin from muscle into the urine, where it occasionally causes acute renal tubular necrosis. Muscle biopsy often shows abnormal storage of glycogen or fats, and specific stains have been developed to identify the enzymes involved and demonstrate their absence in affected persons.

NEOPLASIA

Metastatic tumors from other organs reach muscle by contiguous or blood-borne spread. The cellular pattern is similar to that seen in the organ of origin. Primary muscle tumors are rare and include benign rhabdomyoma and malignant rhabdomyosarcoma.

Rhabdomyoma. Rhabdomyoma is an extremely rare tumor composed of myofibrilar cells without evidence of mitotic change. Surprisingly, it is rarely found in skeletal muscle but may be present in heart, gastrointestinal, or genitourinary tissues.

Rhabdomyosarcoma. There are two major varieties of rhabdomyosarcoma, a highly malignant neoplasm. The first arises in teratomatous tissue that contains striated muscle fibers. It may be in genitourinary or other tissue, but at times it appears in muscle, particularly around the head, neck, orbit, and occasionally the limbs. It is usually encountered as a rapidly expanding, painless mass that appears during the first 2 decades of life.

Biopsy of the lesion shows small, undifferentiated cells, spindle-shaped cells, or, occasionally, a pattern of cells resembling pulmonary alveolar units. Scattered fibers that are attempting to differentiate into myofibrils are usually found throughout the tumor body.

The other form of rhabdomyosarcoma commonly is found in the skeletal muscles of the limbs. It is more commonly encountered in the 5th and 6th decades of life but may appear at any age. There is usually a rapidly growing mass that becomes multilobulated and may outgrow its blood supply, resulting in necrosis and hemorrhage. Biopsy reveals a pleomorphic cell type with rich, acidophilic cytoplasm, frequent deeply staining granules, and bizarre arrangements of delicate fibrils, which have been called "spiderweb cells." Some cells will show attempts at the formation of striations, which shows they are of striated muscle origin.

All rhabdomyosarcomas are highly malignant, and the five-year survival rate has traditionally been less than 10%. Recent aggressive chemotherapeutic measures may improve this prognosis.

SELECTED REFERENCES

Adams RD: Diseases of Muscle: A Study in Pathology, 3rd ed. New York, Harper and Row, 1975

Brooke MH: A Clinician's View of Neuromuscular Disease. Baltimore, Williams & Wilkins, 1977

Dubowitz V: Muscle Disorders in Childhood. Philadelphia, WB Saunders, 1978

Dubowitz V, Brooke MH: Muscle Biopsy: A Modern Approach. Philadelphia, WB Saunders, 1973

Walton JN: Disorders of Voluntary Muscle, 4th ed. London, Churchill Livingstone, 1981

Part Seven

BASIC PROCESSES IN JOINTS

Chapter 16

Histology of Cartilage and Synovium

Charles W. Hooker

GOALS AND OBJECTIVES

Goals: To review the varieties of cartilage in terms of structure, nourishment, growth, and regeneration, with emphasis upon articular cartilage and articular discs; to review the gross and microscopic anatomy of the synovial membrane and the nature and production of synovial fluid

Objectives: On completion of this unit, and using the text as a standard reference, one should be able to recognize, describe or discuss the following:

1. The varieties of cartilage
2. Articular cartilage
3. The physical attributes, maintenance, and regeneration of cartilage
4. Articular discs
5. The synovium
6. The nature, site of production, and function of synovial fluid

OUTLINE

I. Synovial joints
II. Cartilage
   A. Hyaline cartilage
   B. Elastic cartilage
   C. Fibrocartilage
   D. Attributes of cartilage
      1. Articular cartilage
      2. Articular discs
III. The synovium
   A. General description
   B. Types of synovial membrane
   C. Regenerative capacity
   D. Innervation
   E. Synovial fluid

SYNOVIAL JOINTS

The synovial joint, the concern of this section, is in all respects a remarkable structural device. It is the most highly evolved of the several varieties of joint and, in most instances, is specialized to permit free movement. In keeping with this generalization, most of the joints of the limbs are synovial joints, whereas many of the joints in other parts of the body are less movable, and the participating bones are "joined" to each other by fibrous tissue (syndesmoses, as in the sutures of the young skull) or cartilage (synchondroses, as in the sternocostal joints). Certain synovial joints must bear forces of weight that can greatly exceed the weight of the body. Moreover, the force borne may change abruptly from virtually zero to a large figure, as exemplified by the forces at the knee and hip joints of a man of 180 pounds carrying a load of 150 pounds and shifting the force from one lower limb to the other in walking. These joints must bear the stresses produced by movement, stresses that vary with the load being moved. Although synovial joints are categorized as freely movable joints, the movement actually permitted ranges from almost none at the sacroiliac joint, through a simple hinge movement at the interphalangeal joints, to movement in many planes at the shoulder and hip joints. Not the least remarkable of the attributes of the healthy joint is the property of self-maintenance.

The usual synovial joint (Fig. 16-1) involves two bones. The portion of each bone participating in the formation of the joint has a covering of articular cartilage. The participating ends of the two bones and their caps of cartilage project into a space, the synovial cavity, that contains a synovial fluid and that, in healthy joints, is little more than a potential space. The synovial cavity is bounded by the articular cartilages and the synovial membrane. The synovial membrane is the innermost portion of a sleevelike, fibrous capsular ligament extending from one bone to the other. The capsular ligament is reinforced externally, and in some instances internally, by additional ligaments extending from one bone to the other. The remarkable attributes of synovial joints are conferred upon them primarily by the articular cartilages, the synovial membrane, and the synovial fluid. These entities also have in them the seeds of crippling disorders that are a major affliction of mankind. Each of them is reviewed in summary fashion.

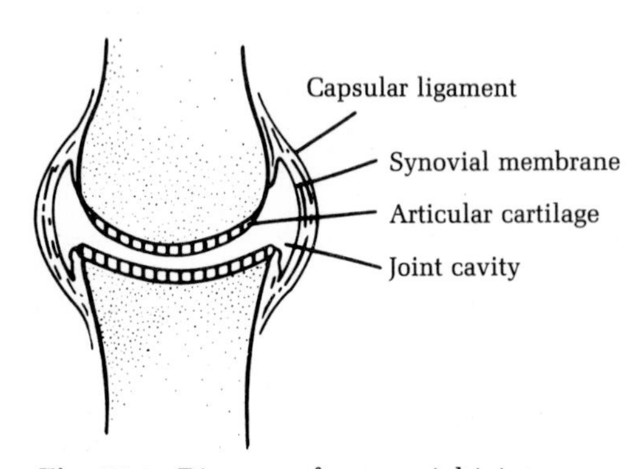

Fig. 16-1. Diagram of a synovial joint.

CARTILAGE

As in all varieties of connective tissue, cartilage is composed of cells and an intercellular matrix that is produced by, or under the influence of, the cells. In terms of the nature of the matrix, three varieties occur: hyaline cartilage, elastic cartilage, and fibrocartilage. All three varieties are capable of meeting stress and bearing weight, but less so than bone.

Hyaline cartilage is the most widespread variety, and its name suggests its glassy appearance. It forms the costal cartilages, many of the cartilages of the respiratory tract, the articular cartilages, the epiphyseal plates, and much of the fetal skeleton that is later replaced by bone. The cells, termed chondrocytes, occupy otherwise empty spaces (lacunae) generously distributed through the matrix. Lacunae and their enclosed cells are essentially spherical in the deep portion, but are flattened and discoidal toward the periphery of the cartilage. Each peripheral lacuna typically houses a single chondrocyte; deeper lacunae usually contain two or more chondrocytes. Each lacuna is immediately surrounded by a capsule of recently formed, territorial matrix that stains more deeply than interterritorial matrix. The free surfaces of most hyaline cartilage (but not articular cartilage) are covered by a layer of fibrous connective tissue, the perichondrium. The deep portion of the perichondrium is composed of small, plump cells, often termed chondroblasts, in a relatively loose connective tissue; the external portion is less cellular and more densely fibrous. Intermediate stages in the transition of perichondrial cells into peripheral chondrocytes may be seen, especially in growing cartilage.

Young chondrocytes and chondroblasts have rounded nuclei, each with one or more nucleoli. The cytoplasm contains a well-developed granular endoplasmic reticulum with moderately distended cisternae, elongated mitochondria, a well-developed Golgi apparatus, varying amounts of glycogen, and occasional lipid droplets. In older chrondrocytes, the endoplasmic reticulum and Golgi apparatus are less prominent, but glycogen and lipid are increased. In both, the surface is irregular with many projecting processes.

Approximately 75% of the matrix is water. A meshwork of collagenous fibrils accounts for about half of the dry weight; the remainder is a nonfibrous filler material. These entities together form a stiff sol. The filler material is composed of glycosaminoglycans with molecular weights up to 40,000, chiefly chondroitin sulphate, keratan sulphate, and hyaluronic acid. The matrix is translucent, and the meshwork of fibrils, visible only after use of special histologic methods, is disposed with regard to the lacunae and to tensional requirements of the cartilaginous mass. The collagenous fibrils differ from collagen in skin and bone in respect to the α chains, and, in general, are of two sizes, fibrils 20 nm or less and fibrils from 50 to 60 nm in diameter. The larger fibrils exhibit a banding pattern like that of collagen in other sites; the thinner fibrils do not exhibit the full band pattern, but may show cross striations suggesting a periodicity of 21 nm. Territorial matrix contains quite fine fibrils in the pericellular halo; a bit further from the cells, more mature fibrils are numerous. Further from the cells, in the interterritorial zone, the fibrils are larger and regularly cross-banded. Cartilage has been compared to the automobile tire whose rubber, like the filler matrix, resists compression and whose cord, like the fibrous component, resists tension. Chondrocytes and chondroblasts are essential in the formation and maintenance of matrix; reciprocally, the matrix is involved in maintenance of the chondrocytes.

Elastic cartilage is essentially hyaline cartilage permeated with elastic fibers that confer resiliency upon the tissue. This variety of cartilage is found in the external ear, the walls of the external acoustic meatus and auditory tube, and the arytenoid cartilages and epiglottis of the larynx.

Fibrocartilage does not have a surrounding perichondrium. It is composed chiefly of bundles of thick, collagenous fibers, between which are unicellular islands of cartilage arranged singly, in pairs, or in chains. Cartilaginous matrix is seen only around each chondrocyte, and a lacuna may be the only apparent evidence of its presence. The collagenous fibers are usually arrayed parallel to the tension on the tissue.

Fibrocartilage is found in certain ligaments; in tendons subject to frictional pressure, as at the point of insertion into bone; in symphyseal joints, as in the intervertebral discs; and in articular discs. The amount of this variety of cartilage increases with age; indeed, it has been suggested that transformation of hyaline cartilage into fibrocartilage is one of the early signs of aging.

Attributes of Cartilage

Hyaline cartilage is the variety of major concern here. One of its more interesting properties is a propensity for becoming impregnated with calcium salts, an attribute strikingly exemplified by the fact that most of the bones appear first as cartilaginous models. Much of the hyaline cartilage of the body ultimately calcifies. When calcification occurs, the chondrocytes die and the matrix disintegrates. Articular cartilage is unusual in that its more superficial zones do not calcify, except in pathologic states such as pseudogout (chondrocalcinosis articularis).

Growth involves either or both of two processes. One is appositional growth, the formation of new cartilage at the surface by cells derived from mesenchymal cells (chondroblasts) of the perichondrium. The other is interstitial growth, increase in the internal mass of the cartilage by activity of chrondrocytes that multiply within their lacunae. Young cartilage grows by both methods; later growth is primarily appositional. Regeneration is slow and involves activity of the perichondrium.

Humoral agents that modify skeletal growth exert this influence to a considerable extent by affecting growth of cartilage. Administration of growth hormone provokes proliferation and increase in size of chondrocytes, along with an increase in the amount of granular endoplasmic reticulum and Golgi material and an increase in the number of mitochondria and micropinocytotic vesicles. The matrix becomes more fibrous. Testosterone and insulin have similar effects. Estrogens, which inhibit growth, promote development of endoplasmic reticulum in chondrocytes and the accumulation of glycogen; the Golgi complex does not enlarge, and synthesis of glycosaminoglycans is inhibited. Administration of cortisol and related substances can result in underdevelopment of cartilage. Thyroxin provokes hypertrophy of chondrocytes but has no effect upon their proliferation.

Although blood vessels may course through it, cartilage usually has no direct vascularization. Nourishment is provided by diffusion from capillaries in the perichondrium and by imbibition. The reality of diffusion is shown by the rapid spread of vital dyes through living cartilage. Diffusion apparently ceases when cartilage calcifies, and death of chondrocytes ensues. Certain large masses of cartilage are reported to have vascular canals that enter from the perichondrium. Such vascular canals may arise preliminarily to ossification in endochondral formation of bone, but in certain instances they appear quite a long time prior to ossification. They are also said to be present in large animals in certain large cartilages that rarely ossify.

Related to the structure of cartilage is the success in its transplantation; homografts have been observed to persist for years. There is evidence that chondrocytes possess histocompatibility antigens; however, these antigens are shielded by the matrix, which prevents both their egress and the access of cytotoxic antibodies of the host.

Cartilage is innervated sparingly, if at all, a circumstance that explains the lack of pain or discomfort in healthy joints subjected to pressure and friction.

Articular Cartilage. The cartilage capping the ends of the bones that form a synovial joint is usually hyaline cartilage that provides both a cushion and a slick surface for movement. The free surface of this cartilage is smooth to the touch and to the naked eye, but at quite high magnification it exhibits many rounded elevations when young and growing, and many shallow pits when mature. The thickness of articular cartilage varies from area to area in a given joint, from joint to joint in the same species of animal, and from species to species. In man it is thickest over the ends of the femur and tibia, ranging from 2 to 4 mm. In health the thickness changes little, despite activity of the joint. The articular cartilage is in reality a persisting end of the cartilaginous model of the bone. When the joint cavity first appears during development, the end of the cartilaginous precursor of the bone is covered with mesenchyme that is much like the perichondrium over the remainder of the model. The terminal covering of mesenchyme disappears, possibly as a consequence of movement of the joint. In any case, the free surface of articular cartilage has perichondrium only at the periphery.

The cells and lacunae of articular cartilage are arranged in three vaguely defined layers. In the superficial layer they are small and flattened, with their long axes parallel to the surface. In the next layer they are a bit larger and rounded, and often arranged in columns at right angles to the surface. In the deep layer they are large. In the deepest portion of the deep layer, the cartilaginous matrix is calcified. During growth, the deep layer is progressively replaced by bone, while the more superficial portions form cartilage that is added to that nearer the surface. The numerous minute elevations on the surface of young cartilage are thought to mark the locations of lacunae near the surface, and the small pits on the surface of older cartilage are thought to be sites of lacunae that have collapsed after death of their contained chondrocytes.

During growth, mitotic figures may be seen in chondrocytes in the intermediate layer of articular cartilage, but not in the superficial layer. Mitosis apparently ceases when growth of the bone ceases. With this means of compensation for wear gone, it is usually assumed that under normal conditions cartilage wears slightly and gradually. Cessation of mitosis and growth may be related to calcification at the interface between cartilage and bone and the failure of diffusion through the calcified cartilage. It has been reported that, relative to the amount of matrix, the number of cells in articular cartilage decreases with age. It is possible, therefore, that production of more matrix by each chondrocyte is a means of compensating for wear.

The collagenous fibers in articular cartilage are masked by the amorphous ground substance in young persons but can be revealed more readily in older persons. They arise in the trabeculae of subchondral bone, aggregate into bundles at the junction of calcified and uncalcified cartilage (the "tidemark"), and course radially toward the surface between rows of lacunae. In the middle zone of the cartilage, these bundles cross each other and then open into a feltwork of fibrils lying parallel to the surface, as though designed to withstand stress (Fig. 16-2). In older persons, the fibrils in both the superficial and middle portions have been found to be compressed and oriented parallel to the surface, and the chondrocytes in both areas appeared to be in various stages of degeneration. These changes may maintain the stiffness and preserve the integrity of aging cartilage.

In other hyaline cartilage, the surrounding perichondrium contains both the capillaries responsible for nourishment of the cartilage and the cells that become involved in appositional growth. Articular cartilage has no more than a peripheral rim of perichondrium on its free surface, and calcification of the portion of the cartilage abutting bone may limit or preclude diffusion from blood vessels supplying subchondral bone. The problem of nourishment is apparently met by the synovial fluid that bathes the cartilage, as shown by the frequent observation that fragments of cartilage, detached by injury or disease and free in the synovial cavity, may survive for considerable periods of time and may even grow. Moreover, withdrawal of synovial fluid often leads to rapid deterioration of the cartilage. Radioactive tracers introduced into synovial fluid are reported to enter the cartilage and diffuse through it with some rapidity. Fluid is expressed from articular cartilage when it is compressed and reimbibed when the pressure is removed. It has been suggested that this compression and release may serve as a pump that facilitates nourishment of the cartilage by synovial fluid.

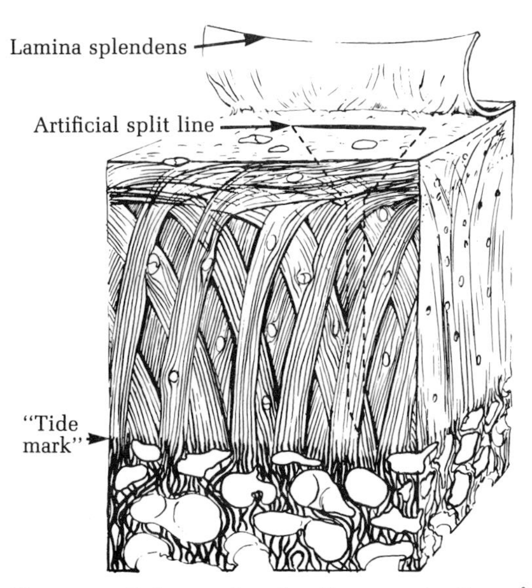

Fig. 16-2. Schema showing the organization of fibrils in human articular cartilage. Below the "tide mark" is subchondral bone. (Minn RJ, Steven FS: The collagen fibril organization in human articular cartilage. J Anat 123:437, 1977, Cambridge University Press)

Regeneration of most cartilage is slow, and is accomplished primarily by growth that requires activity of the perichondrium. Regeneration of articular cartilage is severely limited except at the periphery, where there is perichondrium, and at attachments of synovial membrane. Thus, superficial injuries, except those near the peripheral rim of perichondrium or near an attachment of synovium, remain unhealed for long periods of time.

Not all articular cartilage is hyaline cartilage. In movable joints between bones formed by intramembranous rather than endochondral ossification, the articular cartilages are fibrocartilage. The temporomandibular joint is such a joint.

Articular Discs. Between the articular surfaces of certain synovial joints is an articular disc, a pad of fibrocartilage that blends peripherally with the capsular ligament. In the sternoclavicular and temporomandibular joints, the synovial cavity is separated into two compartments by a complete disc. In the acromioclavicular joint, the articular disc is a wedge-shaped projection into the joint cavity. In the knee joint, the menisci are crescentic articular discs, wedge-shaped in cross section, projecting between the condyles of the femur and the tibia. The articular disc adds its resilience to that of the articular cartilages in cushioning the ends of the bones, and may also assist in maintaining a layer of synovial fluid over the articular surfaces.

THE SYNOVIUM

The synovial membrane is the innermost portion of the capsular ligament of a synovial joint and, together with the articular cartilages, forms the walls of the synovial cavity. It may protrude through gaps in the capsular ligament, and the synovial cavity in many instances is continuous with bursae about the joint. Despite these evaginations, the synovial cavity is a closed cavity. Intraarticular ligaments (such as the cruciate ligaments of the knee joint and the round ligament of the hip joint) and tendons that course through the joint cavity (such as that of the long head of the biceps brachii) are covered with synovial membrane.

The synovial membrane is usually smooth and glistening, and may exhibit infoldings (synovial folds) and slender projections, the larger ones being termed synovial villi. It is richly supplied with blood vessels, lymphatics, and nerves. The richness of blood capillaries and their proximity to the inner surface account for hemorrhage into joints that may follow minor injuries. Although it lines a cavity, the synovial membrane is a sheet of fibrous connective tissue and has no epithelial component. This circumstance is accounted for by the fact that the synovial cavity arises by coalescence of clefts in the mesenchyme between the ends of two prospective bones; the mesenchyme that persists becomes the capsular ligament, including its inner surface, the synovial membrane.

The cells of the membrane, usually called synovial cells, have the appearance of undifferentiated cells and resemble fibroblasts. They tend to be concentrated at the inner surface of the membrane, occasionally to the extent of appearing to constitute a continuous cellular layer. Actually, however, the cells along the inner surface are situated among, rather than on, the fibers, which are also a component of the inner part of the membrane, and are rarely contiguous.

Two types of synovial cells have been described. Type A has a prominent Golgi complex and many smooth-walled vacuoles, but has little rough endoplasmic reticulum. Type B has a scanty Golgi complex and few smooth-walled vacuoles, but much rough endoplasmic reticulum. The Golgi complex appears to be the site of production of hyaluronic acid, which is transported to the fibrous matrix and synovial cavity in large, smooth-walled vacuoles. Accordingly, cells of Type A are probably the producers of the hyaluronic acid of synovial fluid.

Mast cells and macrophages are also numerous in the synovial membrane.

Types of Synovial Membrane. The synovial membrane may lie directly on the inner surface of the capsular ligament or it may be separated from that ligament by intervening tissue. On this basis, three types of synovial membrane can be recognized: fibrous, areolar, and adipose.

The fibrous variety rests directly on the capsular ligament. The cells along the surface facing the joint cavity are widely separated from each other, and are larger and more numerous than the cells deeper in the membrane. This type of synovium is present over intraarticular ligaments and tendons, and in areas in which the synovium is subjected to pressure.

The areolar type is loosely bound to the capsular ligament and is found where it must move freely, as in the suprapatellar pouch of the knee joint. The superficial cells are closely grouped, often in three or four rows of cells, and are in the meshes of collagenous fibers that blend with the fibers binding the membrane to the capsular ligament. This type of membrane usually contains many elastic fibers that may form a distinct layer.

The adipose type, as the name suggests, covers intraarticular fat pads, such as that in the olecranon fossa, where the membrane may appear to be a layer of cells resting on adipose tissue intervening between it and the capsular ligament. Study reveals, however, that the cells lie in the meshes of a thin layer of collagenous fibers, as in the other varieties.

Regenerative Capacity. Transition of synovial cells into chondrocytes is a regular occurrence in the region of attachment of the synovial membrane to the periphery of the articular cartilage. At this zone of transition, a fold of synovium may overlie the articular cartilage for a short distance.

Consistent with the undifferentiated appearance of synovial cells and with their capacity to differentiate into chondrocytes, the synovium is capable of rapid and complete repair or regeneration.

Innervation. The nerves entering the synovium appear to be distributed primarily to the blood vessels, probably as vasomotor and vasosensory nerves. The observation that the synovium is not very sensitive to pain suggests that relatively few of the nerve fibers are pain fibers.

Synovial Fluid. The joint cavity contains a viscous, glairy fluid, the synovial fluid (*syn* means together; *ovum* means egg). Despite its lack of glands and of epithelium, the synovial membrane is the site of production of this fluid.

The fluid is a dialysate or ultrafiltrate of blood plasma plus a mucin, composed chiefly of highly polymerized hyaluronic acid, which is responsible for the viscous quality. Synovial fluid resembles the material in the interstices of loose connective tissue in respect to both components. Inasmuch as the synovial membrane is loose connective tissue and the synovial cavity arises as a space in connective tissue, it seems reasonable to regard synovial fluid, as well as the fluid in tendon sheaths and bursae, as essentially intercellular material of connective tissue. The rich vascularization of the synovial membrane favors formation of this material, and the compactness of the capsular ligament external to the synovial membrane limits spread other than into the joint cavity.

The synovial fluid contains cells whose identities and numbers are different in different joints. Cell counts are reported to vary from 80 to several thousand per mm^3. The cells include monocytes, macrophages, primitive cells, synovial cells, and leukocytes—the cells commonly found in loose connective tissue.

The rate and method of the passage of substances into and out of synovial fluid depend upon the molecular size of the substance. Crystalloids diffuse rapidly in both directions. The same is true of gases, explaining the presence of nitrogen bubbles in joint cavities in caisson disease. Larger proteins appear to leave the fluid by way of the lymphatics, an event requiring a somewhat longer time. Particulate matter is taken up by macrophages, and its egress from the joint cavity is quite slow.

The viscid, slimy nature of synovial fluid prompted early observers to consider this fluid to be primarily a lubricant of the joint. Supporting this view is the report that the coefficient of friction in a dry joint is approximately 14 times that of the same joint containing synovial fluid. It has also been observed that wear of articular surfaces is much increased when the enzyme hyaluronidase is injected into the joint cavity, a finding that suggests that the lubricating component of synovial fluid is its hyaluronic acid. Present concepts of the lubrication of joints are discussed in Chapter 18. Nourishment of the articular cartilage as a function of synovial fluid has already been mentioned. It is probable that this function and the viscoelastic properties of synovial fluid counteract wear of articular cartilage.

SELECTED REFERENCES

Barnett CH: Wear and tear in joints: An experimental study. J Bone Joint Surg 38B:567, 1956

Elliott HC: Studies on articular cartilage. I. Growth mechanisms. Am J Anat 58:127, 1936

Gardner E: Physiology of movable joints. Physiol Rev 30:127, 1950

Ghadially FN, Roy S: Ultrastructure of Synovial Joints in Health and Disease. London, Butterworth & Co, 1969

Honner R, Thompson RC: The nutritional pathways of articular cartilage. J Bone Joint Surg 53A:742, 1971

Meachim G, Stockwell RA: The matrix. In Freeman MAR (ed): Adult Articular Cartilage. Pitman Medical Publishing Co Ltd, Kent, England, 1979

Minns RJ, Steven FS: The collagen fibril organization in human articular cartilage. J Anat 123:437, 1977

Redlar I, Mow VG, Mansell J: Ultrastructural changes in aging human articular cartilage. J Bone Joint Surg 57A:575, 1975

Serafini-Fracassini A, Smith JW: The Structure and Biochemistry of Cartilage. Edinburgh, Churchill and Livingston, 1974

Sokoloff L: The Joints and Synovial Fluid. New York, Academic Press, 1978

Stockwell RA: Biology of Cartilage Cells. Cambridge, Cambridge University Press, 1979

Chapter 17

Chemistry and Biochemistry of Cartilage and Synovial Fluid

Carole J. VanderWiel

GOALS AND OBJECTIVES

Goals: To acquaint the reader with the composition and function of cartilage, with emphasis on the ground substance and the constituents of synovial fluid, and their alteration by disease

Objectives: On completion of this unit, and using the text as a standard reference, one should be able to evaluate, describe, list, or recognize the

1. Main glycosaminoglycans found in cartilage and synovial fluids
2. Physical and chemical properties of the glycosaminoglycans, especially hyaluronic acid
3. Physical and chemical characteristics of the proteoglycans
4. Polyelectrolytic nature of the proteoglycan and its importance in biologic systems
5. Principal constituents of synovial fluid
6. Primary changes in synovial fluid caused by disease of the synovial membrane

OUTLINE

I. Cartilage
   A. Introduction
   B. The ground substance and its components
      1. Water

CARTILAGE

Cartilage is made up of chondrocytes embedded in a woven skeleton of collagen fibers and matrix of ground substance. All cartilages contain approximately 70% water, the proportion being higher in younger animals. The ground substance is primarily glycosaminoglycans, which are long, unbranched carbohydrates made up largely of repeating disaccharide units. These glycosaminoglycans are attached to noncollagenous proteins, forming a complex of protein polysaccharides or a proteoglycan. Therefore, the basic structural unit, referred to as a proteoglycan, consists of a protein core to which many polysaccharide side chains are attached. The distribution of water, proteoglycans, and collagen gives cartilage its tough and resilient properties.

The three different types of cartilage can be recognized by their chemical composition. Fibrocartilage is clearly defined by its orderly arrangement of collagen fibers and a low content of glycosaminoglycans (2% of dry weight). Elastic cartilage is characterized by the presence of a unique protein known as elastin, which comprises about 20% of the dry weight of the tissue. Hyaline cartilage has the highest content of glycosaminoglycans with a higher refractive index in the interfibrillar substance, which renders the collagen fibers histologically invisible. The exact concentrations of individual chemical components can only be approximated, because the tissue content is subject to regional and age variations.

Cartilage is a highly specialized connective tissue containing relatively few cells in a large amount of extracellular matrix. This unusual composition accounts for its distinctive properties. It is essential that cartilage be rigid enough to maintain its shape, as required, for example, in nasal septa, but more resilient than bone to fulfill its role in the skeletal articulations. In the embryonic skeleton, which is constantly changing shape, cartilage is the model for the formation of bone. Cartilage is elastic; its shape may be altered by compression, torsion, or tension, yet it returns to normal when forces causing deformation are removed.

The Ground Substance and Its Components

The ground substance is the medium formed by the various connective tissue cells that secrete soluble collagen, glycosaminoglycans, and proteins. It also contains inorganic and organic components of plasma such as salts, glucose, urea, and plasma proteins. The ground substance of cartilage may be considered the *interieur milieu* surrounding the chondrocytes, and is a mixture of many components. The chondrocyte is the cell responsible for synthesis of both proteoglycan and collagen proteins, using the predicted genetic ribosomal processes. The assembly and sulfation of the proteoglycan macromolecule takes place at the Golgi apparatus. After intracellular assembly of proteoglycan molecules, they are extruded into the matrix for further aggregation.

In general, the functions and attributes of the ground substance may be described as follows:

1. It provides the homeostatic environment for the cells, and is the origin of their needed supplies and the reservoir for their metabolic products.
2. It stabilizes the spatial and functional relationship of the cells.
3. It acts as a barrier to bacterial invasion.
4. It may be altered during growth, dif-

ferentiation, regeneration, and aging, and by hormonal action.

5. It manifests pathologic changes in such diseases as scurvy and rickets, and in collagen diseases.
6. It is susceptible to normal and pathologic calcification.

Water. Cartilage is a hyperhydrated tissue. The water content of the ground substance contributes to its elasticity and resiliency; it also plays an important role in joint lubrication. Although the actual binding of water molecules within cartilage is poorly understood, they appear to be bound to collagen and proteoglycan molecules.

Collagen. Collagen is the primary structural protein of the body and occurs in bone, tendon, and scar tissue as well as in cartilage. Its composition differs slightly in different species, but its general function is the same in all. Most collagens are insoluble in water under physiologic conditions; this property and its fibrous nature give collagen its physiologic uniqueness.

In different tissues, the size of the collagen fibers varies markedly. For example, as measured by light microscopy, the diameter of a tendon fiber may be several hundred microns, whereas in loose connective tissue it may be only 1 μ. However, with the electron microscope, finer fibers called fibrils are noted in all tissues. The diameters of fibrils vary from 20 nm or less to 50 or 60 nm. The arrangement of these fibrils and their size characterizes different tissues.

Cartilage contains type I and type II collagens. Approximately 10% of the wet weight and 50% of the dry weight of cartilage is collagen, which interacts with proteoglycans to provide cartilage with its special properties. The functions of collagen fibers within cartilage are (1) to resist the movement of interstitial water and proteoglycans while preserving their colloidal properties; (2) to provide a taut framework for proteoglycans while it sustains compressional loading; and (3) to anchor the ground substance of articular cartilage to subchondral bone.

Glycosaminoglycans. Glycosaminoglycans, as the name implies, are composed of many saccharide units, usually more than 20; these high-molecular-weight substances do not diffuse through cellulose membranes. The six most common and best-characterized polysaccharides are shown in Figure 17-1.

The structures of these polysaccharides have many things in common. They all appear to be straight chains with no branching. The chains are primarily alterations of two monosaccharide units; one unit is usually an hexosamine. The amino group of the hexosamine is either acetylated (primarily the N-acetyl form) or sulfated. The second monosaccharide unit is either a hexuronate or galactose. All contain fixed negative charges distributed along the length of the chain in the form of anionic groups (COO^- or SO_3O^-), which must be associated with an equivalent number of cations so that they have the properties of polyelectrolytes. Usually the cation is sodium. The polysaccharides also contain small amounts of other components such as amino acids, other saccharide units, and sialic acid.

The Chemistry of Glycosaminoglycans

Two major glycosaminoglycans within the cartilage ground substance are chondroitin sulfate and keratan sulfate. However, their concentration and distribution within the matrix vary considerably according to age, the type of cartilage, and the morphological location within the tissue. Hyaluronic acid is a glycosaminoglycan isolated from synovial fluid.

Chondroitin Sulfate. In chondroitin sulfate, N-acetyl galactosamine alternates with glucuronic acid to form the disaccharide repeating unit of the polymer. The chondroitin sulfates A and C are distinct molecular entities that exhibit different infrared absorption spectra. These differences are attributed to the presence of a sulfate ester group in axial configuration at the carbon atom 4 position of the galactosamine residue of chondroitin sulfate A and in the equatorial configuration of carbon atom 6 of the same residue of chondroitin sulfate C.

Keratan Sulfate. Keratan sulfate has a disaccharide repeating unit consisting of N-acetyl glucosamine alternating with galactose. The amino sugar residue may carry sulfate ester

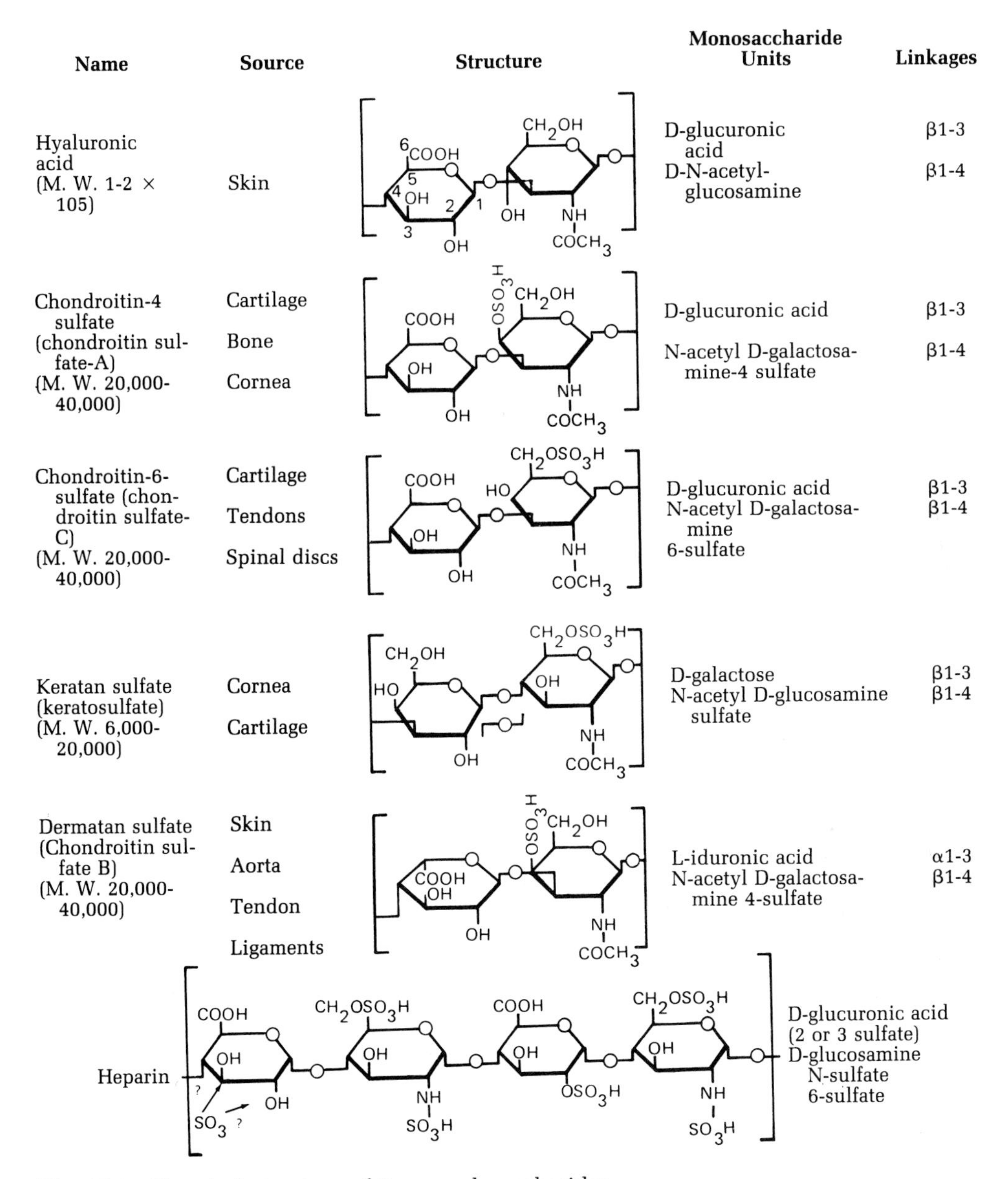

Fig. 17-1. Chemical structure of tissue polysaccharides.

groups bound to carbon atoms 4 and 6; also, the galactose residue may be variably sulfated. Keratan sulfate is more variable than chondroitin sulfate, both in its chain length and in the degree of sulfation.

Hyaluronic Acid. Hyaluronic acid was first isolated from vitreous humor and later from synovial fluid, skin, umbilical cord, hemolytic streptococci, and other sources. In joint fluid, hyaluronic acid arises from the synovial membrane and not from the plasma, and the evidence is strongly in favor of its coming from the lining cell layers. Hyaluronic acid serves as an integral part of connective tissue, and as a lubricant and shock absorber in joints. Its solutions are viscous, and contribute to the lubricating qualities of synovial and other body fluids. Hyaluronic acid in tissue seems to act as a cementing substance and as a tissue barrier permitting metabolites to pass through by diffusion but resisting penetration by bacteria and other infectious agents.

Hyaluronic acid is the only nonsulfated glycosaminoglycan. The repeating disaccharide units are N-acetyl glucosamine and glucuronic acid. Hyaluronic acid occurs in the tissue as single chains and not as multichain proteoglycans. Its carboxyl groups are completely ionized, giving it negative charges at pH 7. Hyaluronic acid is soluble in water, in which it forms highly viscous solutions. The amount in cartilage is variable but usually represents less than 1% of the total uronic acid. Hyaluronic acid can be present in a free state, but it usually exists as a component of the proteoglycan aggregates in cartilage.

Proteoglycans in Cartilage

Structure of Proteoglycans. The proteoglycan is a macromolecule constructed of a protein core to which many glycosaminoglycan chains are attached laterally (Fig. 17-2). The average chain has a molecular weight of one to three million; the protein core has an average molecular weight of 20,000 with about 100 chondroitin sulfate and 50 keratan sulfate chains attached. Thus, about 10% of the weight of the molecule is protein, and 90% is glycosaminoglycans or proteoglycan subunits. The relative proportions of chondroitin sulfate and keratan sulfate vary widely from proteoglycans containing mainly chondroitin sulfate to those having an equal amount of chondroitin sulfate and keratan sulfate.

Within the ground substance of cartilage, the proteoglycan subunits exist as multimolecular aggregates with a molecular weight of approximately 50 million. The proteoglycan subunits have a highly specific interaction with hyaluronic acid and link protein, which leads to a proteoglycan aggregate with increased hydrodynamic size and viscosity. The proteoglycan aggregate has a filamentous backbone of hyaluronic acid to which the proteoglycan subunits are noncovalently bound at regular intervals perpendicular to the backbone. In cartilage, there are more proteoglycans than hyaluronic acid, which allows hyaluronic acid to bind proteoglycans at intervals of 20 nm. Link protein serves to stabilize the aggregate. The negatively charged sulfate and carboxylate groups on both chondroitin sulfate and keratan sulfate repel each other, so that the glycosaminoglycan chains assume a fully extended conformation. Within the proteoglycan subunit, they stand out from the protein core by electrostatic repulsion.

Proteoglycans as Polyelectrolytes. The connective tissue proteoglycans are electrolytes of a special nature. Most electrolytes dissociate into free positive and negative ions, which for the most part are freely mobile in solution and can conduct an electrical current. Chondroitin sulfate exists as anions related to sodium cations. The chondroitin sulfate anions consist of a chain of about 60 repeating units of N-acetylchondrosine sulfate carrying about 120 anionic charges. Thus, a proteoglycan molecule that contains 20 such chains possesses over 2000 anionic charges. There is very little independent motion of these anionic groups, which produces a highly localized density of negative charges—one of the special properties of polyelectrolytes. In proteoglycan subunits, there is further constraint by the attachment to the protein. The polyelectrolyte chain is somewhat stiff and distributes itself throughout a larger volume than an uncharged chain. This volume of solution is called its molecular domain.

These chains have a higher attractive force for counter ions, which also cannot move about as freely as simple electrolytes. In some ways, they appear to be bound to the polyanions, which seems to shield one chain from another to lessen the repulsion between two chains with high negative charges, thus reducing the stiffness of the chain. The proteoglycans behave in a manner analogous to cation exchange resins and are capable of binding protons as well as univalent, divalent, and trivalent metal ions. The binding is usually stronger the higher the cationic charge and the smaller the radius of the cation. Also, the carboxyl anion has a great affinity for the hydrogen ion. These binding affinities account for the metachromatic staining of certain dyes such as alician blue or toluidine blue. The term *metachromasia* means a change in the staining properties of a dye. This change in color is the result of

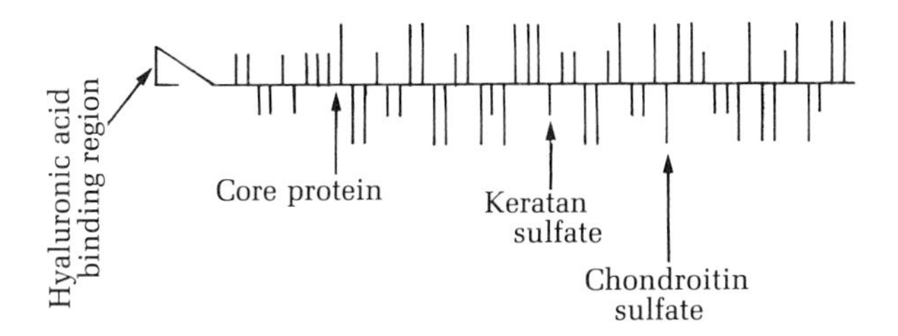

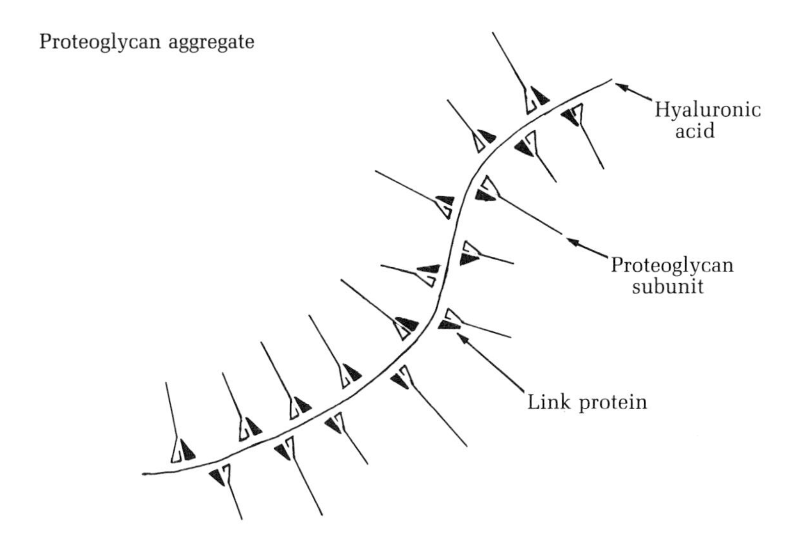

Fig. 17-2. Diagram of proteoglycans in cartilage.

counter-ion binding, and indicates a shift in the wave length of peak absorbency of the dye. In tissue sections, metachromasia results from formation of salts of polyanions (the polyelectrolytes) with a metachromatic dye (the counter ion). The addition of a dilute solution of polyanions to the dye has the same effect as increasing the concentration of dye in solution. In addition, there is polymerization of the dye cations in aqueous solution when crowded together. These two phenomena account for the property of metachromasia, which indicates the presence of polyelectrolytes in a tissue.

Excluded Volume Effect and Sieving Effect. Proteins and uncharged glycosaminoglycans behave in solution as random coils. The chains are flexible and can assume many shapes and conformations. This flexibility is derived from the freedom of rotation of atoms around single covalent bonds. If the chain is large and has bulky groups, the extent of rotation is limited. In proteoglycan chains, there are anionic charges that cause electrostatic repulsion along the chain and between chains. The internal repulsion between anionic charges will lengthen and stiffen the chain. The repulsion between chains also makes stiffer chains that enclose or occupy a larger volume. The larger chain has small openings to allow small molecules to pass through, but, because of its somewhat rigid structure, it does not allow large molecules through. These proteoglycans have been called diffuse molecules and two have properties that are important for connective tissue: the static equilibrium state (excluded volume effect) and the dynamic transport process (sieving effect). The excluded volume effect accounts for the ability of hyaluronic acid in connective tissue to prevent passage of large protein molecules and bacteria. The sieving effect means that transmission of large molecules is retarded to an extent that increases with their size; however, diffusion also depends on the shape of the molecule. These properties regulate the diffusion rates of both nutritive and degraded materials through cartilage.

Degradation. Proteoglycans have a much more rapid turnover than collagen, both during and after growth. Their breakdown is controlled either by enzymes that hydrolyze protein (proteases) or by carbohydrates (saccharases). The proteases are produced by the chondrocytes and different proteolytic enzymes and serve to reduce the viscosity of proteoglycan solutions to varying degrees. For example, the injection of papain, a potent protease, into rabbits' ears results in a prompt drooping of the ears that requires several days for recovery. Proteoglycans disappeared from cartilage and were found in increased amounts in plasma and urine. This finding suggests that the stiffness of cartilage, such as that found in the ear, is dependent on the content of proteoglycans, which, when degraded by papain, leave the cartilage and escape into the bloodstream. With the synthesis of new proteoglycans by the cells, the cartilage becomes stiff again.

Release of lysosomal enzymes into the cartilage matrix is an important mechanism for degradation of cartilage and other connective tissues. A possible sequence of events could be as follows: (1) an intracellular stimulus (by hormones or other agents) releases appropriate degradative lysosomal enzymes from cells into the cartilage matrix; (2) this is followed by degradation of proteoglycans; (3) these degradative products diffuse out of the ground substance into the circulation and are removed by the liver, where degradation is completed. The above sequence can occur in controlled or excessive amounts.

Cartilage Changes With Aging

Cartilage undergoes specific changes with aging that predispose it to increasing fragility, rigidity, and fibrillation. The water content of cartilage, which is 80% to 90% in the fetus, declines to approximately 70% in the human adult. The collagen content increases in the first decade of life, then appears to remain constant. Proportions of individual glycosaminoglycans in cartilage also vary with age. The concentration of chondroitin-4 sulfate steadily decreases with increasing age. The chondroitin-6 sulfate concentration remains constant until after 30 years of age, then increases. In the embryo and during early growth, keratan sulfate is absent. Its concentration rises in the person between 10 and 40 years of age, and thereafter it remains constant at approximately 55% of the total glycosaminoglycan content of the tissue.

SYNOVIAL FLUID

One of the main functions of the lining cells of synovium is to secrete certain components of the synovial fluid. However, in addition to substances secreted by the lining cells, synovial fluid contains proteins that are electrophoretically and immunologically identical to plasma proteins. These proteins come from the blood that circulates in the synovial membranes; however, the concentration and electrophoretic distribution of proteins in synovial fluid differs from that in plasma. The main differences are a lower protein content, a higher percentage of albumin, and a lower percentage of α-2-globulin in the synovial fluid. How the membrane regulates protein concentration is not known. After intravenous injection of various proteins into animal joints, only those of lower molecular weight can be detected, so size is probably a factor in determining diffusion of materials into synovial fluid. The lining cells are an unlikely barrier, since they do not form a continuous membrane. The absence of some proteins from synovial fluid could be due to their exclusion by macromolecules, either at the capillary level, in the intercellular space, or in the synovial fluid itself. The long, extended chains of macromolecules can sterically exclude the entry of a large or asymmetrically shaped protein (e.g., fibrinogen) from the diffuse domain they occupy in solution. Hyaluronate is one diffuse macromolecule that shows an excluded volume effect in the joint.

Some proteins found in synovial fluid do not appear to originate in the plasma. Alkaline phosphatase may arise in part from cartilage; it is also synthesized by lining cells and secreted into the synovial fluid. Also, a cartilage proteoglycan component has been

Table 17-1. Synovianalysis

	DISEASE	APPEARANCE: CLARITY	COLOR	VISCOSITY	MUCIN CLOT	SPONTANEOUS CLOT FORMATION	AVERAGE WBC COUNT (per cu. mm)	POLYS (%)	GLUCOSE-SYNOVIAL COMPARED TO SERUM	CRYSTALS	BACTERIA
Normal		Clear	Straw	High	Good	0	<200	<25%	Equal	0	0
Inflammatory	Rheumatoid	Cloudy	Yellow to greenish	Low	Poor	Moderate	15,000–20,000+	75%	Moderately decreased	Occ. choles.	0
	Gout	Cloudy	Yellow to milky	Low	Poor	Minimal	10,000–20,000	25%–50%	Equal	Urate	0
Septic	Tuberculous	Cloudy	Yellow	Low	Poor	Minimal	25,000	50%–60%	Decreased to absent	0	+
	Pyogenic	Cloudy	Greyish	Low	Poor	Moderate to marked	80,000–200,000	75%	Markedly decreased to absent	0	+
Non-Inflammatory	Osteo-arthritis	Clear	Yellow	High	Good	0-slight	1,000	<25%	Equal	0	0
	Trauma	Serosang. to bloody	Straw to bloody to xanthochromic	High	Good	Slight	<2,000 WBC many RBC's	<25%	Equal	0	0

found that may be a degradation product of cartilage, or it may be synthesized by lining cells. Proteins immunologically identical to plasma proteins may be synthesized in the synovial membrane.

It is well recognized clinically that blood shed into joint fluid, as might occur, for example, following a fracture, does not coagulate well; if clots do form, they are poorly organized and are rapidly removed from the joint fluid. It has been suggested that articular cartilage and synovial membrane release an activator of the proteolytic enzyme plasminogen, which, after its conversion to plasmin, breaks down fibrinogen and prevents the formation of a firm clot. In addition, the synovial fluid tends to wash out whatever clot does form between the fracture surfaces. These mechanisms contribute to the high nonunion rate in intraarticular fractures.

Absorption of Synovial Fluid From Diarthrodial Joints. The synovial membrane can absorb materials injected into the joint, but passage between lining cells is also a major route of elimination. Once within the membrane, substances may enter capillaries or lymphatics, remain in macrophages, or lie free in tissues. Small proteins injected into the joint are removed by way of the lymphatics, but those of higher molecular weight remain in the joint indefinitely. However, particulate matter, such as colloidal mercuric sulfide, which forms aggregates as large as 0.5 μ, is absorbed through the synovial membrane. This observation indicates that size is not the only limiting factor to absorption.

One difficulty in understanding the mechanism of absorption of intraarticular material by synovial membrane is that, regardless of the type of substance injected, an inflammatory response always occurs. Migration of leukocytes between lining cells, edema, and exudation from capillaries obviously affect the process of absorption. Also, marked changes occur within the lining cells.

Alterations in Synovial Fluid Caused by Disease of the Synovial Membrane. Pronounced alterations in the composition of synovial fluid occur when the joint is injured. These changes have been described in over 30 separate disease states; however, they can be considered in three major groups: inflammatory arthritis (rheumatoid, gouty), septic arthritis (bacterial, tuberculous), and noninflammatory arthritis (osteoarthritis, post-traumatic). Analysis of the major constituents of synovial fluid can provide diagnostic leads in these disease categories. Table 17-1 points out the areas and magnitude of these changes.

SELECTED REFERENCES

Freeman MAR: Adult Articular Cartilage. Kent, England, Pitman Medical Publishing Co Ltd, 1979

Serafini-Fracassini A, Smith JW: The Structure and Biochemistry of Cartilage. London, Churchill Livingstone Medical Division, 1974

Simon WH: The Human Joint in Health and Disease. Philadelphia, University of Pennsylvania Press, 1978

Chapter 18

Lubrication of Human Joints

William H. Bowers

GOALS AND OBJECTIVES

Goals: To acquaint the reader with the principles of friction and lubrication as employed in mechanical systems and their application to the lubrication of human joints

Objectives: On completion of this unit, and using the text as a standard reference, one should be able to evaluate, describe, recognize, or list the

1. Mechanical basis for friction forces
2. Differences between friction in solid systems and shear stress in liquids
3. Major modes of mechanical lubrication
4. Methods of achieving and maintaining a lubricant film between surfaces in mechanical systems
5. Disadvantages of mechanical lubrication in human joints
6. Major modes of achieving and maintaining a lubricant film in human joints
7. Role of hyaluronate in diarthrodial joint lubrication (e.g., boundary and "boosted" mechanisms)

OUTLINE

I. Principles of friction and lubrication in mechanical systems
   A. Dry solid friction and coefficient of friction
   B. Liquid shear stress and viscosity
   C. Mechanisms of lubrication
      1. Boundary
      2. Fluid film
         a. Hydrostatic fluid
         b. "Squeeze film"
         c. Hydrodynamic
         d. Elastohydrodynamic

II. Lubrication in human diarthrodial joints
  A. Boundary mechanisms
  B. "Squeeze film"
  C. Self-pressurized hydrostatic (weeping) mechanisms
  D. Elastohydrodynamic mechanisms
  E. Boosted lubrication

PRINCIPLES OF FRICTION AND LUBRICATION IN MECHANICAL SYSTEMS

Lubrication of human joints is a complex interrelationship between joint surface structure and synovial fluid. In recent years, work by many investigators has produced a large amount of data that has been succinctly reviewed by Radin, Frankel, and Burstein.

Human joint lubrication mechanisms can best be understood by first reviewing friction and lubrication concepts in mechanical systems. Unlubricated (dry) surfaces moving on each other at low velocities develop friction forces when the peaks of surface irregularities (asperities) come in contact. These irregularities momentarily fuse, producing cold welds, which are disrupted as movement continues (Fig. 18-1). As the applied load across the surface is increased, the total number of contacts, and thus the area of contact, increases. The friction force is the force that must be developed to disrupt these contact welds and is proportional to the applied load, the proportionality constant being termed *the coefficient of friction*. Except at initial low velocity, the dry friction is relatively independent of velocity. Typical coefficients of friction are about 0.1 to 0.3 for plastic on plastic and 0.3 to 0.8 for metal on metal. The coefficient of friction is thus material property that must be considered, along with the variable of applied force, to determine friction force.

When a lubricant is placed between two dry surfaces, a new dimension is created. Solid friction is relatively independent of velocity of motion, but fluid friction forces are extremely sensitive to velocity and to lubricant film thickness. These two factors are quantitated as the velocity gradient. Shear stress in liquids (analogous to friction forces between dry solids) is proportional to the velocity gradient, the proportionality constant being termed *the viscosity*. The viscosity, like the coefficient of friction, is a material property of the liquid and must also be considered in relation to a second variable, the velocity gradient, in order to calculate the shear stress.

When a lubricant is placed between moving surfaces, two types of fluid lubrication may occur: *boundary lubrication* and *fluid film lubrication*. Machine bearings are usually designed for one type of lubrication or the other, but not for both. In *boundary lubrication* (Fig. 18-2), each bearing surface is impregnated with a thin layer of molecules that slide on each other much more readily than they are sheared off the impregnated surface, as is the case with a Teflon-coated frying pan. Other materials capable of boundary lubrication are graphite, oil, cream, and ink. Boundary lubrication is essentially independent of the physical properties of either the lubricant (e.g., viscosity) or the contacting bodies (e.g., stiffness). In *fluid film lubrication* (Fig. 18-3), the moving surfaces are completely separated by a thick film of lubricant. The resistance to motion arises from the viscosity of the lubricant itself and the relative velocity of the moving surfaces. The load is borne by the pressure generated in this fluid film.

Several methods may be used to maintain thick lubricant films between surfaces. In the first of these, called *hydrostatic fluid lubrication*, the fluid is confined under pressure maintained by a pump external to the system. The Mount Palomar telescope suspension is operated under high load, low relative velocity conditions by this method. As the relative tangential velocity of the two moving surfaces increases, this method is less applicable.

A second method, operative when the surfaces are moving tangentially, is *hydrodynamic lubrication*. Continuous tangential motion of the surfaces maintains a wedge of lubricant between the surfaces. As the velocity of motion between the two surfaces increases, film thickness increases by means of the wedge effect. Because a force is exerted continuously on the moving surfaces to sustain the velocity, energy is put into the surface and hence into the field. The energy is dissipated with the fluid as heat, but, in the process, pressure is created in the fluid layer, which separates the two moving masses dy-

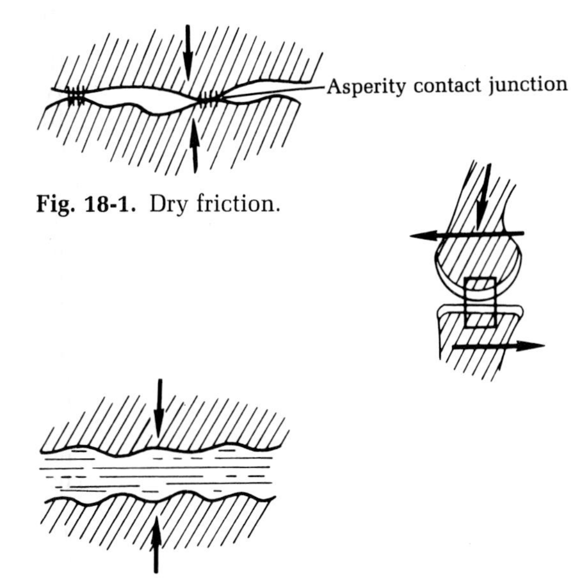

Fig. 18-1. Dry friction.

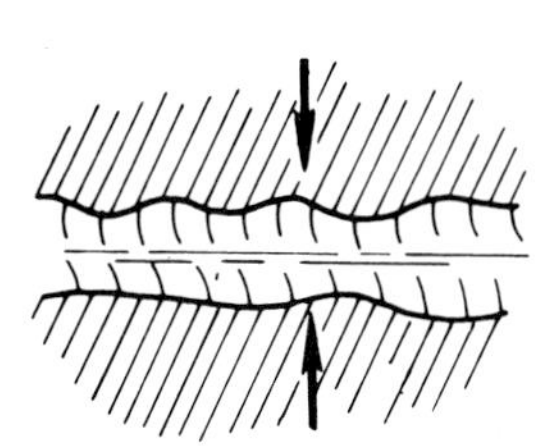

Fig. 18-2. Boundary lubrication.

Fig. 18-3. Fluid lubrication.

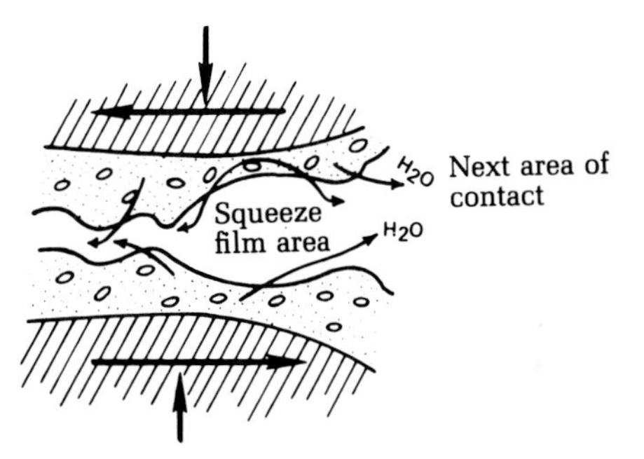

Fig. 18-4. Fluid film lubrication in human joints. The cartilage deforms maximally as pressure increases in the squeeze film. Interstitial fluid flows out of cartlage (*small arrows*) into low-pressure periphery of immediate contact area providing squeeze film for the next contact area. This diagram then depicts a combination of "squeeze film elastohydrodynamic" and "self-pressurized hydrostatic" mechanisms.

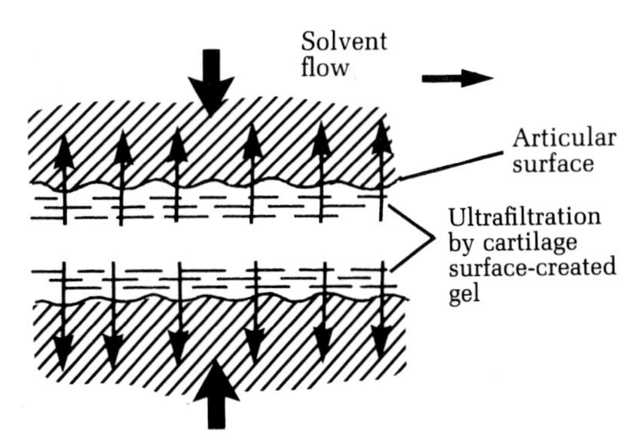

Fig. 18-5. "Boosted" lubrication.

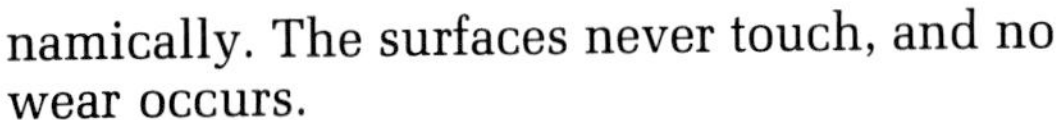

namically. The surfaces never touch, and no wear occurs.

If the surfaces are moving perpendicularly toward each other, the fluid must be squeezed out from the gap between the two surfaces. Again, the viscosity and inertia of the fluid require that pressure be generated in the fluid film to force out the lubricant. This third mode of fluid film lubrication is termed *squeeze film lubrication*. Obviously, the load cannot be supported indefinitely by the squeeze film process. Eventually the film of fluid will be so thin that contact of the asperities on the two surfaces will occur. However, the mechanism is sufficient to carry high loads for short durations.

In squeeze film and hydrodynamic lubrication, the thickness, extent, and load-carrying capacity of the fluid film are determined by the viscosity of the lubricant, the film's geometry (*i.e.*, the shape of the gap between the two surfaces), and the speed of the relative motion of the surfaces. However, if the bearing material is relatively soft, the pressure in the fluid film may cause substantial deformations of the contacting surfaces. These deformations beneficially alter the film geometry and contact area, causing a greater restriction to lubricant fluid escape and therefore resulting in a more substantial and longer lasting film. This fourth type of fluid film lubrication is known as *elastohydro-*

dynamic lubrication. If the soft surfaces are moving tangentially under load, the trailing edges deform, maintaining a pressurized leading wedge of fluid—*sliding elastohydrodynamic lubrication*. If the loaded surfaces are static or slow moving, the soft surface deforms peripheral to the load—*squeeze film elastohydrodynamic lubrication*.

LUBRICATION IN HUMAN DIARTHRODIAL JOINTS

Human joints cannot supply the conditions for hydrostatic or hydrodynamic lubrication as described for mechanical systems. One reason is the requirement for maintenance of the hydrodynamic fluid wedge by unidirectional rotation and velocity. Human joints oscillate slowly; therefore, the fluid wedge quickly deteriorates. The thixotrophic nature of joint fluid compensates somewhat for this deficit, because the lubricating fluid is able to enter the region of hydrodynamic lubrication at much lower velocities. Another difficulty is that the load generated in human joints is insufficient in itself to generate a squeeze film thicker than the height of joint surface irregularities.

The synovial fluid in synovial joints can act, under some loading conditions, as a boundary lubricant for articular cartilage. Furthermore, this lubricating ability is not dependent on the viscosity of the synovial fluid. This mechanism is most important under severe loading conditions. Under less severe conditions, when the loads are lower, oscillatory, and the relative speed of the contacting surfaces is higher, the joint may operate under the fluid film lubrication mechanisms.

Both the sliding and squeeze film elastohydrodynamic lubrication mechanisms are conceptually possible in human joints. The sliding elastohydrodynamic mechanism would function in low load–high velocity situations, such as the swing phase of gait, whereas the squeeze film elastohydrodynamic mechanism would come into play under high load–low velocity situations, such as the stance phase of gait (Fig. 18-4).

The elasticity of cartilage and its small pore size (60 A) provide another lubrication mechanism. Pores of this size allow only small molecules (ions and water) to pass freely while the large mucopolysaccharides remain within the cartilage matrix. When cartilage is compressed, it "weeps" interstitial fluid like a squeezed sponge. As the pressure is increased in the center of the impending area of contact, the cartilage deforms and fluid weeps out at the periphery where pressure is lowest. As translation of the area of impending contact occurs with motion, this fluid quickly becomes part of the joint fluid, generating pressure in the next area of contact. When the load is removed from the articular cartilage, the fluid returns to the interstitium of the cartilage. This mechanism is termed *self-pressurized hydrostatic lubrication* (Fig. 18-4).

Another mechanism by which the cartilage surfaces might be protected has been termed *boosted lubrication*. It becomes progressively more difficult, as the two cartilage surfaces approach each other, for the large hyaluronic acid polymers in the synovial fluid to escape from the gap between the surface. The water and small solute molecules can escape either through the cartilage surface or laterally through the spaces between the two surfaces, but the large hyaluronic acid protein complexes may be too large to escape. This ultrafiltration process can eventually yield a concentrated gel of high viscosity that is probably less than 1 μ thick and has some protective lubrication capability (Fig. 18-5).

SELECTED REFERENCES

Bowden FP, Tabor D: Friction and Lubrication. New York, Barnes & Noble, 1967

Frankel VH, Burstein AH: Orthopaedic Biomechanics. Philadelphia, Lea & Febiger, 1970

Radin EL, Paul JL: A consolidated concept of joint lubrication. J Bone Joint Surg 54A:607, 1972

Swann DA, Radin EL: The molecular basis of articular lubrication. J Biol Chem 247:8069, 1972

Wright V: Lubrication and Wear in Joints. Philadelphia, JB Lippincott, 1970

Part Eight

PATHOLOGIC PROCESSES IN JOINTS

Chapter 19

Osteoarthritis

Michael A. Friedman,
Robert A. Eisenberg,
and Paul H. Wright

GOALS AND OBJECTIVES

Goals: To introduce the reader to the pathology, pathogenesis, clinical, laboratory, and roentgenographic features of osteoarthritis

Objectives: On completion of this unit, and using the text as a standard reference, one should be able to describe or list the following:

1. The pathology of osteoarthritis
2. Two major theories of its pathogenesis
3. The clinical features of osteoarthritis, with particular reference to those that distinguish it from the inflammatory arthritides
4. The pattern of joint involvement in primary generalized osteoarthritis
5. Four common causes of secondary osteoarthritis
6. The principles governing the therapy of osteoarthritis

OUTLINE

I. Epidemiology
II. Pathology
III. Pathogenesis
IV. Clinical features
  A. Primary osteoarthritis
  B. Secondary osteoarthritis
  C. Localized osteoarthritis
V. Roentgenographic aspects
VI. Laboratory aspects
VII. Therapeutic principles

Osteoarthritis is a condition characterized by alterations in joint architecture secondary to cartilage degeneration, together with misdirected bone and cartilage growth. The synonyms *degenerative joint disease* and *osteoarthrosis* underscore the fact that marked inflammation is not a prerequisite for the articular destruction of osteoarthritis.

EPIDEMIOLOGY

The U.S. Department of Health and Human Services estimates that 37% of the U.S. adult population has roentgenographic evidence of osteoarthritis in the hands or feet. The prevalence of osteoarthritis rises strikingly with age. Men and women are affected in nearly equal frequency, but moderate and severe roentgenographic findings are more common in women than men over age 45. The syndrome of *primary generalized osteoarthritis* is found more frequently in women and displays a familial aggregation.

PATHOLOGY

The pathology of the osteoarthritic lesion reflects the gradual processes of destruction and regeneration.

Early in the disease, the articular cartilage loses its glistening appearance. Later, the surface layers flake off while deeper layers develop longitudinal fissures, a process termed *fibrillation*. The cartilage becomes thin and in some areas may be absent. The unprotected subchondral bone becomes sclerotic and polished, resembling ivory. This process is aptly termed *eburnation*. Cysts may form within the subchondral bone; these cysts on occasion communicate with fissures in the overlying cartilage, suggesting either that intrasynovial pressure formed the cyst or that material under pressure within the cyst fractured the overlying cartilage during its escape into the joint space.

Spurlike bony outgrowths covered by hyaline cartilage, *osteophytes*, may develop at the margins of the joint and progressively enlarge (Fig. 19-1). Small bits of cartilage-covered bone, known as *joint mice*, may actually break off into the joint.

Microscopically, the cartilage matrix loses its ability to stain for proteoglycans with alcian blue or safranin-O. There is a diminution of chondrocytes in superficial zones, whereas deeper chondrocytes demonstrate a surprising proliferation in clusters called *brood capsules*, which probably represent an attempt at cartilage repair. Capillary buds penetrate the layer of calcified cartilage. Newly formed sements of cartilage push up from below, splitting and reduplicating the *tidemark*, which is the demarcation between calcified and noncalcified cartilage. Subchondral bone displays thickened trabeculae and microfractures. The synovium is hypertrophied and thrown into villose folds, and the joint capsule is thickened and contracted. A low-grade mononuclear infiltrate may be present.

Ultrastructural characteristics parallel the changes seen by light microscopy. Cartilage with advanced osteoarthritic changes shows numerous degenerating chondrocytes, whereas earlier lesions contain chondrocytes with prominent Golgi apparatus and a rough endoplasmic reticulum, indicative of synthetic activity.

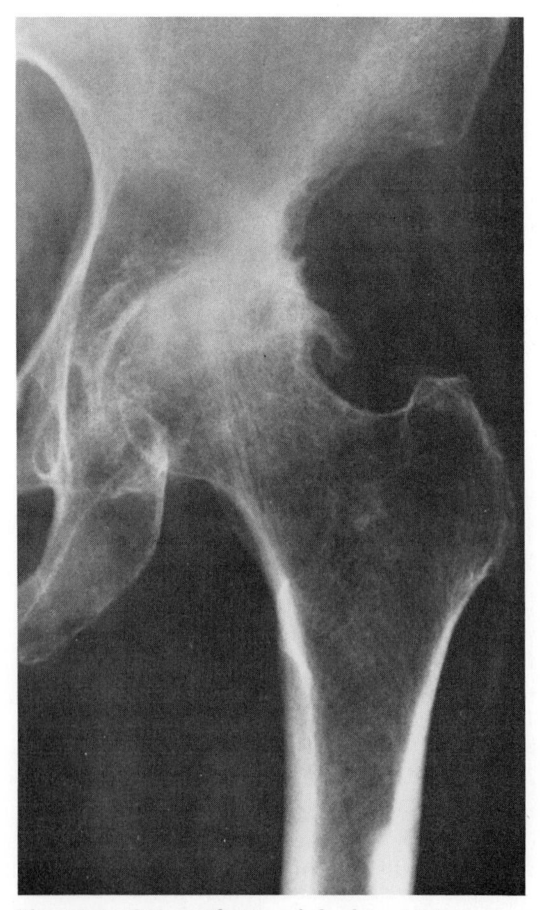

Fig. 19-1. Osteoarthritis of the hip. Note narrowing of the cartilage space superolaterally, subchondral sclerosis, cysts within the head, and the lateral osteophyte.

PATHOGENESIS

Multiple factors may be responsible for creating the osteoarthritic lesion. Cartilage and bone vie for the distinction of being the site of the initial disturbance. According to the cartilage theory, damage to the chondrocyte causes the release of enzymes capable of degrading the matrix proteoglycans. This process must be quantitatively sufficient to overcome the activity of naturally occurring enzyme inhibitors and the enhanced synthesis of new proteoglycans. Changes in the conformational state of the remaining proteoglycans permit the cartilage to swell by imbibing excess water. The biomechanical properties of the cartilage are thus altered, rendering both matrix and chondrocytes more vulnerable to mechanical stress and enzymatic attack.

In support of the cartilage theory is the finding of high levels of cathepsin-D, an acid protease, as well as neutral proteases in osteoarthritic cartilage. These enzymes act to degrade proteoglycans in or near chondrocytes or at more distant matrix sites, according to their *p*H optima. A collagenase has recently been isolated from osteoarthritic cartilage, its activity roughly paralleling disease severity. Various polysaccharidases have been detected in synovial fluid. Although they would be excluded from normal cartilage, they might penetrate fibrillated cartilage and amplify the process of matrix breakdown.

Evidence that enzymatic breakdown occurs is indirect and is derived from studies on biochemical differences between normal and osteoarthritic cartilage matrices. Shortened chondroitin sulfate chains have been extracted from osteoarthritic cartilage. There may be differing relative concentrations of chondroitin sulfate and keratan sulfate between normal and osteoarthritic cartilage, but current data are not consistent as to which glycosaminoglycan predominates in which condition. The proteoglycan subunits in osteoarthritis are less aggregated than in the normal state. Two mechanisms for this alteration have been observed. In one, a defect in the link protein or the hyaluronate binding region of the core protein prevents the noncovalent binding of proteoglycans to hyaluronic acid. In the other, the abnormality lies in the hyaluronic acid itself, and the proteoglycans retain the ability to aggregate with exogenous hyaluronate.

The major uncertainty in these studies is whether matrix abnormalities represent enzymatic degradation or the *de novo* synthesis of impaired matrix constituents. Indeed, an alternate version of the cartilage theory defines the primary alteration as disruption of the collagen framework. Proteoglycans would consequently be leached out of the cartilage, and enzymatic proteoglycan destruction need not be postulated.

According to the bone theory, mechanical stress is dissipated by microfracturing of the subchondral bone. With subsequent healing, the trabeculae harden. As more shock-absorbing function falls upon the articular cartilage, degeneration ensues.

In either case, it is clear that mechanical stress, if not causal, is related in some way to the development of osteoarthritis. Such factors as handedness and occupational task patterns influence the distribution of involved joints. Osteoarthritis has been produced in experimental animals by surgical procedures designed to create joint instability. After severing the anterior cruciate ligament in the dog, for example, typical osteoarthritic changes occur in the knee, including decreased proteoglycan aggregation. Obesity may play a role in the development of osteoarthritis, but this issue is far from being settled. The increased prevalence of osteoarthritis with age could be due to age-specific changes in the ability of cartilage to withstand stress in addition to the effect of increased cumulative physical insults acquired by older joints.

CLINICAL FEATURES

Primary Osteoarthritis

Primary osteoarthritis is that which develops in the absence of a well-defined predisposing disease.

The syndrome of *primary generalized osteoarthritis* has a characteristic pattern of joint involvement. The patient, typically a woman in the fifth or sixth decade of life, notices the gradual onset of pain in the distal interphalangeal (DIP) joints. Aggravating nocturnal fingertip pain and paresthesias may develop. Cystic swellings containing gelatinous hyaluronic acid appear on the dorsolateral aspects of these joints; these are the harbingers of knobby excrescences of bone and cartilage termed *Heberden's nodes* that form at these sites. Similar enlargements at the proximal interphalangeal (PIP) joints are known as *Bouchard's nodes*. In some patients, the onset of primary osteoarthritis is more abrupt, with painful erythema of one or more DIP joints. This acute stage may last up to several months. Mimicking an acute inflammatory disorder, this mode of onset has been given the name *inflammatory osteoarthritis*.

With either presentation, a chronic stage is usually reached that is marked by a reduction in inflammatory manifestations but with loss of finger joint mobility. Other joints, especially those that bear weight, may become increasingly painful. A fairly characteristic deformity of the hand develops. The phalanges often deviate radially at the interphalangeal joints. In rare instances, bony ankylosis at these joints supervenes. The metacarpophalangeal (MCP) joints are typically spared. Disease of the saddle-shaped joint between the trapezium and the metacarpal of the thumb, the first carpometacarpal (CMC) joint, leads to pain and tenderness at the base of the thumb. Adduction, flexion, and volar subluxation of this joint narrows the web space between the thumb and index finger. Bone hypertrophy develops, and the hand assumes a square contour. The trapezioscaphoid joint may also become involved, but the remainder of the wrist articulations are typically spared (Fig. 19-2).

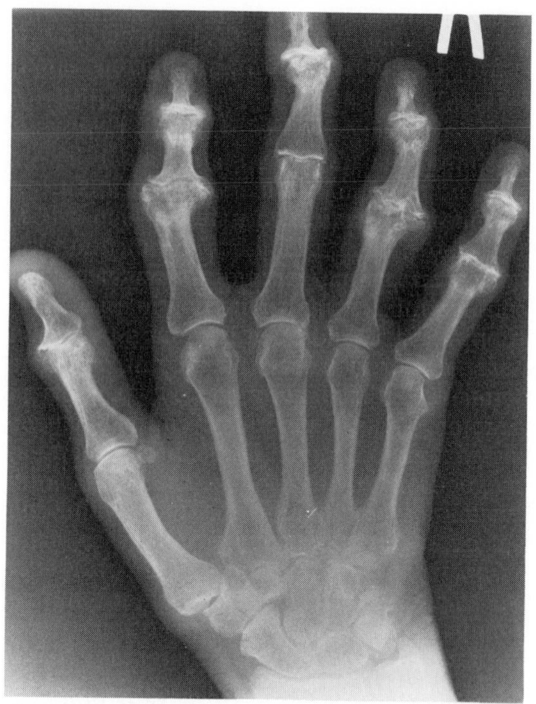

Fig. 19-2. Osteoarthritis of the hand. Note extensive involvement of the IP joints (with relative sparing of the MCP joints) and soft-tissue swelling at the DIP (Heberden's nodes) and PIP (Bouchard's nodes) joints.

Hips are less frequently involved than knees. The particular vulnerability of the knee to degenerative changes may be explained, at least in part, by certain unique biomechanical features of the knee.

1. Unlike the hip, the knee has relatively little bony stability or protection.
2. Since it rests at the end of the two longest lever arms in the body, the knee is subject to great angular stresses.
3. As a result of the muscle forces acting across the joint, any load transmitted through the knee during weight-bearing is about three times as great as the body weight being transmitted.

Preexisting valgus deformities or, more commonly, varus deformities increase the weight-bearing load and degenerative changes in the lateral or medial compartment of the joint. Foot involvement commonly affects the first metatarsophalangeal (MTP), first tarsometatarsal (TMT), and subtalar joints, the ankle joint usually being spared. Spinal involvement occurs at the intervertebral facets, usually in association with degenerative changes in the corresponding discs.

The prolonged joint stiffness upon arising that is typical of inflammatory arthritis is rare in osteoarthritis. Usually the patient experiences brief morning stiffness that reappears after a period of inactivity. The cause of this *gel phenomenon* is obscure.

Osteoarthritis is subject to intermittent exacerbations, although they are not as severe as those of rheumatoid arthritis. These flares may in some cases be due to inflammation induced by trivial trauma to an already compromised joint, or they may result from associated pseudogout.

Secondary Osteoarthritis

A variety of diseases and conditions predispose a person to osteoarthritis, some of which are considered here (see list below). The roles of trauma and developmental hip abnormalities are discussed in the preceding section.

Conditions Predisposing to Osteoarthritis

Trauma
Inflammatory arthritis
CPPD deposition disease
Osteonecrosis
Recurrent hemarthrosis
Neuropathic (Charcot's) arthropathy
Excessive use of intraarticular steroids
Heritable disorders of connective tissue
Developmental skeletal abnormalities
Ochronosis
Hemochromatosis
Wilson's disease

A form of generalized osteoarthritis may be seen in conjunction with calcium pyrophosphate dihydrate (CPPD) deposition disease, even in the absence of recurrent attacks of pseudogout. It affects joints not usually involved in primary generalized osteoarthritis, such as wrists, MCPs, shoulders, and ankles. Osteoarthritis also develops in several systemic disorders including acromegaly, Wilson's disease, hyperparathyroidism, hemochromatosis, and ochronosis. The latter condition is interesting in that it is an example of a biochemical insult to cartilage. Neuropathic (Charcot's) arthropathy is a severe form of degenerative arthritis occurring in joints deprived of proprioceptive or pain innervation, the most common underlying conditions being tabes dorsalis, syringomyelia, and diabetes mellitus. Many heritable connective tissue disorders are also associated with premature joint degeneration.

Localized Osteoarthritis

Isolated osteoarthritis of the hip is a significant cause of disability in the elderly. It presents either unilaterally or bilaterally, with pain on weight-bearing felt in the groin, buttock, medial thigh, greater trochanteric region, or knee. The patient limps to diminish the mechanical stress on the joint and thereby lessen pain. Most distressing is the development of pain during sleep, when the protective function of muscular splinting is absent. The gel phenomenon, discussed above, plays a prominent role in this picture. Once thought to be a primary form, osteoarthritis of the hip has been shown to develop in most cases as a result of preexisting abnormalities. In addition to such obvious hip pathology as congenital hip dysplasia, aseptic necrosis of the femoral head, or an old slipped capital femoral epiphysis, previously unrecognized subtle alterations of the acetabulum may play a role in its pathogenesis.

Localized osteoarthritis may follow repetitive occupational trauma or certain fractures. Examples of the former are wrist, elbow, and shoulder osteoarthritis in pneumatic drill operators and ankle osteoarthritis in ballet dancers. Interphalangeal osteoarthritis has been reported following frostbite injury.

Chondromalacia patellae is a form of osteoarthritis confined to the patellofemoral joint of adolescents or young adults. Pain under the patella with activity or prolonged flexion and an annoying grating sensation are the main symptoms.

Osteoarthritis affects the apophyseal joints of the spine. In the cervical spine, upward projections of the posterolateral vertebral bodies articulate with the adjacent vertebral body. Osteophytes from these *uncovertebral joints of Luschka* can impinge on nerve roots, causing radicular pain and sensory or motor deficits.

Shoulder pain may be due to osteoarthritis of the acromioclavicular or sternoclavicular joints. The glenohumeral joint is not as frequently affected.

ROENTGENOGRAPHIC ASPECTS

The loss of articular cartilage is seen roentgenographically as a nonuniform narrowing of the joint. In the hips, this change takes place either superolaterally or medially. Initial narrowing in the knees is usually confined to a single compartment. Eburnation can be recognized by increased radiodensity of subchondral bone. Osteophytes appear at the joint margins. Heberden's nodes, however, may not be as visible roentgenographically as one might expect from their clinical appearance because of their large cartilaginous component. Cysts are frequently seen as radiolucent areas in the subchondral bone, most commonly in the hip (Fig. 19-1). In some cases of inflammatory osteoarthritis, erosions of subchondral bone occur in the interphalangeal joints of the fingers, but the juxta-articular osteopenia of rheumatoid arthritis is absent.

Diffuse idiopathic skeletal hyperostosis (DISH, or senile ankylosing hyperostosis of Forestier and Rotes-Querol) is worthy of mention here because of its superficial roentgenographic resemblance to osteoarthritis. It is predominantly a disease of men, which, although usually first recognized in the elderly, probably develops slowly throughout adult life. Spinal stiffness and miscellaneous skeletal complaints are associated with flowing osteophyte formation that predilects the right side of the vertebral bodies. Osteophytes are also seen at extravertebral sites, particularly the margins of large joints. Notable are the absence of disc and joint narrowing and the subchondral bone changes of osteoarthritis.

LABORATORY ASPECTS

Synovial fluid from osteoarthritis is transparent and of good viscosity, and contains less than 3000 white cells per mm^3. It may be present in copious amounts. Osteoarthritis produces no alterations in routine laboratory tests; abnormal findings demand an alternate explanation.

THERAPEUTIC PRINCIPLES

There is currently no pharmacologic intervention that interrupts, retards, or prevents the fundamental pathologic processes that occur in osteoarthritis. Until our understanding of the pathogenesis of osteoarthritis is more complete, the principles of treatment are to reduce physical stress on joints and minimize the impact that pain and limitation of joint motion have on the patient's quality of life. It would seem rational to treat any conditions associated with secondary osteoarthritis, but the effect of such treatment on the natural history of osteoarthritis remains conjectural. Reassurance, patient education, and counseling on vocational, social, and sexual matters are important in the overall management of the patient with osteoarthritis.

Pain is treated by analgesic anti-inflammatory agents and physical modalities such as hot paraffin hand soaks, vapor-coolant spray, heat, and transcutaneous nerve stimulation. Psychopharmacologic regimens may be required in cases of refractory pain, but the routine use of narcotic analgesics is to be avoided. There is no indication for systemically administered corticosteroids. Intra-articular steroids, however, may benefit flares of osteoarthritis, but excessive use of this modality can accelerate cartilage destruction.

Physical stress on joints is lessened by daytime rest periods and by weight reduction when necessary. Physical and occupational therapy help in the preservation of joint range of motion, in the protection of joints through muscle strengthening, and by instructing patients in more efficient ways to perform daily tasks. Walking aids, splints, self-help devices, and home modifications are also of value in maintaining a patient's independence.

Painful or dysfunctional joints that are refractory to nonoperative management may benefit from a surgical approach. Operative alternatives include debridement, osteotomy, replacement arthroplasty, and arthrodesis. Debridement or osteotomy are often preferable for limited or localized changes; replacement or arthrodesis are "end-of-the-road" procedures for patients disabled by more extensive joint destruction. When skillfully performed in properly selected cases, surgery can be an extremely beneficial modality in the overall management of osteoarthritis.

SELECTED REFERENCES

Ehlich GE: Inflammatory osteoarthritis. I. The clinical syndrome. J Chronic Dis 23:317, 1972

Hadler NM, Gillings DB, Imbus HR et al: Hand structure and function in an industrial setting. Arthritis Rheum 21:210, 1978

Howell DS, Woessner JF, Jimenez S et al: A view on the pathogenesis of osteoarthritis. Bull Rheum Dis 29:996, 1978–1979

Kellgren JH, Moore R: Generalized osteoarthritis and Heberden's nodes. Br Med J 1:181, 1952

McCarty DJ (ed): Arthritis and Allied Conditions, 9th ed, pp 1135–1189. Philadelphia, Lea & Febinger, 1979

Resnick D, Shapiro RF, Wiesner KB et al: Diffuse idiopathic skeletal hyperostosis (DISH) [Ankylosing Hyperostosis of Forestier and Rotes-Querol]. Semin Arthritis Rheum 7:153, 1978

Schwartz ER, Greenwald RA: Experimental models of osteoarthritis. Bull Rheum Dis 30:1030, 1979–1980

Chapter 20

Rheumatoid Arthritis and Other Chronic Inflammatory Arthritides

Philip L. Cohen

GOALS AND OBJECTIVES

Goals: To introduce the reader to the pathogenesis, pathology, clinical and laboratory features, and therapeutic principles of rheumatoid arthritis and other chronic inflammatory arthritides

Objectives: On completion of this unit and using the text as a standard reference, one should be able to evaluate, describe, list, or recognize the following:

1. The theories of the pathogenesis of rheumatoid arthritis
2. Immunologic and pathologic findings in rheumatoid arthritis and their relationship to the clinical and laboratory findings
3. The rationale for three general therapeutic approaches to the treatment of rheumatoid arthritis
4. General features of the spondyloarthropathies and related seronegative chronic arthritides

OUTLINE

I. Rheumatoid arthritis
   A. Epidemiology
   B. Pathogenesis
   C. Pathology
   D. Clinical aspects

E. Laboratory aspects
F. Roentgenographic aspects
G. Therapeutic principles

II. Spondyloarthropathies and related chronic seronegative arthritides
A. Ankylosing spondylitis
B. Reiter's syndrome
C. Psoriatic arthritis
D. Arthritis related to inflammatory bowel disease

This chapter will consider the common inflammatory polyarthritides of unknown etiology: rheumatoid arthritis, the spondyloarthropathies, and related chronic seronegative arthritides.

RHEUMATOID ARTHRITIS

Rheumatoid arthritis (RA) is a chronic polyarthritis with a relapsing–remitting course. It is usually symmetrical and associated with rheumatoid factor (see below), and there is evidence of systemic inflammation. Although predominantly a disease of joints, RA is a systemic disorder that may affect skin, blood vessels, eyes, pleura, lungs, peripheral nerves, and exocrine glands.

Epidemiology. RA is a common illness, affecting 1% to 3% of the adult population. There is a female predominance of about 3 to 1, and the disease occurs worldwide. The peak age of onset is between 35 and 45 years. The course of the illness is highly variable. In one large series of patients followed for 10 to 15 year periods, 50% to 70% were considered still able to work full time, and the incidence of crippling was only about 10%.

Pathogenesis. Although RA remains a disease of unknown cause, much recent evidence points to a combination of genetic and environmental factors in its etiology. It has been established that the HLA-D locus antigen Dw4 is significantly more common in RA patients than in the general population. This genetic marker, located in the putative immune response region of the human HLA complex, may render rheumatoid patients particularly susceptible to illness induced by an environmental agent or agents. Recent data indicate that patients with rheumatoid arthritis are more likely than normal individuals to have antibodies to antigens thought to be encoded for by Epstein-Barr (EB) virus, and that rheumatoid peripheral blood lymphocytes readily undergo transformation into EB virus-containing cells. These data form the basis of the argument that the EB virus plays a role in the pathogenesis of RA. Other appealing evidence comes from the study of animal models of polyarthritis. It is possible to induce a relapsing–remitting arthritis with features remarkably similar to rheumatoid arthritis by giving rodents bacterial cell wall products. The resulting illness may be due to the inflammatory reaction provoked by nondegradable and persistent bacterial residues. Other agents that have been proposed as the cause of rheumatoid arthritis include the mycoplasmas, the chlamydiae, and a host of other bacteria and viruses.

Whatever the initiating process, the immune system is involved in the rheumatoid inflammatory process. About 80% of rheumatoid patients have antibodies to the Fc region of IgG. This antibody, called rheumatoid factor, initially thought to be unique to rheumatoid arthritis, is now known to occur in the serum of some patients suffering from a variety of inflammatory diseases, such as subacute bacterial endocarditis, schistosomiasis, leprosy, osteomyelitis, and other chronic infections; it is also found in some patients with connective tissue diseases other than RA and occasionally in normal people, especially the aged. Nevertheless, the finding of rheumatoid factor is a useful diagnostic test for rheumatoid arthritis, and the titers in rheumatoid arthritis are usually much higher than those in other inflammatory illnesses. Although it is clear that the mere presence of this antibody in the serum does not cause disease, persuasive evidence indicates that rheumatoid factor, locally produced within the joint, can form immune complexes that then fix complement and effect a strong inflammatory response. Whether the action of immune complexes within joints is adequate to account for the destruction observed is uncertain. Although clinical laboratories measure IgM rheumatoid factor, other classes of rheumatoid factors have been described. It is generally believed that complexes of IgG rheumatoid factor with IgG can deposit in blood vessels and lead to vasculitis.

Pathology. In rheumatoid arthritis, the normally delicate synovial membrane becomes infiltrated with macrophages, lymphocytes, plasma cells, and granulocytes. Germinal centers are seen occasionally. The microscopic appearance of the rheumatoid synovium is not unique to RA; similar changes occur with other inflammatory arthritides. The rheumatoid nodule with its fibrinoid center, palisades of epitheloid cells, and mantle of lymphocytes usually distinguishes RA pathologically from other arthritides.

In severe disease, the rheumatoid synovial membrane undergoes gross hypertrophy and may erode articular cartilage and bone. These phenomena are probably mediated by lysosomal hydrolases released by granulocytes and macrophages. Progressive bone and cartilage damage and chronic swelling reduce the ability of joints to withstand the stresses of normal use, which leads to further destruction. Long-standing rheumatoid inflammation may lead to total loss of cartilage, joint deformation, and, eventually, fibrous or bony ankylosis.

Through similar inflammatory changes, tendons may become weakened or displaced, causing imbalance of the forces that maintain alignment of complex joint systems such as those in the hand, leading to malalignment and subluxation. Occasionally, outright tendon rupture occurs.

Clinical Aspects. Symmetrical polyarthralgias, morning stiffness, and fatigue are early symptoms that may progress to include limitation of motion owing to pain or joint destruction. There is little problem in diagnosis in the presence of rheumatoid nodules or typical deformities, but the diagnosis of RA may be subtle in early cases. Although RA may involve any synovial joint, there is a predilection for the wrists and hands. Longstanding joint and tendon inflammation gives rise to characteristic deformities such as ulnar deviation, and swan-neck and boutonnière deformities of the fingers. The American Rheumatism Association has established criteria for the diagnosis of rheumatoid arthritis, which are presented on p. 240.

Although RA is primarily a disease of joints, extraarticular manifestations may be prominent in some patients, notably those with high-titer rheumatoid factor. Specific organs may be involved in or affected by the rheumatoid inflammatory process: the heart (pericarditis, cardiomyopathy, and valvular incompetence caused by nodules); the lungs (pleurisy, parenchymal nodules, and interstitial fibrosis); the eyes (scleritis, and occasionally scleromalacia perforans); the nervous system (mononeuritis multiplex, and peripheral compression syndromes such as median neuropathy); the kidneys (amyloid deposition); and the hematopoietic system (anemia, Felty's syndrome, splenomegaly, and leukopenia). In addition, vasculitis associated with RA may give rise to skin lesions, leg ulcers, necrotizing arteritis of the viscera, digital infarctions, and fever. Sjögren's syndrome, or sicca syndrome, occurs in about 15% of RA patients and is due to infiltration of exocrine glands with lymphocytes. Although usually presenting as keratoconjunctivitis sicca and xerostomia, lymphoid infiltration of parenchymal organs may occur, and patients are greatly at risk for development of lymphoid malignancies.

Laboratory Aspects. The diagnosis of RA is greatly aided by the presence of rheumatoid factor, but its absence does not rule out the diagnosis, and its presence does not make the diagnosis certain. Active rheumatoid disease is frequently, but not always, accompanied by an elevated erythrocyte sedimentation rate. Most patients ultimately develop a normochromic, normocytic anemia, and a few may manifest antinuclear antibodies, usually of low titer.

Analysis of synovial fluid is extremely useful in distinguishing early RA from noninflammatory and infectious arthritides. The joint fluid from patients with RA is sterile, and has a pleocytosis (usually polymorphonuclear), increased protein, and decreased viscosity and complement.

Roentgenographic Aspects. Early changes in RA are limited to the soft tissues, and appear as fusiform swelling and joint effusion. Deossification, initially juxta-articular, may become more generalized as the disease progresses. Cartilage destruction produces narrowing of the joint. Erosion of bone occurs characteristically in the metaphyseal region underlying collateral ligament attachments. Malalignment, displacement, and ankylosis

American Rheumatism Association Diagnostic Criteria for Rheumatoid Arthritis

A. Classical rheumatoid arthritis (seven of the following criteria must be present and, for criteria 1-5, signs or symptoms must be continuous for at least 6 weeks)
   1. Morning stiffness
   2. Pain on motion, or tenderness in at least one joint*
   3. Swelling (soft tissue thickening or fluid, not bony overgrowth alone) in at least one joint*
   4. Swelling of at least one other joint* (any interval free of joint symptoms between the two joint involvements may not be longer than 3 months)
   5. Symmetrical joint swelling
   6. Subcutaneous nodules*
   7. Typical roentgenographic changes
   8. Presence of rheumatoid factor
   9. Poor mucin precipitate from synovial fluid
   10. Characteristic histologic changes in synovium
   11. Characteristic histologic changes in nodules

B. Definite rheumatoid arthritis (five of the above criteria required)

C. Probable rheumatoid arthritis (three of the above criteria required)

D. Possible rheumatoid arthritis (two of the following criteria are required, and total duration of joint symptoms must be at least 3 weeks)
   1. Morning stiffness
   2. Tenderness or pain on motion with a history of recurrence of persistence for 3 weeks*
   3. History or observation of joint swelling
   4. Subcutaneous nodules*
   5. Elevated sedimentation rate or C-reactive protein
   6. Iritis (pertinent only for juvenile rheumatoid arthritis)

E. Exclusions (any patient having any of the clinical findings below is excluded from the classification scheme)
   1. Typical rash of systemic lupus erythematosus
   2. High concentration of LE cells, or other clear-cut evidence of lupus
   3. Histologic evidence of periarteritis nodosa
   4. Clinical features of dermatomyositis, scleroderma, rheumatic fever, gouty arthritis, infectious arthritis, Reiter's syndrome, shoulder-hand syndrome, hypertrophic osteoarthropathy, neuroarthropathy, alkaptonuria, sarcoidosis, multiple myeloma, erythema nodosum, leukemia or lymphoma, or agammaglobulinemia

*Observed by a physician (condensed from official criteria in McCarty DA (ed): Arthritis. Philadelphia, Lea & Febiger, 1979)

of the joint mark end-stage rheumatoid disease (Fig. 20-1).

Therapeutic Principles. Anti-inflammatory agents, remittive agents (see below), corticosteroids, physical therapy, and reconstructive surgery comprise the medical approaches to therapy in RA.

Salicylates remain the most useful drugs in the treatment of RA. Since many patients do not tolerate the high doses required (5 g–6 g per day), the introduction of a variety of alternative nonsteroidal anti-inflammatory drugs has been welcomed. Use of these agents is largely empirical at present; there are large individual variations in patient responsiveness, and trial and error is often the only means of finding a suitable agent.

Gold, penicillamine, azathioprine, cyclophosphamide, and antimalarials are the only drugs that may favorably alter the natural history of RA, and are thus referred to as remittive agents. These agents are used in progressive or severe forms of RA; the serious associated side-effects must be weighed against any possible benefit. It is occasionally necessary to employ corticosteroids to alleviate intractable joint inflammation or vasculitis in RA; however, the use of steroids entails the risk of iatrogenic Cushing's syndrome and should be minimized. Intraarticular instillation of steroids is useful in the management of disease that is worst in a single joint; repeated injections increase the risk of articular cartilage damage from the catabolic effects of local steroids.

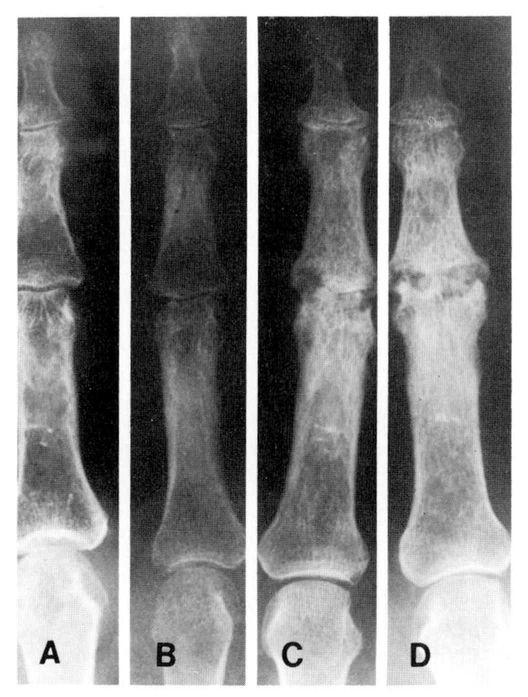

Fig. 20-1. Rheumatoid arthritis of the finger joints. (*A*) Symptoms present for 3 mo. There is diffuse osteoporosis, which is relatively greater near the joint surfaces. Small periarticular erosions are also present. (*B*) Symptoms present for 2 yr. The periarticular erosions are larger, especially at the proximal interphalangeal joint, and the cartilage space is thinned. (*C*) Symptoms present for 54 yr. The marginal erosions at the proximal interphalangeal joint are much larger and the cartilage space is markedly narrowed. (*D*) Symptoms present for 12 yr. The proximal interphalangeal joint is completely destroyed by the rheumatoid process.

Physical therapy to maintain strength and joint function is vital in RA. Its major goal is the preservation of joint motion and the prevention of deformity. During exacerbations, splinting may be briefly necessary for pain. Long-term splinting, especially of the wrists and hands, may prevent contracture and deformity.

Although there are many operative procedures that may be done for diseased or deformed joints, those that preserve or enhance motion are preferred in RA because of the tendency toward progressive loss of motion that occurs in this disease. In general, surgery should be considered for any rheumatoid patient persistently disabled by joint pain, deformity, or instability in spite of adequate nonoperative management. The procedures most frequently employed are synovectomy and joint replacement. To be most effective, synovectomy must be done before significant damage of the articular surfaces has occurred. It is of particular value in the knee and metacarpophalangeal joints, although the major benefit is pain relief rather than improved motion.

Joint replacement is carried out for end-stage disease and, like synovectomy, is most appreciated for its pain-relieving effect.

SPONDYLOARTHROPATHIES AND RELATED CHRONIC SERONEGATIVE ARTHRITIDES

Ankylosing spondylitis, Reiter's syndrome, and the spondylitis associated with psoriasis and inflammatory bowel disease constitute the spondyloarthropathies. These entities share a predilection for inflammation of the axial skeleton, absence of rheumatoid factor, and the tendency of inflamed areas to heal with fibroblastic proliferation followed by new bone formation. Most patients have the HLA-B27 phenotype. The pathogenesis of these disorders is unknown except for Reiter's syndrome, which is generally believed to result from an aberrant host response to a pathogenic microorganism.

Ankylosing spondylitis is an illness of young to middle-aged men that is characterized by the insidious onset of pain and stiffness in the lower back associated with gradual loss of spinal mobility. Not infrequently, frank inflammatory arthritis of large joints such as the hip occurs; the illness may also cause inflammation in the uveal tract of the eye and in the intima of the aorta. The disorder has a tendency to progress slowly, with diminished mobility of the spine and sacroiliac joints.

Reiter's syndrome is characterized by arthritis of large joints (particularly knees and ankles), uveitis, skin lesions, and urethritis. In a variety of this illness seen more commonly in Europe, there is diarrhea instead of urethritis, and *Shigella*, *Yersinia*, and *Salmonella* have been indirectly implicated in its pathogenesis. There is a tendency toward exuberant periostitis, particularly in the heel. Although some patients have only one episode of this illness, the majority of patients have recurrent attacks, and some develop ankylosing spondylitis.

A small percentage of patients with psoriasis develop arthritis. Most commonly, this is an asymmetrical oligoarthritis, which occasionally is quite destructive. Some patients, however, develop a unique inflammatory arthritis involving the distal interphalangeal joints. Another small group develops a spondylitis that does not differ greatly from ankylosing spondylitis, and which is associated with the HLA-B27 antigen. Activity of skin lesions is thought to correlate with activity of peripheral, but not axial, arthritis.

Inflammatory bowel disease is associated with a peripheral arthritis, which reflects the activity of the bowel disease and is frequently associated with erythema nodosum. Some patients also develop a spondylitis whose activity is independent of the bowel disease. Most of these patients are HLA-B27 positive.

SELECTED REFERENCES

McCarty DA (ed) Arthritis. Philadelphia, Lea & Febiger, 1979

Paget SA, Gibofsky A: Immunopathogenesis of rheumatoid arthritis. Am J Med 67:961, 1979

Ragan CA, Farrington E: The clinical features of rheumatoid arthritis. JAMA 181:663, 1962

Chapter 21

Crystal-Induced Arthritis

Gary E. Ragan and John B. Winfield

GOALS AND OBJECTIVES

Goals: To acquaint the reader with the pathophysiology and clinical manifestations of crystal-induced arthritis and to provide an understanding of the bases for various modes of therapy

Objectives: On completion of this unit, one should be able to describe, list, or recognize the

1. Clinical forms of gout and pseudogout
2. Processes of crystal deposition, displacement, phagocytosis, and clearance from the articular region
3. Pathophysiology of crystal-induced inflammation
4. Rationale and indications for pharmacologic intervention in terms of biochemical and metabolic considerations

OUTLINE

I. Articular crystals
II. Gout
  A. Clinical perspectives
  B. Diagnosis
  C. Hyperuricemia
  D. Pathophysiology
  E. Therapeutic principles
III. Pseudogout
  A. Clinical perspectives
  B. Pathophysiology
  C. Therapeutic principles
IV. Other crystals

ARTICULAR CRYSTALS

Although crystal-induced arthritides have been distinguished as separate clinical entities for several decades, only recently have they been defined pathophysiologically. The paradigm, and historically most notable, of these is gout, an acute, intermittent arthritis secondary to monosodium urate (MSU) crystal-induced inflammation. However, it is now recognized that other crystals may nearly as often play an important role in rheumatic complaints, disability, and medical economics.

Crystalline species that have been implicated as a cause of arthritis include MSU, calcium pyrophosphate dihydrate (CPPD), apatite, and, ironically, the crystalline corticosteroid ester preparations that are injected intraarticularly to inhibit inflammation. Other crystalline species of less clear clinical relevance that are found in synovial fluids include cholesterol, cysteine, various calcium salts, and crystallizing immunoglobulin, which is found in a rare type of systemic gammopathy. Although the pathophysiology of crystal-induced inflammation and subsequent joint complaints is believed to be similar regardless of the species of crystal, a number of morphologically similar crystalline substances have been injected into animal joints without precipitating inflammation.

Crystal-induced arthritides may be primary without definable metabolic abnormality or familial tendency. They also occur with greater than chance frequency in the setting of other diseases that may be relatively asymptomatic. For this reason, physicians must always "look beyond" the painful joint and consider the possibility of associated diseases or extraarticular manifestations of the crystal-induced disease.

GOUT

Clinical Perspectives. The classic caricature of the glutton with his grog-blossom face from alcohol abuse and exquisitely painful, carefully wrapped great toe stricken by gout certainly still exists. However, the modern-day presentation of gout is changing dramatically. Once rarely seen in females and certain ethnic groups, gout now occurs in all members of modern society. Although basically a severe monoarticular arthritis lasting for days to weeks, polyarticular arthritis without podagra (gout of the first metatarsophalangeal joint) is not rare and can closely mimic other forms of arthritis.

Attacks of gout usually begin between the ages of 30 and 50. Patients may complain of very mild attacks developing without provocation that abate without specific treatment. In certain instances, patients may be misdiagnosed because of low-grade, persistent, polyarticular involvement suggesting rheumatoid arthritis or related disorders.

At the present time, it is estimated that approximately a half million patients have gout in the United States. Following the first attack, two thirds of these patients will develop a second attack within 1 year; within 2 years, three fourths will suffer a second attack. One tenth of these patients will not have a second attack for the following 10 years. Following the first few episodes, however, recurrences are more frequent.

The term *gout* refers to articular disease or MSU deposits (tophi) in soft tissues. Nephrolithiasis is the major extraarticular manifestation. Only a small minority of patients with gout develop obvious tophi, but many ultimately develop renal stones. Pure uric acid stones are found 80% of the time, and uric acid is probably the nidus for calcium phosphate and oxalate calculi in the remainder. In about half the patients with gout, symptoms from renal stones actually precede the arthritis. Common chronic diseases associated with gout include alcoholism, obesity, hypertension, coronary artery disease, and hypertriglyceridemia. On the average, a family history of gout can be obtained in less than half the patients.

Diagnosis. The diagnosis of gout is made by observing (with plane polarized light microscopy) negatively birefringent, needle-shaped MSU crystals engulfed by polymorphonuclear leukocytes (PMNs) in a synovial fluid aspirate. The diagnosis is particularly firm when many crystals are found in a single PMN, an almost invariable finding during the first few days of an attack. It should be remembered that extracellular crystals frequently persist in the synovial fluid for many years following an attack of acute gouty arthritis. A less satisfactory diagnosis can be made on the basis of a typical clinical picture with a compatible history, or on the basis of response to a standard therapeutic regimen. With rapid destruction of a gouty joint (e.g., by intraarticular infection), crystalline deposits may be released into the synovial fluid, leading to diagnostic confusion.

Laboratory studies may also be a source of confusion. An elevated serum uric acid level is not in itself diagnostic of gout and should not play a pivotal role in the differential diagnosis. Leukocytosis, with a shift in the differential to more immature PMNs, an elevated erythrocyte sedimentation rate, and the presence of serum acute phase reactants (*i.e.*, laboratory correlates of infectious arthritis) may all be present in acute gout. Although the degree of inflammation may be impressive, with synovial fluid leukocyte counts approaching those seen in septic arthritis, the viscosity of the synovial fluid is characteristically less that that encountered in pyogenic or chronic inflammatory arthritides.

Hyperuricemia. In most animals, urate is an intermediate metabolite catabolized by uricase in the elimination of excess nucleic acid purines and nitrogenous waste products through production and excretion of allantoic acid. Man lacks the enzyme uricase, and uric acid is the end product requiring excretion. Gout is, therefore, exclusively a disease of man. The metabolic pathways leading to the production of uric acid are shown in Figure 21-1.

Dietary sources contribute partially to urate production, but endogenous overproduction is more important in the pathogenesis of hyperuricemia in gout. Precursors are committed to inosinic acid formation at the rate-limiting reaction between phosphoribosyl pyrophosphate (PRPP) and glutamine, predominantly in the liver. This is an important step; however, increased availability of PRPP and glutamine, and increased activity of the controlling enzyme, PRPP amidotransferase, have all been implicated in urate overproduction. Activity of this enzyme is under negative feedback modulation by purine nucleosides, an aspect of *de novo* synthesis discussed later.

Another important feature of purine biosynthesis is the salvage of purine bases that would otherwise be converted to urate and lost for nucleic acid synthesis in nonhepatic tissue. In these cells, hypoxanthine and guanine are "salvaged" by the enzyme hypoxanthine–guanine–phosphoribosyl transferase (HGPRTase). Decreased or absent activity of HGPRTase, seen in the Lesch-Nyhan syndrome and in certain relatives of patients with this disease, leads to markedly increased *de novo* urate production, probably because of the known overabundance of the PRPP not used in salvaging purine bases.

The biochemical hallmark of gout is hyperuricemia. In the steady state, the serum urate level reflects the balance between input from endogenous urate production and diet, and output from intestinal disposal, re-

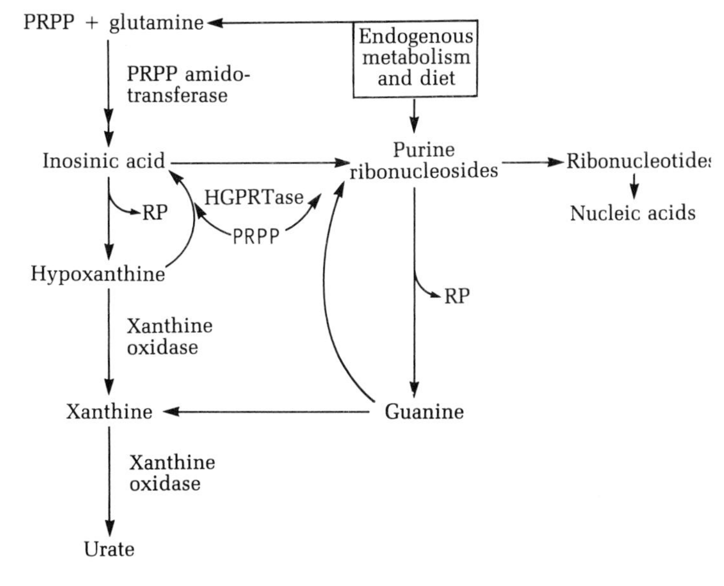

Fig. 21-1. The pathway for urate and purine ribonucleoside (adenine and guanosine) production. Phosphoribosyl pyrophosphate (PRPP) receives an amido group from glutamine at the rate-limiting and irreversible first step toward *de novo* synthesis of the basic purine ring structure. Inosinic acid may then either lose the ribose–phosphate moeity and become oxidized to urate or may be made available for nucleic acid synthesis. Hypoxanthine–guanine–phosphoribosyl transferase (HGPRTase) "salvages" the ring structures for economy of nucleic acid synthesis in nonhepatic tissue by catalyzing the return of the ribosyl phosphate group.

nal excretion, and soft tissue absorption. It is helpful to classify the causes of hyperuricemia as *primary* (an idiopathic or inborn error of metabolism leading only to hyperuricemia) and *secondary* (an acquired or inborn error of metabolism leading to a spectrum of diseases, one of which is gout). For an individual patient with gout, multiple factors probably interact to determine the severity of the disease.

More than 95% of the total number of patients with gout have primary hyperuricemia. These patients exhibit overproduction of endogenous urate regardless of dietary intake, but, in the majority, the exact biochemical defect is unknown. Specific enzyme deficiences have been identified in only a few patients. Patients with primary gout also have a defect in renal handling of urate, since as a group they excrete 40% less urate in the urine for any given level of serum urate. For a patient with gout to eliminate the same amount of urate through the kidneys as a normal person, the serum urate must be, on the average, almost 2 mg/dl higher. Only 20% of patients with primary gout actually excrete more urate than do age-matched controls. In the remainder, urinary excretion is in the normal range or actually decreased, despite hyperuricemia.

In normal persons, roughly 0.5 g per day of urate is produced, most of which is eliminated in the urine. The total body burden (miscible pool) for these persons at any given time averages 1 g. In patients with gout without tophi, this pool may expand to 4 g because of the chronic net retention of urate. In patients with advanced gout and tophus formation, the miscible pool may be expanded 15 to 30 times normal, or even higher, because the crystalline urate deposits deep within tophi, containing as much as one kg of urate, do not participate in daily metabolism.

A small number of patients with gout have underlying secondary hyperuricemia. Acquired chronic problems that may tip the body balance of urate toward soft tissue MSU deposition and arthritis include increased nucleic acid turnover (especially myeloproliferative diseases), certain inborn errors of metabolism (Lesch-Nyhan syndrome and von Gierke's disease), and acquired renal disease leading to underexcretion of uric acid. A frequently encountered clinical entity in the southeastern United States is lead nephropathy in "moonshine" drinkers (saturnine gout).

In the kidney, urate is filtered initially by the glomerulus. Excretion can be reduced by simple reduction of renal mass or blood flow. After filtration, urate is reabsorbed by active transport along the tubule, especially in the proximal portion. Urate also is secreted at various sites in the tubule. Competition for these sites by similar molecules may lead to hyperuricemia, as occurs in metabolic acidosis (lactate), ketosis (ketogenic acids), and certain drugs (salicylate).

Pathophysiology. Most researchers agree that the earliest pathologic finding in the natural history of gouty arthritis is the deposition of MSU crystals in synovial and periarticular tissue rather than their formation by precipitation in synovial fluid, although this event may occur as well. Such deposits (microtophi) are found routinely in pathologic specimens of gouty joints. Factors related to microtophus formation may include the reduced solubility of MSU at the periphery of the body because of lower temperatures; recurrent trauma (house painters may develop tophi where their anterior shins rub against the rungs of a ladder); differential ultrafiltration of urate and water from the pressure of weight bearing (the MTP joint is said to incur the highest force per unit area of any joint); and genetic or age-induced alterations in the binding affinity of urate to glycoproteins in the connective tissue matrix.

As deposits form, the crystals are partially displaced, degraded, or removed regularly. If crystals are freed into the joint space sufficiently rapidly by any of a variety of physical or metabolic changes (e.g., trauma, microfractures, enzymatic "strip-mining," tissue necrosis, and rapid dissolution of tophi as a result of drug therapy), inflammatory arthritis ensues. Intraarticular injections of pure MSU crystals induce an identical arthritis in humans. Why most acute attacks end spontaneously after several days is still conjectural, but it is presumably related to the reduction of synovial fluid crystal population by the inflammatory response itself.

Urate crystals have many interesting properties that are thought to be related to their ability to promote inflammation (Fig. 21-2). Through electrostatic interactions, various proteins found in synovial fluids adsorb to the surface of MSU crystals. IgG is bound in such a way that the Fc portion is available to PMN surface Fc-receptors, promoting adherence and phagocytosis. Hageman factor, C1, C3, and C4 can also be directly bound and activated, amplifying the inflammatory response. Whether other synovial proteins play assisting or inhibiting roles is unknown.

During acute attacks, MSU crystals are often several times longer than the PMN and are sharp-ended, raising the possibility of incomplete phagocytosis and membrane rupture, allowing lysosomal contents to be regurgitated and cellular contents to be liberated. Fully phagocytosed MSU crystals are membranolytic to phagolysosomes, leading to elevated synovial fluid levels of lysozyme and cytoplasmic PMN components during attacks of gout.

A glycopeptide with a molecular weight of 8400 daltons, termed crystal chemotactic factor, is released from PMNs on exposure to MSU crystals. This substance attracts other PMNs into the synovial fluid from the circulation prior to inflammatory vasodilation, with resultant intense PMN infiltrations.

Therapeutic Principles. Therapy of gout is based upon several of the well-defined pathophysiologic abnormalities in this disorder. There are two primary goals: (1) to abort or prevent the acute attack; (2) to decrease the miscible pool of urate either by increasing excretion or decreasing production.

The phlogistic response to MSU crystals can be interrupted with joint rest, application of cold packs (hot packs routinely worsen attacks), anti-inflammatory drugs, or administration of colchicine. The mechanism of colchicine action in gout has only recently been elucidated. Colchicine inhibits PMN microtubular function and migration, but only at toxic concentrations, and it is a very weak antiinflammatory agent. A more important action may be inhibition of MSU-induced chemotactic factor release by PMNs. Colchicine may have other effects as well, including reduction of the level of the connective tissue matrix substance, uronic acid, which is elevated in the serum of patients with gout but not in those with hyperuricemia alone. In addition to the treatment of acute gout, prophylactic administration of low doses of colchicine is effective in reducing the frequency of multiple attacks.

For patients who continue to have frequent attacks, tophi at a relatively young age, renal stones of any type, extreme hyperuricemia, or a strong family history of gout, efforts to reduce the expanded miscible pool

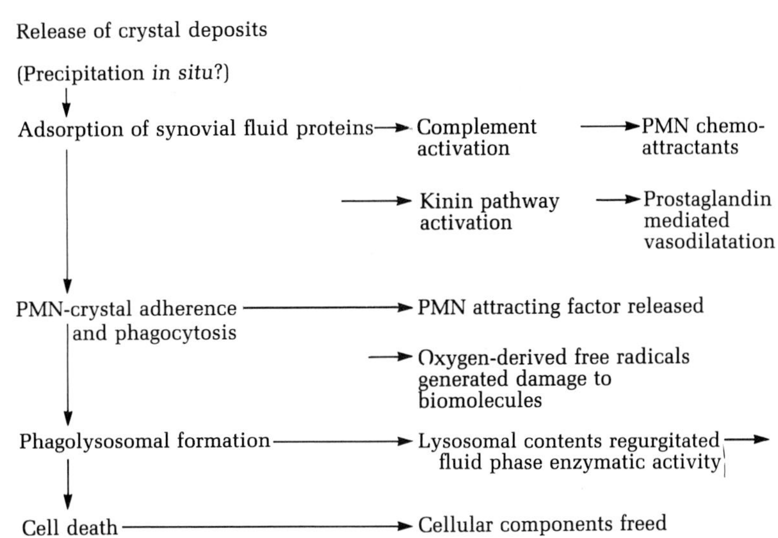

Fig. 21-2. The proposed sequence of events in crystal-induced arthritis is shown in the left hand column proceeding from crystal release into synovial fluid to PMN cell death. The phlogistic consequences of these steps are shown on the right, including enhanced PMN migration into joint fluid and periarticular vasodilatation with subsequent signs of inflammatory arthritis. This model accounts for the synovial fluid findings during acute attacks of low hemolytic complement levels and elevated levels in the fluid of PMN lysosomal and cellular enzymes.

of urate usually are required. For patients with relatively normal urinary urate excretion, uricosuric agents (e.g., probenecid) are used and do not appear to increase a patient's risk of stone formation. These drugs block renal tubular resorption of uric acid, thus increasing net excretion. For patients with a history of renal stones or elevated urinary urate excretion rates, uricosurics may promote nephrolithiasis and are contraindicated unless measures are taken to promote uric acid solubility in the urine.

Originally synthesized for use as a purine antimetabolite for cancer chemotherapy, allopurinol may be administered on a long-term basis to patients with gout to block purine degradation. Allopurinol and its metabolite, oxypurinol, are converted *in vivo* to purine ribonucleoside analogs; they slow *de novo* synthesis of purines by feedback inhibition at the initial rate-limiting step of synthesis governed by the enzyme PRPP-amidotransferase. Allopurinol and oxypurinol also effectively block the enzyme xanthine oxidase.

Allopurinol is not a uricosuric agent *per se*. However, with inhibition of xanthine oxidase, there is a net increase in blood levels of xanthine and hypoxanthine. These compounds are highly soluble in urine and are cleared rapidly by the kidney, so that plasma solubility limits are not approached. Rare cases of renal stones containing urate precursors or oxypurinol have been described, as have asymptomatic noninflammatory deposits in muscles of patients on long-term allopurinol therapy.

For all patients with gout, regardless of whether it is primary or secondary, it is of value to remove factors that commonly precipitate attacks (e.g., an alcoholic debauch). The common advice to moderate dietary purine and caloric intake is probably of little value in the treatment of gout *per se*, but may do wonders for the associated obesity and hypertension.

PSEUDOGOUT

Clinical Perspectives. Pseudogout is the term used to describe the acute arthritis caused by CPPD crystal-induced inflammation. Indeed, this disease, which brings at least half as many patients to physicians as does gout, may perfectly mimic gout during an acute flare. As in gout, both sexes may be affected but with a much closer male to female ratio. Ethnic and familial predilections have been described in addition to the more common idiopathic cases. Although gout usually begins to be symptomatic before age 50, pseudogout attacks occurring before age 50 are uncommon and should alert the physician to look for an associated disease such as hyperparathyroidism, hypothyroidism, hemachromatosis, ochronosis, and even gout. The clinical course is quite variable; certain patients have only an occasional, self-limited attack, whereas others rapidly develop progressive joint destruction. Typically, however, pseudogout masquerades as an attack of gout that is milder and that takes somewhat longer to develop its intensity.

As in gout, the diagnosis of pseudogout is made by polarizing light microscopy of synovial fluid. Crystals may be more difficult to detect than MSU crystals because of their smaller size, more typical intraphagolysosomal location, lower population, and less brilliant colors. In contrast to MSU crystals, CPPD crystals show weak positive birefringency and have squared ends.

The same caveat regarding diagnostic confusion issued for gout applies to pseudogout. Calcium pyrophosphate crystals may exist in joint fluid asymptomatically or as a result of processes that disrupt deposition sites. Polyarticular attacks may exhibit fever and laboratory evidence of a systemic inflammatory response suggesting infection.

Pathophysiology. The earliest event in the natural history of pseudogout appears to be an alteration in the integrity of joint cartilage, identified by changes in histochemical staining characteristics. Crystalline formation follows because of poorly defined interactions with constituents of the altered cartilaginous matrix. Deposits do not grow sufficiently large to be detected by physical examination but, if extensive, may be seen as linear or punctate radiodensities in the articular cartilage, or, less commonly, in the cartilage of tendons and ligaments (chondrocalcinosis).

Trafficking of CPPD crystals through the joint space occurs as in gout. Attacks of experimental pseudogout can be produced by intraarticular instillation of purified crystals or, in joints known to have CPPD deposits, by lavage with fluids (saline, magnesium solutions, buffered EDTA) that dissolve these crystals. The latter procedure was once suggested as a therapeutic maneuver on the erroneous assumption that crystals formed *in situ* during an attack. This approach was quickly abandoned because attacks were routinely exacerbated.

CPPD crystals bind synovial fluid proteins and interact with PMNs in a fashion similar to MSU crystals. *In vitro* experiments indicate that CPPD crystals are less potent than MSU in evoking an inflammatory response, a finding that coincides with the generally milder clinical characteristics of pseudogout.

Therapeutic Principles. Therapy for pseudogout is directed at minimizing inflammation and discomfort during the acute episode. The usual therapeutic modalities include placing the affected joint at rest, administration of a nonsteroidal anti-inflammatory agent (e.g., indomethacin), and joint aspiration. Colchicine does not generally induce the rapid reduction of acute inflammation seen in pseudogout. To date, there is no agent available to mobilize CPPD deposits. Correction of an associated metabolic disturbance does not necessarily reverse the arthritis, presumably because the cartilaginous changes are irreversible.

OTHER CRYSTALS

Monoarticular arthritis, bursitis, and periarthritis syndromes associated with calcium deposits are common clinical problems for which crystal-induced inflammation seems likely. Through the use of transmission and scanning electron microscopy, electron probes, and x-ray diffraction analysis, other calcium-containing crystals have been identified in inflamed joints and bursal fluids, and have been found deposited as tophus-like structures in periarticular regions.

Crystals of apatite, the principal mineral of normal bone, are too small to be seen by routine light microscopy, and no routinely available chemical assay for their presence in synovial fluid exists. Clumps of these crystals may be inferred by special stains using the light microscope, or they can be seen in PMNs directly with the electron microscope. Purified crystals produce inflammation when injected into a joint. A presumptive diagnosis may be made on the finding of a gout-like clinical pattern, periarticular calcium on the roentgenogram, absence of other causes of acute arthritis, and observation of purple, rounded inclusions in PMNs. Apatite crystal arthritis may be more common than is generally appreciated.

The fourth crystal species known to produce an inflammatory synovitis is the iatrogenically introduced corticosteroid ester. Although infrequent and only mildly symptomatic, the post-injection flare of arthritis occurs within hours after the injection and subsides within a few days, although crystals of steroid esters may be found in joint fluid for several months following injection. In contrast, infection introduced by needle insertion does not become symptomatic until days later and does not abate without prompt treatment.

Cholesterol crystals do not induce inflammation but are encountered occasionally under polarizing light as platelike structures noted during a search for other crystals. Cholesterol crystals usually occur in the setting of a chronic and intense synovitis, for example, that of rheumatoid arthritis, and have no clinical significance.

SELECTED REFERENCES

McCarty D (ed): Arthritis and Allied Conditions, 9th ed. Philadelphia, Lea & Febiger, 1979

Proceedings of the second conference on gout and purine metabolism. Arthritis Rheum 18 (6: suppl), 1975

Proceedings of the Conference on Pseudogout and Pyrophosphate Metabolism. Arthritis Rheum 19 (3: supplement), 1976

Wallace S: The treatment of gout. Arthritis Rheum 15:317, 1972

Chapter 22

Musculoskeletal Complications of Hemophilia

Walter B. Greene and R. Beverly Raney

GOALS AND OBJECTIVES

Goals: To introduce the reader to the principles of diagnosis and treatment of the musculoskeletal complications of hemophilia

Objectives: On completion of this unit, and using the text as a standard reference, one should be able to list or describe the

1. Mode of inheritance and the clotting factor that is deficient in each of the two hemophilioid disorders responsible for most damage to joints and other structures of the musculoskeletal system
2. Gross and histologic changes produced in synovium, cartilage, and bone by repeated intraarticular bleeding
3. Symptoms and signs seen in acute, subacute, and chronic hemarthropathy
4. Extraarticular manifestations of hemophilia on the musculoskeletal system
5. Principles of management of acute, subacute, and chronic hemarthropathy

OUTLINE

I. The hemophilioid disorders: hemophilia A and B
   A. Diagnosis
   B. Treatment
II. Hemophilic arthropathy
   A. Pathologic changes
   B. Clinical stages
      1. Acute hemarthrosis
      2. Subacute hemarthropathy
      3. Chronic hemarthropathy
III. Extraarticular lesions

THE HEMOPHILIOID DISORDERS: HEMOPHILIA A AND B

Hereditary defects of coagulation, commonly referred to as hemophilia, may cause musculoskeletal problems associated with spontaneous or easily elicited hemorrhage into muscles or joints. Repeated intraarticular bleeding may cause joint destruction, and the cumulative result may be more catastrophic for the affected person than the deformities and disabilities produced by septic or rheumatoid arthritis. To prevent or minimize the musculoskeletal deformities caused by these diseases, the physician must be knowledgeable of their causes, their pathologic and clinical manifestations, and their treatment.

Although any abnormality of molecular structure or deficiency in the coagulation cascade (Fig. 22-1) may cause a clotting defect, most musculoskeletal problems result from a deficiency of either factor VIII or factor IX. The other coagulation defects are associated with easy bruising, epistaxis, menorrhagia, gingival bleeding, and other hemorrhagic problems, but unless the affected persons sustain significant trauma or undergo surgery, their limbs and joints are frequently spared.

Classical hemophilia (hemophilia A) results from a physiologic deficiency of factor VIII clotting activity. The inheritance pattern is sex-linked recessive, and although female carriers may have abnormal coagulation studies or even a mild bleeding diathesis, only affected males generally demonstrate bleeding problems. An affected male will have normal sons and daughters who are carriers. Therefore, the clinical problems with bleeding will skip generations.

The severity of hemophilia A depends upon the level of factor VIII clotting activity. *A severely affected patient* has a factor VIII activity level of less than 1% and characteristically bleeds into joints or muscles spontaneously or with minimal trauma. *Moderately involved patients* have between 1% and 5% factor VIII activity; in this group, spontaneous hemorrhage is infrequent, but joint or muscle bleeds may occur with minor

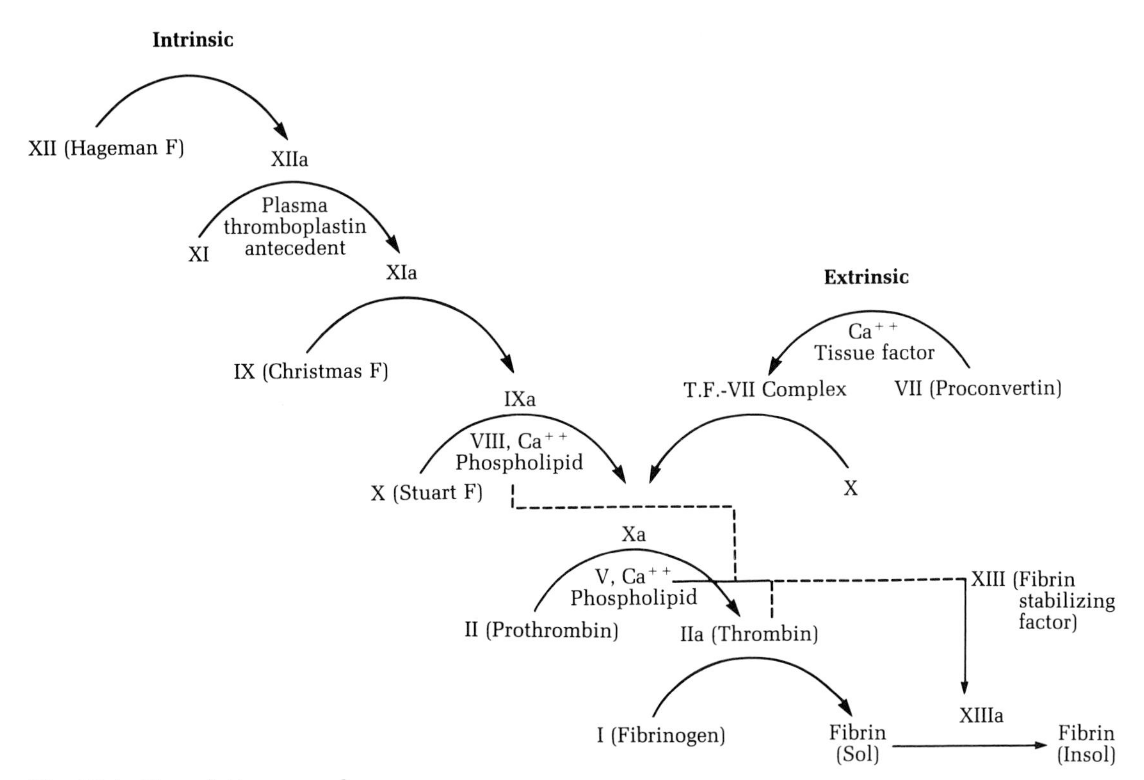

Fig. 22-1. Coagulation cascade.

trauma. *Mildly affected patients* have more than 5% factor VIII levels and usually bleed only with more severe trauma or during surgery.

Present evidence indicates that hemophilia A is not caused by an absence or absolute deficiency of factor VIII, but results from an abnormal molecule making up part of the VIII clotting factor. In support of this theory, most hemophilia A patients have normal or increased amounts of factor VIII antigen. In approximately 15% of classical hemophiliacs, antibodies to the factor VIII antigen develop; these patients are said to have an inhibitor to the usual replacement therapy. They are refractory to the usual therapy, treatment of their hemorrhagic episodes is sharply limited, and reconstructive surgery is contraindicated.

Hemophilia B, or Christmas disease, results from a deficiency of clotting factor IX. Although not as common as hemophilia A, factor IX deficiency is similar in that both diseases have sex-linked recessive inheritance, vary from mild to severe, frequently exhibit spontaneous muscle or joint hemorrhages, and commonly produce crippling arthritides.

Diagnosis. Before effective therapy can be instituted, the cause of the clotting abnormality must be elucidated. A detailed family history is important, but in 25% of hemophilia A patients the disease is the result of a new mutation. The diagnosis of hemophilia A is confirmed by an abnormal partial thromboplastin time, a normal bleeding time, and, most importantly, by a low level of factor VIII activity. Von Willebrand's disease, which infrequently causes musculoskeletal problems, may also exhibit low levels of factor VIII activity. Von Willebrand's disease is differentiated by its autosomal dominant transmission, long bleeding time, decreased factor VIII antigen level, and decrease in ristocetin-induced platelet aggregation. The diagnosis of hemophilia B is confirmed by an abnormal partial thromboplastin time and a low factor IX activity.

Treatment. Appropriate replacement of the missing clotting factor remains the *sine qua non* for treatment of any hemorrhage in the hemophilic patient. Prior to the development of concentrated replacement products, large volumes of plasma infusion were necessary to effect hemostasis. Such large infusions were commonly associated with circulatory overload and, in essence, precluded any reconstructive surgery. Although replacement therapy may still be complicated by hemolytic anemia, hepatitis, or allergic reactions, the use of clotting factor concentrates has greatly enhanced the treatment of patients with clotting deficiencies. Hemorrhagic episodes can now be treated without volume overload problems, and elective surgery can be undertaken to alleviate the deformity and pain of disabling arthropathy. Moreover, many hemorrhages can now be treated with infusions given at home by the patient or his parents; thus, bleeding can be controlled earlier, the incidence of major hemorrhagic emergencies can be reduced, and the patient can lead a more normal life.

HEMOPHILIC ARTHROPATHY

Hemophilia is most crippling when repeated bleeding into a joint produces arthritis. Prior to the development of adequate replacement therapy, most severe hemophiliacs suffered destruction of one or more joints by early adolescence. Even with the use of today's home therapy, disabling arthritis is a frequent occurrence. By far the most commonly affected joint is the knee, followed in frequency by the elbow, ankle, shoulder, hip, and wrist.

Pathologic Changes

After a joint bleed, or hemarthrosis, the synovium must absorb the degradation products of the blood. Repeated hemarthroses, particularly when they occur within a short time span, cause synovial hypertrophy and inflammation. Some hemophiliacs develop florid synovial hypertrophy after only two or three joint bleeds, whereas others seem to be more resistant and require more hemarthroses to develop significant synovial changes. This individual variation in the development of synovitis has led some authors to suggest that, in hemophilic arthropathy, an autoimmune mechanism may be involved with antigen–antibody formation induced by a product of red cell breakdown.

Early hemophilic arthropathy is characterized by synovial hypertrophy; its pathologic picture is similar to that of rheumatoid arthritis. The synovium shows marked vascular hyperplasia, hemosiderin deposits, infiltration by chronic inflammatory cells (lymphocytes, plasma cells, and giant cells), and the gradual development of fibrous tissue. Hemosiderin-stained pannus begins to creep over the joint surfaces. Constant oozing of blood from the highly vascular and friable synovium tends to perpetuate the synovial inflammation. The hypertrophied synovium also produces large quantities of hydrolytic enzymes that not only sustain the inflammatory state but also promote fibrillation and subsequent erosion of the articular cartilage.

The later stages of hemophilic arthropathy include degenerative changes somewhat similar to those seen in osteoarthritis. Thinning and erosion of the articular cartilage are, in large part, caused by the altered configuration and mechanics of the joint. Progressive fibrosis of the synovium may contribute to joint contracture and restriction of joint motion.

Clinical Stages

Hemophilic arthropathy usually manifests itself in one of three typical forms: acute hemarthrosis, subacute hemarthropathy, and chronic hemarthropathy.

Acute Hemarthrosis. In acute hemarthrosis, pain is the early and predominant symptom. Caused by the effusion and synovitis, an aura of pain may be perceived by the patient even before the clinical signs of hemarthrosis appear. The physical signs are swelling, tenderness, fluctuation, increased local heat, and impaired mobility. An acute hemarthrosis may, of course, occur in joints affected by subacute or chronic hemarthropathy.

Treatment of an acute hemarthrosis consists of replacement of the missing clotting factor to approximately 40% of normal levels. Adjunctive therapy, such as compressive dressings, immobilization by splints, elevation, and joint aspiration, is frequently useful to decrease pain and reduce the incidence of recurrent bleeds. After 1 to 2 days of protecting the joint, range of motion and strengthening exercises can begin.

Subacute Hemarthropathy. The patient with subacute hemarthropathy has synovial hypertrophy and frequent bleeds in the affected joint. Destruction of the joint, atrophy of the surrounding muscles, and joint contractures frequently begin during the subacute stage. Roentgenographic changes include osteopenia of the epiphyses associated with synovial hyperemia, squaring of the epiphyses, widening of the intercondylar femoral notch, and early cystic changes in subchondral bone (Fig. 22-2). To diminish the synovial hypertrophy and stop progressive joint destruction, treatment for this stage is designed to reduce the frequency of hemorrhage and to correct contractures and muscle atrophy. If such measures are unsuccessful, surgical removal of the synovium may be helpful.

Chronic Hemarthropathy. Continued progression of hemarthropathy leads to further degenerative changes. As the articular cartilage becomes fibrillated and eroded, the pa-

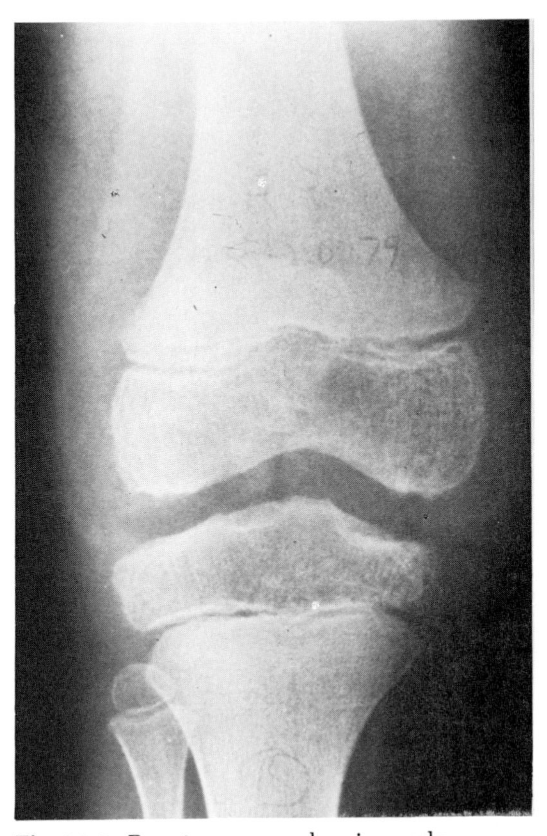

Fig. 22-2. Roentgenogram showing early changes of hemophilic arthropathy with osteopenia, widening of intercondylar notch, and minimal erosive and cystic changes.

tient develops more pain, restricted motion, and deterioration of function. Posterior subluxation of the tibia is frequently associated with chronic hemarthropathy of the knee. Roentgenographic changes include irregular articular surfaces, narrowing of the cartilage space, osteophytes, and subchondral cysts. (Fig. 22-3).

Objectives in the orthopaedic treatment of chronic hemophilic arthritis are correction of deformity, maintenance of such correction, improving motion, and restoration of weakened muscles to normal strength. Often useful for these purposes are selected exercise programs, traction, casts, braces, and operative procedures. The details of treatment must always be suited to the needs of the individual patient. For example, the flexed, weak knee of hemophilic arthritis can often be straightened and strengthened by nonoperative means with marked improvement in the patient's ability to stand and to walk. For the adult patient with severe arthropathy, surgical replacement of the joint or other reconstructive procedures have been helpful in alleviating pain and improving function.

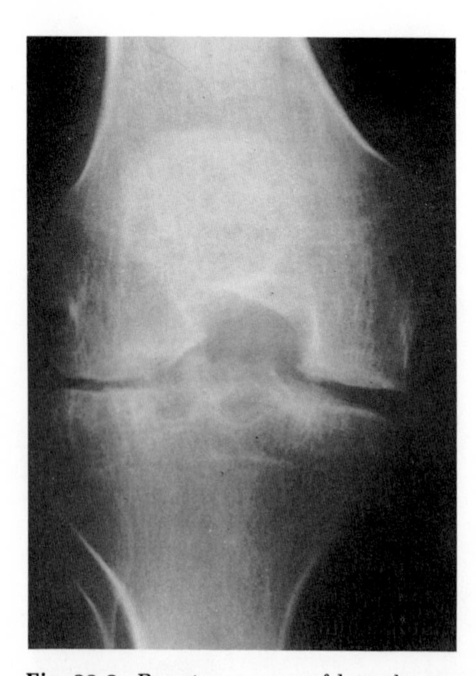

Fig. 22-3. Roentgenogram of late changes of hemophilic arthropathy with narrowing of cartilage space, more advanced cystic changes in the subchondral bone, squaring of epiphyses, and small osteophytes.

EXTRAARTICULAR LESIONS

Extraarticular bleeding may affect muscles, nerves, blood vessels, and even bones. Commonly, it interferes with local physiologic processes by the pressure, tension, and ischemia created by a slowly expanding hematoma.

Intramuscular hematomas that fail to resorb quickly or completely lead to fibrosis and contracture, cyst formation, or myositis ossificans. Bleeding into muscle areas occurs most commonly in the calf, where it may cause severe equinus deformity. Bleeding into the sheath of the iliacus muscle frequently causes paralysis of the femoral nerve and a flexion contracture of the hip. Bleeding into the soft tissues of the forearm may produce ischemic paralysis and Volkmann's contracture. Even ischemic gangrene may result from the pressure of hemorrhage on blood vessels. Localized bleeding about a bone that begins apparently as subperiosteal hemorrhage may, if unchecked by hematologic treatment, lead to a process of bone destruction and new bone formation culminating in the formation of a large cystic mass, or *hemophilic pseudotumor,* which may be curable only by radical excision or amputation. With improved coagulant therapy, pseudotumors are becoming much less frequent.

Fractures in hemophilic patients are especially common in the distal half of the femur, where the bone may be atrophic from disuse and under especial stress because of stiffness of the knee. As a rule, fractures in hemophilia heal normally. In their treatment, care must be taken to prevent ischemia from vascular compression by expanding hemorrhage beneath an unyielding cast. For this reason, plaster splints are safer than cylindrical casts.

SELECTED REFERENCES

Arnold WD, Hilgartner MN: Hemophilic arthropathy: Current concepts of pathogenesis and management. J Bone Joint Surg 59A:287, 1977

Blatt PM, Zeitler KD, Roberts HR: Hemophilia and other hereditary defects of coagulation. In Conn HC, Conn RB (eds): Current Diagnosis. Philadelphia, WB Saunders, 1980

Part Nine

TRAUMA

Chapter 23

The Systemic Response to Trauma

George Johnson, Jr.

GOALS AND OBJECTIVES

Goals: To introduce the reader to the physiologic and biochemical consequences of trauma, and to correlate these abnormal biochemical and physiologic effects with the overall health of the patient

Objectives: On completion of this unit, and using the text as a standard reference, one should be able to evaluate, describe, list, or recognize the basic neuroendocrine and metabolic events that occur in a patient who has been severely injured

OUTLINE

I. Extent of injury
   A. Grading of trauma
   B. Accretion of biologic components
      1. Threshold stimuli
      2. Threatening challenges
      3. Tissue-killing injuries
II. Phases of convalescence
   A. First phase injury
      1. Clinical
      2. Neuroendocrine
      3. Metabolism and biochemistry
      4. Biochemical mediators
      5. Wound
      6. Clinical management
   B. Second phase-turning point
   C. Third phase-muscular strength
   D. Fourth phase-fat gain
   E. Goal of therapy

A 19-year-old college student rides his motorcycle down a steep incline, hits a large rock, and is thrown 30 feet, landing on his side. He sustains multiple pelvic fractures and a fractured femur.

The local injury to soft tissue and bone is comprehensible, but what happens to the *milieu interieur*, or internal environment, referred to by Bernard 125 years ago? Are the "homeostatic" mechanisms encountered able to preserve this internal environment with the major psychological and physical insult that has occurred, or does the resulting "emergency reaction" of Cannon or "alarm reaction" of Selye cause internal chaos?

Moore, Gelin, and Egdahl have attempted to give an orderly picture of the body's internal reaction following trauma. The various periods described do not, however, occur in an orderly fashion; rather, the nervous and humoral pathways evoked depend on the physical and emotional states of the individual patient, as well as the type and site of injury and a complex and interrelated series of reactions. Thus, it is not possible to predict precisely the response of a given patient to trauma.

EXTENT OF INJURY

Attempts to grade trauma on a scale of 10 may be of some benefit to the student or investigator in trying to describe the magnitude of trauma. Unfortunately, a specific injury or operation does not always fall within a predicted grade, causing the system to be chaotic at times. Moore recognized three degrees of injury. The first of these, the threshold stimulus, is minor in extent, transient in duration, and merely initiates endocrine and metabolic changes. Fever, pain, cold, fatigue, anesthesia, and starvation are characteristic threshold stimuli. The second grade of trauma is a threatening challenge to the maintenance of homeostasis, as might occur with severe injury, bleeding, or anoxia. The third category includes tissue-killing injury, which is characterized by extensive tissue injury, invasive sepsis, or profound shock.

PHASES OF CONVALESCENCE

Moore has described four phases of convalescence from injury. The *first* or injury phase, lasts from 2 to 4 days, depending on the extent of trauma. Clinically, the patient has a rapid pulse, feels ill, desires to sleep, does not want to be disturbed, and avoids strong light. This phase is marked initially by an emergency reaction period, in which fear, pain, and apprehension stimulate the hypothalmic–pituitary–adrenal "stress axis." Epinephrine and norepinephrine are secreted in response to stimulation of the adrenal medulla, although the amount is variable. The patient is pale and apprehensive, and exhibits tachycardia, sweating, and vasoconstriction.

Afferent impulses from the area of trauma acting through the stress axis stimulate the release of ACTH, which is secreted in amounts proportionate to the degree of trauma. ACTH stimulates the production of corticoids, which are necessary for the normal response to trauma. Since the action of corticoids is widespread, it is difficult to define the precise mechanisms by which they maintain homeostasis. They have an anti-inflammatory action, decrease capillary permeability, exert a stabilizing influence on cell membranes, stimulate gluconeogenesis from protein, cause peripheral vasodilatation, exert an ionotropic action, and have a profound effect on water and electrolyte balance.

Renin secretion is usually increased, probably as a result of decreased perfusion pressure in the afferent arterioles of the renal cortex. Renin activates the conversion of angiotensinogen to angiotensin. Aldosterone secretion is increased from the renin–angiotensin pathway, directly from ACTH, or from an elevated serum potassium. Antidiuretic hormone is released owing to stimulation of the supraoptic nucleus, or as a result of hypovolemia. Growth hormone, under control of a hypothalamic center, is increased as a result of hypoglycemia, insulin, and neural impulses.

Thus, the humoral alterations occurring in response to trauma are directed toward conservation of water and salt, maintenance of blood pressure, gluconeogenesis, glycolysis, mobilization of carbohydrates, and lipolysis. The neuroendocrine response may be altered in various ways by hypovolemia, acidosis, alkalosis, infection, emotional trauma, anoxia, starvation, hypoglycemia, poison, alcohol, temperature, and anaphylaxis.

Widespread metabolic and biochemical changes occur during the injury phase. Tissue catabolism results in cellular breakdown, which leads to an increase in urinary nitrogen and potassium. Aldosterone secretion leads to an increase in urinary potassium and a decrease in urinary sodium. The carbohydrate that is readily available as glycogen is rapidly depleted during this phase, and the body turns to protein and fat for its energy source. Water may be lost into the area of trauma. The urine output is decreased, probably owing to a decrease in extracellular fluid and increased secretion of ADH. A tendency toward acidosis is noted, usually from inadequate tissue perfusion. As anoxia develops, metabolism is not carried through the tricarboxylic cycle, and lactic acid is produced, with a decrease in high-energy phosphates.

A series of biochemical mediators from the traumatized area are released, although more slowly than the neural mediators. These mediators include lysosomes, kinins, polypeptides, adenosine diphosphate, collagen, potassium, and endotoxins—mostly substances from cellular destruction. Although some of these substances enhance local hemostasis, inflammation, and repair, they may have deleterious effects on the body as a whole. For example, the release of adenosine diphosphate and collagen invoke platelet adhesiveness with local hemostasis, but if this process becomes more generalized and the body's fibrinolytic system is blocked, disseminated intravascular coagulation may occur and hypofibrinogenemia and thrombocytopenia develop. This local aggregation of platelets, fibrinogen, fibrin and fat may form a plug in the microcirculation that moves to the lung, perhaps causing systemic hypoxia. This process may in turn alter cellular function throughout the body.

Local cellular injury may cause a release of lysosomal enzymes, which may cause cellular damage and malfunction of tissue distant from the site of primary trauma.

Vasoactive substances such as histamine, serotonin, epinephrine, and prostaglandin may significantly alter blood flow through the capillary beds, although the interplay and variation of these substances make it difficult to describe their precise roles. Endotoxins from the various bacteria in the intestinal tract may be absorbed, producing cellular damage and adverse physiologic reactions. Cellular damage leads to an increase in the concentration of serum potassium, which causes increased myocardial irritability.

Although not included in this scheme, additional factors that should be remembered are the loss of fluid and blood into the injured area. Blalock and associates in 1930 demonstrated that the major cause of death in severe blunt trauma was hypovolemia. Also, the movement of fluid and electrolytes from one compartment (intracellular, interstitial, and intravascular) to another may be markedly influenced by hemodynamic or metabolic changes that occur as a consequence of the trauma. Thus, Shires and associates have noted an increase in cellular sodium and water associated with a change in the intracellular transmembrane potential in hemorrhage shock.

During this early phase, the wound lacks tensile strength, being composed primarily of serum and cellular debris. The clinical management of this phase of injury depends on a number of variables but in general is aimed at maintaining blood and fluid volume, correcting acid–base abnormalities, and preventing sepsis.

Satisfactory management during the injury phase allows one to mobilize the patient and progress toward the *second phase* of convalescence. During this period, the patient begins to feel considerably better. The endocrine abnormalities return to normal. Marked catabolism ceases and nitrogen equilibrium is restored. There is a diuresis of water and salt. Urinary potassium and fat oxidation decrease.

Management during this phase includes return to oral intake and mobilization of the patient. If adequate caloric intake is not restored by oral therapy, hyperalimentation should be given by the intravenous route. In fact, some traumatologists currently start intravenous hyperalimentation following resuscitation of the patient with extensive trauma in whom it is anticipated that oral intake will be delayed.

The *third phase*, or muscle strength phase, is marked by continued improvement of the patient. Endocrine function returns to normal, nitrogen balance becomes positive, and weight gain begins. Pain in the wound decreases and tensile strength increases with the development and maturation of fibrous tissue. The wound becomes red and raised.

The *fourth phase*, or fat gain phase, develops weeks following injury. The patient feels well during this period. Although it is unusual for the wound to break down at this time, it can disrupt if there is a protein or vitamin C deficiency. During this phase, the patient must be cautioned against overeating and obesity.

Thus trauma, whether from accidental injury or operation, creates a local insult; perhaps just as importantly, it stimulates a diffuse and widespread series of reactions, primarily through the neuroendocrine system, that attempt to maintain body homeostasis. The exact sequence of events, the interplay of the various reactions, and the exact responses that occur are somewhat unpredictable, but it is obvious that all organs and systems are involved. Knowledge of the reactions involved is essential to the appreciation of the potential abnormal systemic effects of massive trauma. Such understanding is necessary as a guide to the therapy of an injured patient such as the 19-year-old student in a motorcycle accident.

SELECTED REFERENCES

Blalock A: Experimental shock: Cause of low blood pressure produced by muscle injury. Arch Surg 20:959, 1930

Gelin L: Reaction of the body as a whole to injury. J Trauma 10:932, 1970

Hume DM, Edahl RH: The importance of the brain in the endocrine response to injury. Ann Surg 150:697, 1959

Moore FD: Homeostasis: Bodily changes in trauma and surgery. In Sabiston DC: Textbook of Surgery: The Biological Basis of Modern Surgical Practice, pp 26–64. Philadelphia, WB Saunders, 1972

Shires GT: Principles and management of hemorrhagic shock. In Shires GT (ed): Care of the Trauma Patient, pp 3–51. New York, McGraw-Hill, 1979

Chapter 24

The Local Response to Trauma

Paul H. Wright and H. Robert Brashear

GOALS AND OBJECTIVES

Goals: To introduce the reader to the changes that occur in bone, cartilage, and tendon as a result of trauma, and to describe the responses of these tissues to injury

Objectives: On completion of this unit, and using the text as a standard reference, one should be able to evaluate, describe, recognize, or list the following:

1. Three phases of wound healing, and two histologic and physiologic features of each
2. Two requirements for satisfactory tendon healing
3. The unique characteristics of the healing of injuries to articular cartilage
4. The phases of fracture healing, in chronologic order, compared with those of soft tissue wounds
5. The histologic differences between fractures that are rigidly immobilized and those in which motion between the two fragments is permitted
6. Four factors that impair or retard bone healing
7. The systematic and local factors that impair wound healing

OUTLINE

I. Soft-tissue injury
   A. Cleanup phase
   B. Repair phase
   C. Maturation phase
II. Factors that influence wound healing
   A. Local factors
      1. Degree of trauma
      2. Contamination
      3. Infection
      4. Extent of wound
   B. Systemic factors
      1. Protein deficiency
      2. Hormonal influence
      3. Ascorbic acid deficiency
III. Healing of tendon
   A. Special requirements of tendons
   B. Healing process

The body's response to tissue injury is governed by many factors, including the extent, duration, and type of injury. For example, mechanical injury, which is dealt with here, may vary from the clean incision of a surgeon's knife to the severe crush injury of a hand caught in a machine press. The tissue reaction differs quantitatively and qualitatively, and each type of tissue has characteristic responses that differ from those of other tissues. Nevertheless, certain responses are common to all tissue injury and, to an extent, to all types of injury.

The reaction to injury may be divided into three functional periods, although there is considerable overlap in each. The first, or cleanup, phase begins very shortly after the hemorrhage, edema, and clot formation that follows injury and is concerned with the removal of cellular debris and substances that behave as foreign material. This phase must be reasonably effective in order for the second, or repair, phase to proceed. In this period, characterized by the abundant production of fibrous tissue, there is an attempt by the organism to restore the damaged tissue to a functional state. The skin defect seals, the cut tendon ends unite, and broken ends of the bone are joined together, which results in quick and abundant restoration of anatomical integrity; however, repair tissue may be disorganized and have poor mechanical properties, which requires the third and final phase of healing, that of maturation, reorganization, and remodeling. In this relatively long and slow period, the tissue becomes organized, compact, and functionally efficient. Fractured bones regain supportive strength, and lacerated tendons regain tensile strength. The extent and success of the remodeling phase depends upon the degree of original injury, the physiologic response potential of the injured tissue, the age of the patient, the type of treatment, and many other factors.

SOFT-TISSUE INJURY

Before considering the healing process in such specialized tissues as bone, cartilage, and tendon, it is helpful to study a classic example of wound healing as seen in the simple, clean, incised surgical wound.

The *cleanup phase* includes the immediate consequences of the insult. In the localized area of the surgical incision, tissues are cut, blood vessels are interrupted, and cell membranes are ruptured or traumatized. The immediate wound area contains cellular debris and blood products, which stimulate a localized inflammatory response by which these toxic materials and debris are removed. The inflammatory response involves a series of chemical reactions interrelated with other physiologic responses.

Several mediators are involved in the inflammatory response, depending on the type and degree of injury. Histamine and serotonin are released from basophils, mast cells, and platelets simultaneously with the tissue injury. These substances increase vascular permeability and dilatation, enabling polymorphonuclear leukocytes to migrate into the area of traumatized tissue. Within a few minutes to hours after injury, additional mediators of inflammation are released, including the kinins, which cause pain by stimulating nerve endings. Prostaglandins become involved about 2 to 6 hours after injury. One function of the prostaglandins is chemotaxis, the attraction of more cells by migration to the injured tissue. By the end of the first 24 hours, the granulocytes are followed by lymphocytes, monocytes, and later by macrophages. These cells, especially the granulocytes, release lysosomal enzymes, which are capable of cleaving all types of macromolecules. One or more of the lysosomal enzymes release arachidonic acid, the precursor for prostaglandin synthesis, from cell membranes. Thus, the inflammatory response can be sustained and toxic materials broken down enzymatically. Cellular elements then remove the breakdown products and prepare the wound for the repair process.

Cellular activity is evident by the second day from mitoses in fibroblasts and endothelial cells in the connective and vascular tissue adjacent to the wound. By the third day, fibroblasts are seen in the traumatized tissue, and small capillary buds are present at the periphery. Thus, the inflammatory process, which includes the mobilization of cellular and vascular elements that carry out the repair phase, lasts for 3 or 4 days.

In the *repair phase,* the capillaries grow into the traumatized area, and fibroblasts begin to produce collagen. Collagen production is rapid and abundant, reaching a peak during the second week and slowing down by the 14th day. Although the collagen produced is somewhat disorganized with respect to the ultimate function of the tissue, its abundance is a safety factor. For example, dermal sutures can usually be safely removed during the second week following an incision, even though the collagen has not matured to produce the eventual tensile strength of mature scar tissue (the scar at 2 weeks is usually quite vascular and reddened).

The *maturation phase* generally begins about 2 weeks after the injury and lasts several months or even years. Collagen synthesis continues at a slower rate than during the repair phase. During maturation and remodeling, the synthesis and breakdown of collagen approach a steady state. Collagen fibers become mature and oriented along the lines of tension, promoting functional efficiency. Intra- and intermolecular cross-linking of collagen increases and adds to mechanical efficiency. Vascularity diminishes during the maturation phase, and many of the new and dilated capillary loops within the scar tissue become obliterated.

FACTORS THAT INFLUENCE WOUND HEALING

Although there are many factors that can retard wound healing, there is no consistently effective means of increasing the rate of healing. Those factors that tend to delay wound healing may be conveniently divided into local and systemic effects.

At the local wound level, the degree of trauma is an important determinant of the rate of healing. The more severe the trauma, the more extensive the tissue disruption and the greater the requirement for cleanup, repair, and maturation. Contamination of a wound by foreign material imposes an additional load on the tissue response to injury and prolongs the cleanup process. Infection severely taxes, and may prevent, complete wound healing. Trauma may be associated with impairment of the blood supply to the injured part, leading to additional tissue death from ischemia, which requires larger cleanup and repair processes in the face of a marginal blood supply. This dangerous combination of injured tissue and ischemia increases the chance of infection, especially by clostridial organisms. Impaired local blood supply is a frequent problem in the lower limbs of diabetics, and wound healing in these patients is often slow.

Systemic factors do not usually affect wound healing greatly; however, surgeons are beginning to realize the importance of adequate nutrition for a maximum healing response. For example, certain chronically malnourished individuals, such as alcoholics, display poor healing of fractures. Experimentally, severe protein depletion delays healing, and this delay can be even more specifically tied to an inadequate supply of the amino acids methionine and cysteine. Extensive studies of the effects of various hormones on wound healing have shown that ACTH and cortisone have an adverse effect. Not only do these hormones diminish the inflammatory response to trauma, but fibroplasia is partially suppressed, and the gain in wound tensile strength is retarded.

One of the most striking adverse effects on healing of wounds is produced by a deficiency of abscorbic acid. Although acute scurvy is rare today, the older literature contains many descriptions of wound disruption or delayed healing in scorbutic patients. The relationship of scurvy to wound healing and collagen synthesis has been extensively documented in studies on experimental animals. Ascorbic acid is important to the formation of collagen, and impairment of collagen synthesis may have disastrous consequences on the healing of a wound.

The healing process in the soft-tissue

wound described above and the factors, local and systemic, that impede healing also apply to the repair of more specialized tissues, although there are differences in the cellular and extracellular responses of these special tissues. Because of differences in blood supply, tissue composition, and functional requirements, the healing of tendon, cartilage, and bone differs significantly enough from the basic processes of tissue repair to warrant separate consideration.

HEALING OF TENDON

Tendons have a somewhat limited blood supply and high functional demands. The great bulk of the tissue mass of tendon consists of bundles of longitudinally oriented collagen fibers. Between the bundles are sparsely placed, flattened, and rather dormant fibrocytes. The vascular supply to tendons is meager, the most important being the mesotenon. The functional requirements of tendons are two: great tensile strength and the ability to glide for a considerable distance through the surrounding tissue. These two requirements pose a problem in tendon healing, for, in one sense, they are diametrically opposed. Great tensile strength requires an abundance of collagen, the formation of which during healing may result in adhesions to surrounding tissue, which impairs the gliding function.

The generalized scheme of healing of tendon is similar to that of soft tissue wounds. Following a clean laceration, an inflammatory exudate develops between the cut ends, followed by an influx of macrophages and later of fibroblasts and capillary buds. These new cellular elements are derived from the surrounding soft tissue and synovial sheath rather than from the cells of the tendon itself. In the fibroblastic repair phase, the collagen formed is at first somewhat randomly oriented and even perpendicular to the line of the tendon. During the maturation phase, these fibers become arranged parallel to the line of tendon pull. The new collagen fibers interdigitate and connect with preexisting tendon fibers. During the fibroblastic repair phase, especially during the second week, the vascular fibrous tissue fuses the tendon and surrounding tissue into a single mass; but during the third week, as reorganization and maturation take place, the tendon separates to a varying degree from the surrounding tissues (Fig. 24-1). It is the extent to which this separation occurs, and, conversely, the density of the adhesions that remain, that determine the future gliding function of the tendon.

As with cutaneous wounds, collagen formation begins at 4 to 5 days, and tensile strength increases steadily thereafter. Strength is not sufficient to permit strong tendon pull for 4 to 5 weeks, and during the first 3 weeks

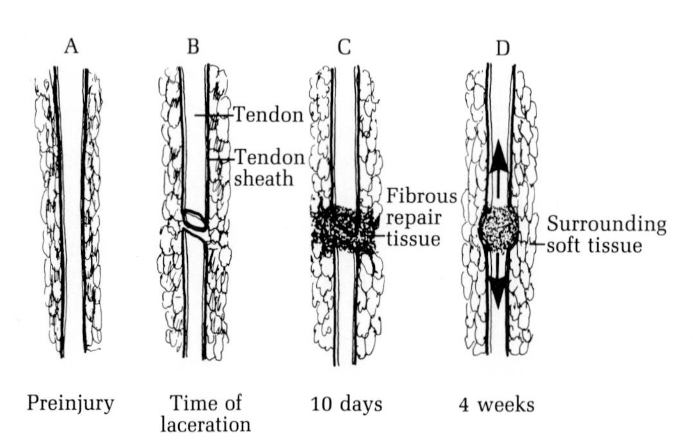

Fig. 24-1. Healing of lacerated tendon. (*A*) Before injury the tendon and tendon sheath are intact, providing tensile strength and the ability to glide through the surrounding soft tissues. (*B*) Sharp laceration interrupting the tendon and tendon sheath, as well as some of the surrounding soft tissues. (*C*) The fibroblastic repair phase is seen about 10 days following injury. Vascularized fibrous tissue fuses the tendon and surrounding soft tissue into a single mass. (*D*) The maturation phase occurs about 4 weeks following injury. As reorganization occurs, the healing tendon separates from the surrounding tissue and gliding ability returns.

there is danger that muscle contraction will pull the tendon ends apart. Should this happen, the tendon will heal in a lengthened state, usually with the formation of an excessive amount of scar tissue and adhesions. Where the tendon passes through a tight fibrous tunnel, such as in the distal palm, adhesions are particularly devastating and may render the tendon functionless. The clinical management of tendon injuries requires considerable sophistication to achieve optimal results.

HEALING OF CARTILAGE

Articular cartilage differs from other tissues in its mechanism of nutrition, which occurs by diffusion of materials through several millimeters of matrix. The four main components of articular cartilage are chondrocytes, collagen, protein polysaccharide, and water. In adult cartilage, the cellular turnover rate is exceedingly low, as is the turnover of the collagen component. Protein polysaccharide, however, is being constantly synthesized and presumably degraded. The absence of vessels within cartilage and the low mitotic activity of its cells impose severe limitations on the healing ability of this tissue; indeed, some traumatic defects in cartilage apparently never heal. The repair of articular cartilage has been the object of numerous studies. Unfortunately, because of considerable variation in the degree and type of healing, there is disagreement as to just how this repair takes place.

When articular cartilage is injured, the type of healing that will take place is influenced by the depth of the injury. If the defect is limited to cartilage, no blood vessels are severed, and the reaction is much less intense than if the injury extends through the cartilage into underlying bone, as occurs in intraarticular fractures (Fig. 24-2).

Defects of or injuries to cartilage that do not extend to the underlying bone heal very slowly and incompletely. Following such an injury, there is necrosis of a few cartilage cells immediately adjacent to the lesion and a loss of mucopolysaccharide from this area. This loss is usually found to extend about 1 mm from the walls of the cartilage defect. The defect fills with fibrin, but the inflammatory response, in the absence of blood vessels, is limited. Between 48 hours and 2 weeks, there is mitotic activity in the cartilage cells adjacent to the defect. This activity increases the number of cartilage cells around the injury, but there is no clearcut evidence that these cells ever enter the defect or contribute significantly to its healing. This increased mitotic activity ceases at about 2 weeks, a time when the lesion is far from healed.

In time, the cartilage defect is filled or partially filled with cells that are elongated and fibrous in appearance. Their origin has been debated, but they probably arise from the flattened cells of the superficial zone of the articular cartilage, which apparently, under the stimulus of injury, can act as a perichondrium. These cellular elements within the cartilage defect may remain fibrous or,

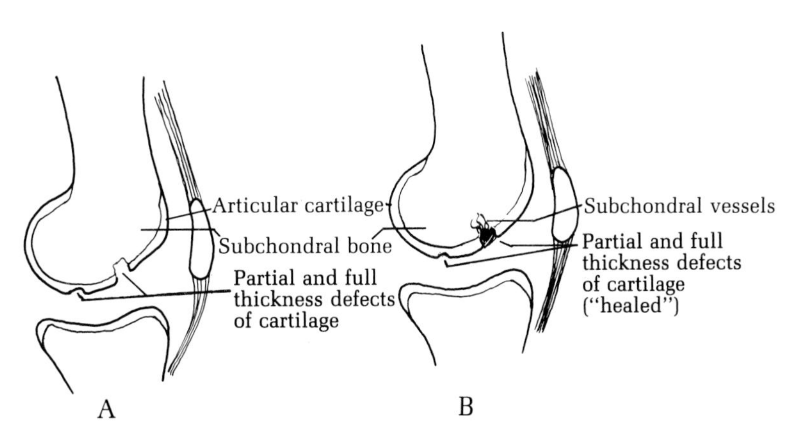

Fig. 24-2. Healing of articular cartilage injury. (*A*) Degrees of injury: The lower defect extends only partway through the cartilage. The upper defect extends completely through the cartilage and into the subchondral bone. (*B*) Healing of injury: Healing is less complete in the partial thickness defect. The full thickness injury is vascularized by subchondral vessels, which enhances healing.

with the accumulation of extracellular matrix, take on the appearance of fibrocartilage; in unusual circumstances, they may even become hyaline cartilage. The factors that determine whether healing will be by fibrous tissue, fibrocartilage, or hyaline cartilage remain a mystery.

If the injury to cartilage extends into the underlying bone, the response is quite different. In this situation, vascular tissue derived from the bone and marrow is available to the cartilage wound. The defect is immediately filled with blood, which clots. There is the same necrosis of cartilage cells adjacent to the injury that is seen in the superficial defect. By 48 hours, there is an ingrowth of vascular granulation tissue from the marrow into the cartilage defect. This process is followed by the accumulation of increasing amounts of fibrous tissue and collagen. Bone formation occurs up to the level of the previous subchondral bone but not into the area of the articular cartilage. In time, the surface of the defect is covered by several layers of flattened cells, presumably derived from the superficial layer of cells of the adjacent intact cartilage. The bulk of the defect is filled with granulation tissue from the underlying bone. This tissue becomes progressively more fibrous and less vascular and, in time, may become fibrocartilaginous; rarely is normal hyaline cartilage formed.

Since the injured cartilage is not replaced by normal articular tissue, the weight-bearing and gliding properties of the damaged tissues are not as good as those of normal hyaline cartilage. Such damaged areas withstand wear poorly and become the focus of degenerative changes, the extent of which depends largely upon the size and irregularity of the defect produced by the injury. In fractures that involve joints, accurate reduction of the articular surfaces is important to minimize these degenerative changes.

HEALING OF BONE

The healing of a fracture is, in many respects, similar to the healing of a soft-tissue wound. The cleanup, reparative, and remodeling phases can be readily recognized, but because of the special nature of this tissue, there is considerable overlap of these phases, and the entire process usually takes longer than soft-tissue healing (Fig. 24-3). Furthermore, the requirements of bone healing differ from those of soft-tissue healing in that not only is tensile strength needed, but torsional, bending, and compressive strengths are also required. Fractures vary in severity from undisplaced cracks to severely displaced fractures in which there is extensive soft-tissue injury and associated instability of the fracture fragments. The undisplaced fracture usually has intact surrounding soft tissues, such as periosteum, which provide stability.

The events that take place in the healing of the fracture involve a number of tissues, including the cortex, periosteum, endosteum, marrow, and soft tissues adjacent to the fracture. When a bone is broken, periosteum is usually ruptured and vessels in the marrow, cortex, and surrounding soft tissue are torn, and hemorrhage ensues. This hemorrhage and the resulting clot are usually contained in the region of the fracture by attachments of muscle, periosteum, and connective tissue. The fibrin strands in the clot serve as scaffolding for the ingrowth of vessels during the early reparative process. There has been much debate as to the importance of this clot in fracture healing; some investigators consider it essential; others look upon the clot as a passive obstruction to the ingrowth of new tissue. There is some evidence to support both sides of this issue, but it seems unlikely that the clot plays a very active role in fracture healing.

As in the case of soft-tissue injury, there is a variable amount of cell death and debris in the fracture area that must be removed. The usual inflammatory reaction to trauma ensues, with dilatation of vessels in tissues about the fracture and outpouring of an exudate, including polymorphonuclear cells and macrophages. The bone immediately adjacent to the fracture invariably dies and must be removed in the cleanup process. The removal of bone debris, which is carried out by osteoclasts, takes considerably longer than the removal of soft-tissue debris and may not be completed for many weeks after the injury.

Within 48 hours following injury, vascular tissue begins to invade the fracture area. The source of most of these new vessels is the soft tissues surrounding the fracture, but

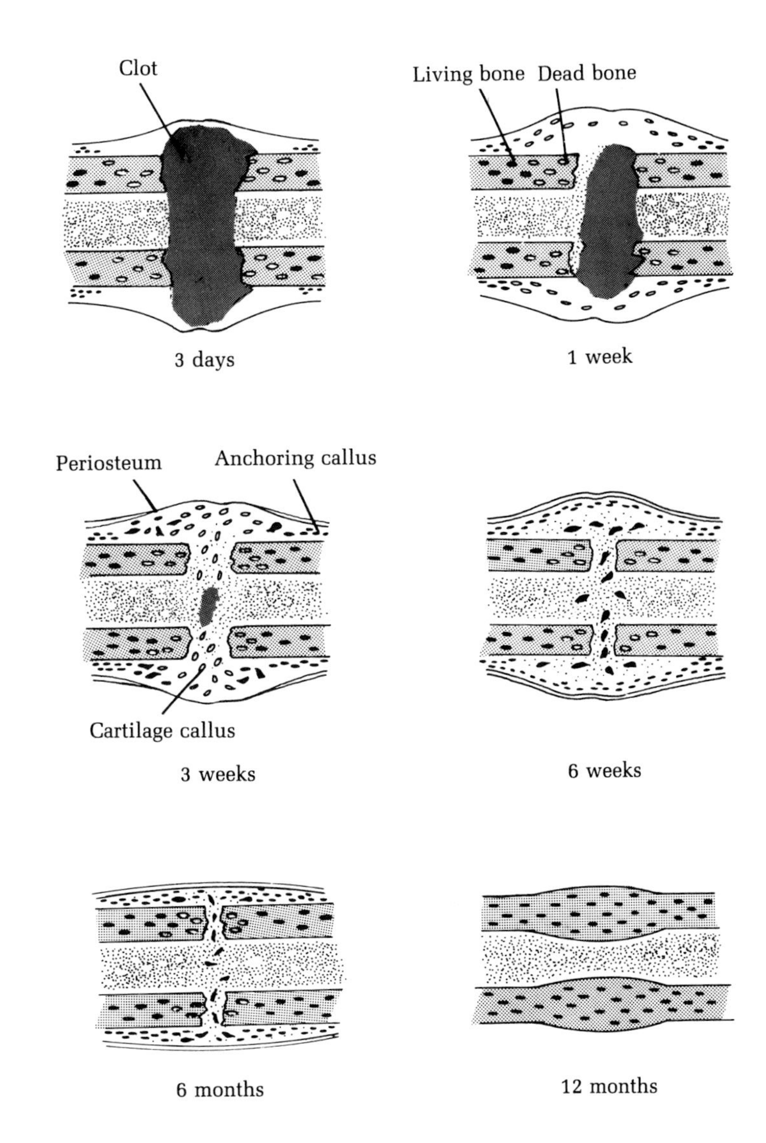

Fig. 24-3. Stages of fracture healing.

vessels of the marrow cavity also contribute. The blood flow of the entire bone increases following a fracture of any portion of the bone. Trauma and hemorrhage always result in some elevation or stripping of the periosteum from the bone. This mechanical disturbance is a stimulus that activates the bone-forming cells of the periosteum not only at the fracture site but also at a considerable distance from it. Mitoses in these cells become evident within several days; over the following days and weeks, these cells produce new subperiosteal bone along the outer surface of the shaft. This bone ultimately acts as an anchor for the callus that will bridge the fracture gap. In the region of the fracture, these activated periosteal cells, along with similar cells from the endosteum and marrow, join the fibrous and vascular invasion of the clot to form the callus surrounding the broken bone.

Callus may be defined as the fusiform mass of repair tissue that envelops the broken ends of a fractured bone. The pluripotential cells of the callus are mesenchymal in origin. These cells are capable of producing collagen, fibrous tissue, cartilage, and bone. The regulatory mechanisms that determine the precise amount of each tissue formed during healing of a fracture are not completely understood, but include movement, pH, oxygen tension, electrical properties, cyclic nucleotides, and other parameters. The usual progression of callus formation in the repair phase is from the production of fibrous tissue to cartilage and finally to bone through the process of enchondral bone formation. Early callus is soft, friable, and easily disrupted, which may impair reestablishment of the microcirculation across the fracture. When the microcirculation of the callus is reestablished early, the pluripotential callus cells may produce bone directly. With either mechanism, this new bone is called *woven* or *fiber bone* and has a disorganized structure. With the accumulation of additional collagen, cartilage, and bone, the callus becomes firmer, more resilient, and able to withstand mild stresses. As the fracture ends become securely united, Wolff's law comes into play for the final maturation or remodeling phase. During the remodeling phase, the woven bone is gradually replaced with organized, efficient *lamellar bone,* and the callus concomitantly becomes smaller and more compact. If remodeling progresses efficiently and long enough, the callus completely disappears, and the healed fracture cannot be distinguished from normal bone.

Many variables can affect the size, cellular composition, and physiology of the healing callus, including those that affect wound healing in general. One factor that can affect callus formation is the location of the fracture; a fracture through a region composed primarily of cancellous bone, such as the metaphyseal region of the proximal tibia, may heal securely with little external callus, whereas a fracture through a well-vascularized cortical bone, such as the clavicle, often heals with abundant callus formation. Cancellous bone fragments usually heal when in direct contact but have less potential than cortical fragments for bridging a fracture with callus. Fractures in areas of poor blood supply, such as the middle or distal thirds of the tibia, usually heal slowly. In regions where immobilization and apposition of the fracture fragments are difficult to maintain, such as the mid-shaft of the humerus, healing may also be somewhat delayed. Although promoting the formation of more callus, motion may impair fracture healing by increasing the ratio of cartilage to bone in the callus. In cases where there is little or no motion at the fracture site, there may be very little external callus formation. For example, fractures that are secured surgically with rigid metal plates and screws may heal with no external callus ever visible on roentgenograms. Thus, the method of treatment can affect callus formation.

Other factors having an adverse influence on healing are the presence of additional fracture fragments and extensive soft-tissue damage, both of which reflect greater trauma.

The time required for fracture healing varies with many factors, including the age of the patient and the type of bone involved. As a general rule, children heal faster than adults, and cancellous bone heals faster than cortical bone. The location and severity of a fracture and the type of treatment are also important determinants, as evident in the discussion on callus formation.

Occasionally, the healing process is not entirely successful. A fracture may heal solidly in nonanatomical position, which is termed a *malunion.* When a fracture does not heal by bone union it is regarded as a *nonunion;* the tissues attempt to clean up the debris and repair the fracture, but the effort is ultimately unsuccessful. The fracture gap of a nonunion is filled with dense fibrous and fibrocartilaginous tissue, and the ends of the bones usually become very hard and sclerotic. Occasionally in such instances, the repair efforts produce a *pseudarthrosis,* or false joint, in which the fibrous tissue in the fracture site may contain a fluid-filled space that resembles a joint. An established nonunion has very little potential for achieving bone union without some type of additional stimulus. Bone grafting is one such stimulus; another is stimulation by electrical currents. As knowledge of fracture healing and cellular physiology increases, other methods of stimulating fracture healing will undoubtedly become available.

SELECTED REFERENCES

Brighton CT, Black J, Pollack SR (eds): Electrical Properties of Bone and Cartilage. New York, Grune & Stratton, 1979

Charnley J: The Closed Treatment of Common Fractures, 3rd ed. Edinburgh, Churchill Livingstone, 1974

Florey HW: General Pathology, 4th ed, Chap 17. Philadelphia, WB Saunders, 1970

Muller ME, Allgower M, Schneider R et al: Manual of Internal Fixation, 2nd ed. New York, Springer-Verlag, 1979

Peacock EE: Surgery and Biology of Wound Repair. Philadelphia, WB Saunders, 1970

Robbins SL, Angell M: Basic Pathology, Chap 2. Philadelphia, WB Saunders, 1971

Rockwood CA Jr, Green DP: Fractures. Philadelphia, JB Lippincott, 1975

Chapter 25

Principles of Diagnosis and Treatment of Musculoskeletal Trauma

Frank C. Wilson

GOALS AND OBJECTIVES

Goals: To introduce the reader to the principles of diagnosis and treatment of musculoskeletal trauma

Objectives: On completion of this unit, and using the text as a standard reference, one should be able to evaluate, describe, list or recognize the following:

1. Eight special roentgenographic techniques and the role of each in the diagnosis of musculoskeletal injury
2. The priority of treatment by organ systems
3. The four elements of fracture treatment
4. Three general types of fracture treatment and the indications for each
5. Four differences between fractures in children and fractures in adults
6. Eight complications of fractures and the cause(s) of each

OUTLINE

I. Diagnosis of musculoskeletal injury
   A. History
   B. Physical examination
   C. Special diagnostic techniques
      1. Routine roentgenograms

2. Stress roentgenograms
3. Dye studies: myelography, cystography, arthrography, angiography
4. Scanograms
5. Radionuclide bone scans
6. Computerized axial tomography
7. Arthroscopy
8. Electromyography and nerve conduction studies
9. Chemical determinations

II. Definitions and terminology

III. Treatment
   A. Priority of treatment by organ systems
   B. Initial care of the patient
   C. Definitive fracture treatment
      1. Goals of fracture treatment
      2. Recognition
      3. Reduction
      4. Retention
      5. Rehabilitation
      6. Open fractures
      7. Fractures in children

IV. Complications of fractures

DIAGNOSIS OF MUSCULOSKELETAL INJURY

The diagnosis of injury to the musculoskeletal system is made on the basis of historical and physical findings and the use of special diagnostic techniques.

History. The history should include a careful description of the events leading to and producing the injury. In addition to its medical importance, such information may be of considerable value if litigation follows. Knowledge of the mechanism of injury is useful in determining therapy, since the reduction of fractures depends upon a *reversal of the injuring forces.* The time lapse between injury and treatment is also important, especially in the management of open fractures or those associated with vascular damage.

Physical Examination. Examination of the injured patient should include a rapid evaluation of the entire patient prior to concentration on a specific area or injury. In particular, the respiratory and cardiovascular systems should be assessed. For example, if a myocardial infarction or stroke preceded the fall that produced a fractured hip, the cardiovascular system should be thoroughly evaluated and stabilized prior to definitive treatment of the fracture. Next, careful assessment of the *neurovascular status* of the limb distal to any injury must be made. Failure to recognize vascular or neurologic deficits may result in loss of the limb or its function. The absence of arterial circulation distal to the site of an injury is a particularly ominous finding and requires immediate attention to preserve the viability of the limb. The initial treatment usually includes reduction of a displaced fracture or dislocation. At the site of injury, a search should be made for tenderness, swelling, instability, crepitus, and deformity (findings that are commonly present with fractures, although one or more may be absent).

Special Diagnostic Techniques. Special diagnostic techniques that may aid in the evaluation of musculoskeletal injuries are roentgenography, arthroscopy, electrodiagnostic studies, and laboratory determinations.

Bone is uniquely suited to *roentgenographic examination.* Skeletal tissue casts a sharp image that is in distinct contrast with the surrounding soft tissues because bone absorbs a higher proportion of the roentgenographic beam than the soft tissues; therefore, few of the rays are transmitted to the film, and a white image is left after processing. Failure to recognize normal findings may lead to diagnostic error. For example, nutrient foramina or epiphyseal plates may be misinterpreted as fracture lines. For an adequate study, roentgenograms should be taken in at least two projections, usually anteroposterior and lateral.

Ligamentous injury may be demonstrated by *stress roentgenograms,* in which the part distal to the joint is deviated away from the side of the ligament being tested. For example, to test the integrity of the medial collateral ligament of the knee, the tibia is forced into valgus while the femur is held steady. Ligamentous disruption is indicated by abnormal widening of the medial side of the knee joint. Soft tissue lesions, such as muscle or tendon disruptions, may also be seen on roentgenograms using underexposure techniques. Overpenetration, the reverse of underexposure, may be used for better visualization of hyperostotic areas.

Various *dye studies* in which contrast media are injected into the spinal canal, urinary tract, joints, or blood vessels also may afford valuable diagnostic information. The injection of dye into the spinal canal is known as *myelography* and is useful in determining the presence and location of intraspinal pathology. The urinary tract may be evaluated using *intravenous pyelography* (the intravenous injection of dye that is rapidly excreted by the kidneys), or by retrograde injection of dye through the urethra (*cystography* or *urethrography*). These studies may be helpful in evaluating the urinary tract after injury to the pelvis. *Arthrography* is performed by injecting contrast material into joints. It has been most useful in diagnosing meniscal injury in the knee and tears of the rotator cuff in the shoulder. The circulation of a limb or organ can be studied by roentgenograms taken after dye is injected into the arterial or venous tree, a technique known as *angiography*.

Serial roentgenograms may be useful in determining the rate of growth in a particular bone or limb. These films, known as *scanograms*, permit a more accurate assessment of growth rates following injury than is possible by clinical measurement and therefore may be important in the follow-up of fractures in children.

Another roentgenographic technique that may be helpful in studying the effects of trauma on bone is radionuclide bone scanning. *Technetium bone scans*, which reflect bone metabolism and circulation, may be used to elucidate an occult fracture, which, if present, is seen as an area of increased isotope uptake ("hot" scan). These scans are also used in the diagnosis of certain complications of fractures, such as avascular necrosis, which produce an area of decreased uptake ("cold" scan).

Computerized axial tomography is a noninvasive radiologic technique that often provides better pathologic definition of spinal and pelvic trauma than conventional roentgenograms, and, for this reason, is employed frequently to facilitate the diagnosis and management of these injuries.

Arthroscopy is also a valuable diagnostic modality. The arthroscope, which permits direct visualization of the interior of large joints, may elucidate intraarticular pathology; it may also be used to remove fragments of bone, cartilage, or synovium.

Electrodiagnostic studies, such as electromyography (the measurement of action potentials in muscles) and nerve conduction studies (the measurement of nerve conduction time or velocity), may be helpful in the diagnosis and study of neurologic injury. Nerve conduction velocity may be diminished or absent following injury of a peripheral nerve. Denervation produces electrical changes in muscle known as fibrillation or denervation potentials. The number and type of action potentials generated by a muscle may also be used as an index of nerve regeneration.

Chemical determinations are sometimes useful in the diagnosis of injury or its complications. The presence of fat droplets in blood aspirated from a joint, for example, may indicate a fracture entering the joint. Fat droplets in the urine and sputum, an elevated serum lipase, or a lowered Po_2 following a fracture suggest fat embolism.

DEFINITIONS AND TERMINOLOGY

Certainly a fracture is more than a broken bone, since its effects are not limited exclusively to bone. A fracture also damages nearby soft tissues, both directly and indirectly (e.g., edema), and it affects the endocrine, metabolic, and emotional state of the injured person as well. To be comprehensive, the definition of a fracture must include not only a loss of bone continuity but also regional, systemic, and psychological effects.

Fractures may be classified as *open* (compound) or *closed* (simple), depending upon whether or not they communicate with the external environment. Fractures involving more than two fragments are said to be *comminuted*. It is also important to note the number of fragments, direction of the fracture line (transverse, oblique, or spiral), and the relationship of the fracture fragments to one another (angulation, rotation, overriding, or distraction), because these factors have prognostic and therapeutic significance.

Other musculoskeletal tissues that may be injured are ligaments and muscles. A partial tear of a ligament is referred to as a *sprain;* a similar injury in muscle or tendon is a *strain.*

TREATMENT

Before the treatment of a specific injury is undertaken, all other organ systems should be assessed, and more life-threatening injuries treated first. The general order of priority in treatment is as follows:

1. Respiratory system
2. Cardiovascular system
3. Neurologic system
4. Abdominal organs
5. Urologic system
6. Musculoskeletal system

After initial assessment, the principles for preservation of life and prevention of further damage are as follows:

1. Keep the airway patent.
2. Control hemorrhage, usually with pressure; cover wounds with clean cloths.
3. Prevent motion of the injured spine.
4. Splint injured extremities, including the joints above and below a fracture.
5. Transport gently; avoid unnecessary haste.

The goal of fracture treatment is bone union, normal anatomy and function, and the absence of symptoms—all accomplished in the shortest possible time.

Basically, fracture therapy consists of the following:

1. Recognition, or diagnosis
2. Reduction of the fracture
3. Retention of the reduction
4. Rehabilitation of the injured part

The *diagnosis* may be suspected from the physical findings but is confirmed by roentgenograms of the affected part. A high index of suspicion is desirable; it is preferable to err on the side of taking negative roentgenograms than to overlook a fracture by failing to take them.

Reduction of the fracture refers to elimination of the fracture deformity. It involves an understanding of the deforming forces and may be accomplished by closed manipulation, traction or operative treatment. In general, when an acceptable reduction can be obtained by manipulation, it is the preferred method of treatment. Where comminution exists, it is often impossible to achieve accurate reduction by either manipulation or open reduction, and traction is the method of choice. Traction also reduces the effect of deforming muscle forces, which, in an area of large muscle mass such as the thigh, may be a significant factor in preventing reduction by other means. Open reduction is required where precise restoration of anatomy is essential, as in intraarticular fractures, or with fractures in which satisfactory reduction cannot be obtained or maintained by closed methods.

Retention refers to the maintenance of reduction and may be accomplished by external immobilization devices such as plaster casts, braces, or splints; by traction, which may be applied to either skin or bone; or by internal fixation devices such as screws, plates, wires, or pins. Internal fixation is selected as the treatment of choice in a fracture when the advantages of this method outweigh the risks involved, as in the patient with a hip fracture whose survival may depend upon the ability to get out of bed.

Rehabilitation after fracture healing is necessary for the mobilization of stiffened joints, strengthening of atrophied muscles, and restoration of function to the injured part.

Open (compound) fractures differ from closed injuries in several important respects. One is the presence of an open wound; another is bacterial contamination. These differences necessitate an initial approach based on an attempt to convert the contaminated open wound to a clean operative wound. This task is impossible if the length of time between injury and treatment has permitted invasion of the surrounding tissues by contaminating organisms, which occurs within about 12 hours of injury. A wound treated within this period by adequate debridement and irrigation may be expected to heal as a clean operative wound. If the wound cannot be adequately debrided, it is irrigated and left open so that free drainage may occur. Thus, the initial treatment of open fractures is devoted to the wound; definitive treatment of the fracture may have to be deferred until the status of the wound is clear. Human tetanus antitoxin and antibiotics are usually employed in the treatment of open fractures, although not as a substitute for surgery.

Fractures in children also have certain unique features. Healing is more rapid and remodeling more extensive because of the higher levels of circulating growth hormone. The more growth remaining in a bone—that is, the younger the child—the greater the potential for bone remodeling, and therefore the more deformity that can be accepted following a given fracture. Other factors that affect the remodeling capacity of a given fracture are its proximity to the epiphyseal plate and the direction of the deformity. Fractures near the epiphyseal plate or with deformity in the plane of motion of the joint have greater remodeling potential. Rotation is the deformity least corrected by growth; therefore, rotational displacement should be corrected by reduction.

Although growth potential enhances remodeling of fracture deformities, a fracture may affect longitudinal growth by causing either lengthening or shortening of the bone, depending on the location of the fracture. Fracture healing results in hyperemia of the part that may stimulate growth in the epiphyseal plate. If the fracture involves the epiphyseal plate, it may injure the proliferating cartilage cells, resulting in slowing or cessation of growth in all or part of the plate, and a shortened or deformed limb.

Because of the excellent healing and remodeling powers of children, open reduction, especially with internal fixation, is required much less often than in adults.

COMPLICATIONS

The complications of fractures include the following:

1. Nonunion
2. Delayed union
3. Malunion
4. Neurologic injury
5. Injury to the vascular tree
6. Growth disturbance
7. Avascular necrosis
8. Infection
9. Tendon injury
10. Myositis ossificans
11. Post-traumatic arthritis
12. Embolization of fat or blood thrombus
13. Sudeck's atrophy

Union does not necessarily occur in a certain number of weeks or months following a fracture. As stated, fracture healing depends on a great many variables; however, delayed union may be said to occur when, after a reasonable period of immobilization, bone union has not taken place. The fracture line may increase in width, but sclerosis of the bone ends at the fracture line is not present. Nonunion is a roentgenographic diagnosis characterized by failure of bone trabeculae to bridge the fracture site. Nonunions are characterized by a diminished blood supply to the fracture site, which may result from poor immobilization that allows the fracture fragments to shear off newly formed capillaries growing into the fracture callus. As a rule, if the hematoma is undisturbed and the bone ends rigidly long enough, the fracture will heal.

Malunion refers to union with deformity, which usually results from inaccurate reduction. Injury to regional nerves or vessels may be produced by the fracturing force, sharp bone ends, or swelling. Avascular necrosis of one of the fracture fragments may occur if that fragment is deprived of its blood supply by the fracture or its treatment. An example of this complication can be seen following femoral neck fractures in which the blood supply to the femoral head is damaged, and the femoral head dies, either partially or totally, as a result. Infection may follow either open fractures or the open treatment of fractures. As a rule, acute infections respond to antibiotic administration, whereas chronic lesions often require operative debridement of dead and avascular tissue in addition to chemotherapy. The most serious infections result from clostridial organisms, which may proliferate in ischemic tissue to produce a virulent myositis that may result in loss of life or limb.

Division of a tendon by a fracture fragment is infrequent, largely because of the elasticity of the musculotendinous unit; however, tendon gliding may be impaired by fracture healing, and late rupture sometimes occurs in tendons moving over bone irregularities produced by the healing process.

Myositis ossificans is the formation of bone in muscle and is thought to result from the seeding of a muscle with endosteum or periosteum following injury to an adjacent bone. It may resolve spontaneously with rest of the part; if however, it does not, and if by its position it causes interference with function, it can be operatively removed after the bone becomes mature. Post-traumatic arthritis may follow fractures involving the articular surface of joints. This risk is reduced, although not eliminated, by anatomical reduction of such fractures. Sudeck's atrophy is a vasomotor disorder associated with intense pain and spotty osteoporosis. It is usually relieved by resumption of normal activity, although sympathetic interruption is occasionally required.

SELECTED REFERENCE

McLaughlin HL: Trauma. Philadelphia, WB Saunders, 1959

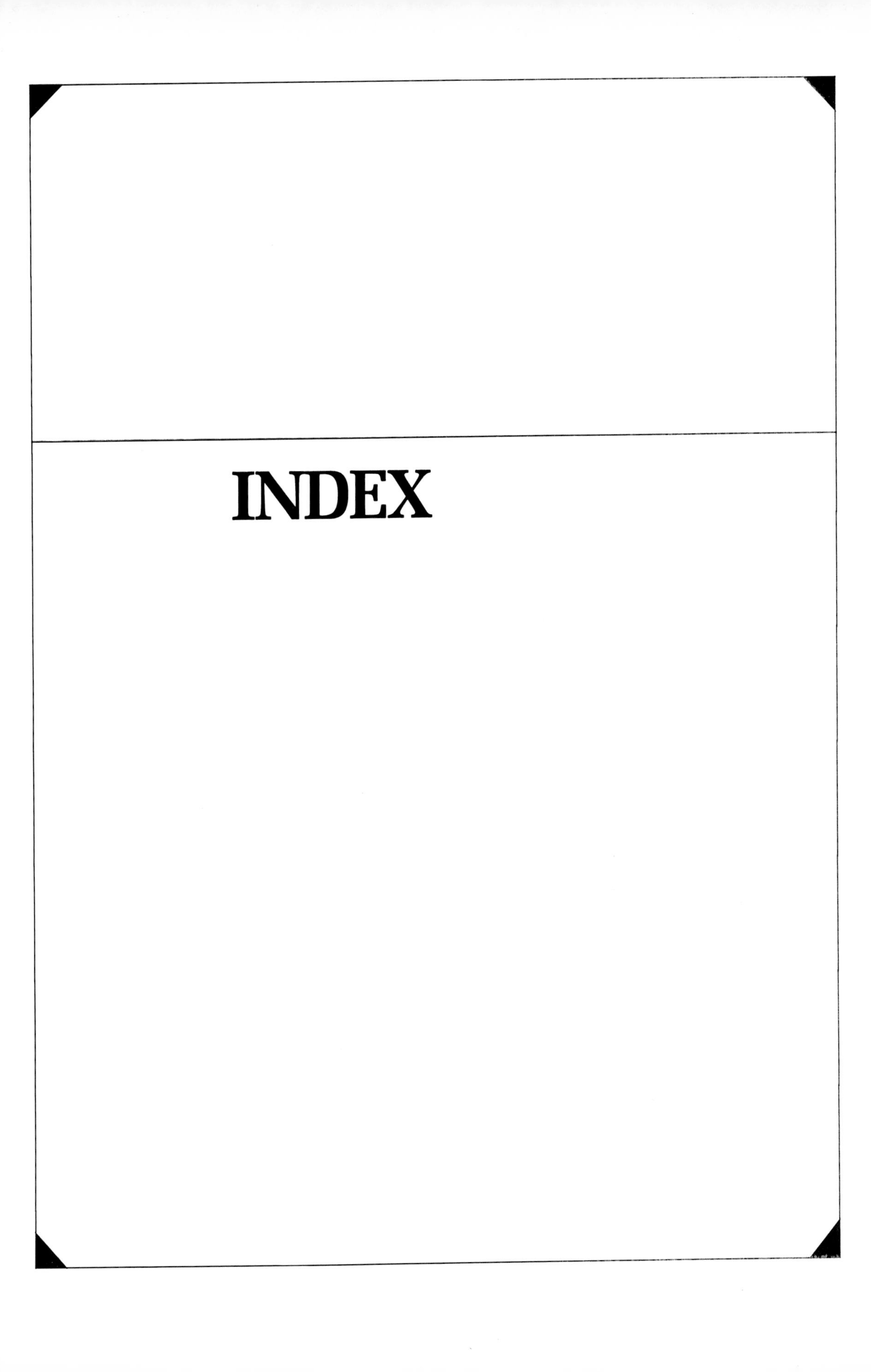

INDEX

Index